PUBLIC HEALTH

Local and Global Perspectives

Third edition

Public Health: Local and Global Perspectives presents a comprehensive introduction to public health issues and concepts in the Australian and international contexts. It provides students with fundamental knowledge of the public health field, including frameworks, theories, key organisations and contemporary issues.

The third edition features a new chapter on the public health workforce and the importance of advocacy in the profession and a thorough update that includes current research and case studies. Discussion of the COVID-19 pandemic and other contemporary public health issues offers students the opportunity to apply theory to familiar examples. Each chapter contextualises key concepts with spotlights and vignettes, reflective questions, tutorial exercises and suggestions for further reading.

Written by an expert team of public health professionals, *Public Health* is an essential resource for students.

Pranee Liamputtong is a medical anthropologist and Professor of Behaviour Sciences at the College of Health Sciences, VinUniversity, Vietnam.

Cambridge University Press acknowledges the Australian Aboriginal and Torres Strait Islander peoples of this nation. We acknowledge the traditional custodians of the lands on which our company is located and where we conduct our business. We pay our respects to ancestors and Elders, past and present. Cambridge University Press is committed to honouring Australian Aboriginal and Torres Strait Islander peoples' unique cultural and spiritual relationships with the land, waters and seas, and their rich contribution to society.

PUBLIC HEALTH

Local and Global Perspectives

Third edition

EDITED BY
Pranee Liamputtong

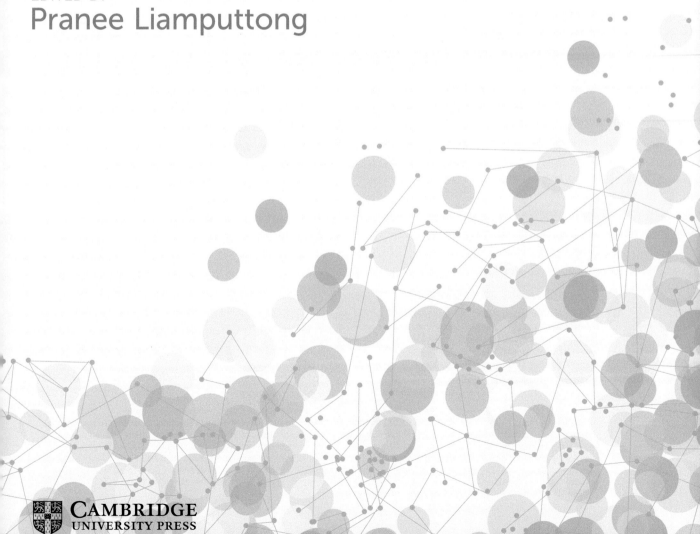

CAMBRIDGE
UNIVERSITY PRESS

CAMBRIDGE
UNIVERSITY PRESS

University Printing House, Cambridge CB2 8BS, United Kingdom

One Liberty Plaza, 20th Floor, New York, NY 10006, USA

477 Williamstown Road, Port Melbourne, VIC 3207, Australia

314–321, 3rd Floor, Plot 3, Splendor Forum, Jasola District Centre, New Delhi – 110025, India

103 Penang Road, #05–06/07, Visioncrest Commercial, Singapore 238467

Cambridge University Press is part of the University of Cambridge.

It furthers the University's mission by disseminating knowledge in the pursuit of
education, learning and research at the highest international levels of excellence.

www.cambridge.org
Information on this title: www.cambridge.org/9781009048569

First published 2016
Second edition 2019
Third edition 2022

Cover designed by Anne-Marie Reeves
Typeset by Straive

A catalogue record for this publication is available from the British Library
A catalogue record for this book is available from the National Library of Australia

ISBN 978-1-009-04856-9 Paperback

Additional resources for this publication at www.cambridge.org/highereducation/isbn/9781009048569/resources

In loving memory of my youngest daughter
Emma Inturatana Rice
who will forever be in my heart

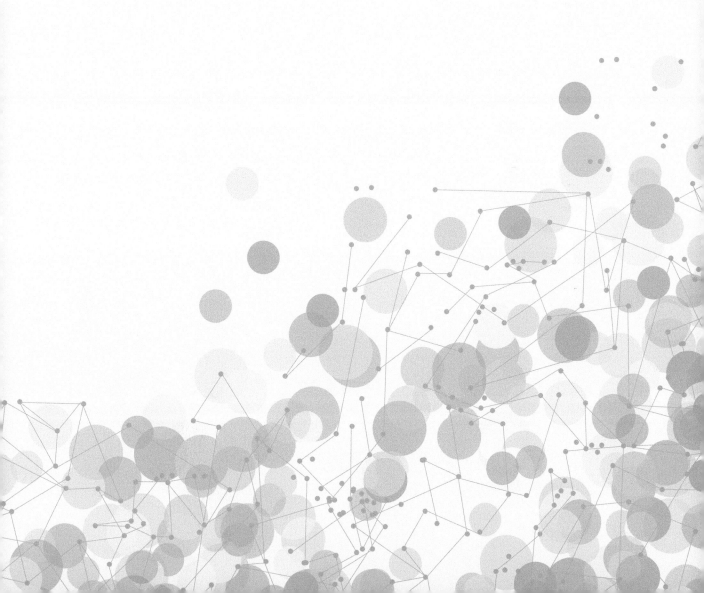

Contents

Preface   *page* xv
Contributors   xvii
Acknowledgements   xxii

Chapter 1 Public health: An introduction to local and global contexts   1
Pranee Liamputtong

   Introduction   2
   What is public health?   3
   The health of Australians   5
   Public health: Global concerns   7
   Social model of health and the new public health   12
   Health inequality and social justice   14
   Summary   17
   Tutorial exercises   17
   Further reading   18
   References   18

Part 1 Historical and theoretical perspectives   23

Chapter 2 Historical and contemporary principles and practices of public health 25
Rebecca E. Olson and Paul Saunders

   Introduction   26
   Ancient to medieval Europe: Sports, swamps and citizens   27
   Modern European history part one: Statistics, socialism and science 29
   Modern European history part two: Economics and excretory ducts   31
   Early Antipodean health   32
   The Antipodean public health story: 'Old public health'   34
   The Antipodean public health story: 'New public health'   36
   Summary   38
   Tutorial exercises   39
   Further reading   39
   References   39

Chapter 3 Health promotion principles and practice: Addressing complex public health issues using the Ottawa Charter   43
Bernadette Sebar, Kirsty Morgan and Jessica Lee

   Introduction   45
   Building healthy public policy   46

Creating supportive environments   48

Strengthening community action   50

Developing personal skills   52

Re-orienting health services   54

Summary   57

Tutorial exercises   57

Further reading   58

References   58

Chapter 4   Primary health care and community health   62
Lawrence Tan and Jennifer Reath

Introduction   63

Definition and concept of PHC and community health   64

Understanding the context of PHC and community health within Australian and global
    healthcare systems   67

Effective models of care within PHC   71

Challenges and future directions in PHC   74

Summary   80

Tutorial exercises   80

Further reading   80

References   81

Chapter 5   Public health ethics   86
Jane Williams and Stacy M. Carter

Introduction   87

What is public health ethics?   88

Consequentialist approaches to public health   89

Liberty and paternalism: The role of the state in public health   91

Justice   94

Equality and equity   95

Putting it all together: Can public health ethics frameworks help?   97

Summary   100

Tutorial exercises   100

Further reading   101

References   101

Chapter 6   Advocacy and the workforce   104
Gemma Crawford, Jonathan Hallett, Tina Price, Toni Hannelly and Christina Pollard

Introduction   106

Building capacity for public health   106

A workforce for the public's health   108

Public health: A political priority?   112

What is public health advocacy?   113

Summary   121

Tutorial exercises   121

Further reading   122

References   122

Part 2   Determinants of health   127

Chapter 7   Social determinants of health   129
John Oldroyd

Introduction   130

Where is health created?   132

Health inequities   134

Ethnic disparities in health   135

Social justice   137

The social gradient in health   138

A key social determinant of public health from *The Solid Facts*   140

Summary   143

Tutorial exercises   143

Further reading   144

References   144

Chapter 8   Behavioural, nutritional and environmental determinants and
public health   147
Jonathan Hallett, Gemma Crawford, Christina Pollard and Toni Hannelly

Introduction   148

Behavioural determinants of health   151

Nutritional determinants of health   153

Environmental determinants of health   155

Summary   159

Tutorial exercises   159

Further reading   160

References   160

Chapter 9   Individual decision-making in public health   164
John Bidewell

Introduction   165

Social and individual determinants of health   166

Perceptions, cognition, affect and choice   167

Theories of individual behaviour   168

Health as chosen or determined   176

Summary   178

Tutorial exercises   178

Further reading   179

References   179

Chapter 10   Political determinants of public health   182
Marguerite C. Sendall

    Introduction   184
    Government's role in health   185
    Australia's healthcare system   187
    The policy environment   189
    Evidence for policy   191
    Ethical advocacy   193
    Summary   196
    Tutorial exercises   197
    Further reading   197
    References   197

Chapter 11   Human rights, social justice and public health   200
Ann Taket

    Introduction   201
    What are human rights?   202
    Why are human rights important to public health practitioners?   206
    Holding governments to account   208
    Human rights and empowerment   211
    Summary   213
    Tutorial exercises   213
    Further reading   214
    References   214

Part 3   Public health and research   217

Chapter 12   Qualitative research methodology and evidence-based practice in
public health   219
Pranee Liamputtong and Zoe Sanipreeya Rice

    Introduction   220
    Qualitative research   221
    The nature of qualitative research   222
    Why qualitative research in public health?   224
    Evidence-based public health and qualitative research   227
    Summary   231
    Tutorial exercises   231
    Further reading   232
    References   232

Chapter 13   Assessing the health of populations: Epidemiology in public health   236
Patricia Lee

    Introduction   238
    Highlights of the definition of epidemiology   238

Frequency of disease occurrence   240

Descriptive epidemiology: Time, personal and place characteristics   243

Epidemiological study designs   246

Measures of association   252

Summary   255

Tutorial exercises   255

Further reading   256

References   256

Chapter 14   Planning and evaluation of public health interventions   258
Stuart Wark

Introduction   259

Why plan? Development of a public health intervention   260

The role of evaluation   269

Summary   273

Tutorial exercises   273

Further reading   274

References   274

Part 4   Public health issues and special populations   277

Chapter 15   The health of children: The right to thrive   279
Lisa Gibbs, Elise Davis, Simon Crouch and Lauren Carpenter

Introduction   280

Prevention of overweight and obesity in childhood   281

Child oral health   283

Children in same-sex parent families   286

Children and mental health   288

Summary   291

Tutorial exercises   292

Further reading   292

References   292

Chapter 16   Adolescence, health, social problems and public health   297
Jessica Heerde and Sheryl Hemphill

Introduction   298

Internalising and externalising problems   299

Homelessness   302

Alcohol, tobacco and other drug use   304

Bullying and cyberbullying perpetration and victimisation   306

Summary   309

Tutorial exercises   310

Further reading   310

References   310

Chapter 17   Healthy ageing   314
Elizabeth Cyarto and Frances Batchelor

    Introduction   315
    What is healthy ageing?   316
    The health of older people   322
    Barriers and enablers to healthy ageing   325
    Summary   327
    Tutorial exercises   327
    Further reading   328
    References   328

Chapter 18   The health inequities of people with intellectual and
developmental disabilities: Strategies for change   331
Teresa Iacono and Christine Bigby

    Introduction   332
    The effects of health inequities   333
    Reasons for health inequities   335
    Barriers to care   338
    Creating a responsive healthcare system   340
    Summary   343
    Tutorial exercises   343
    Further reading   344
    References   344

Chapter 19   The health of indigenous peoples   348
Sharon Chirgwin and Diane Walker

    Introduction   349
    Factors influencing the health of indigenous peoples of the world   349
    The effects of social determinants on indigenous health   352
    The complexities of indigenous health in today's world   355
    Characteristics of successful programs and approaches   358
    Summary   360
    Tutorial exercises   360
    Further reading   361
    References   361

Chapter 20   The health of migrants and refugees   364
Celia McMichael

    Introduction   365
    Social determinants of migrant health   366
    Contemporary migration flows   367
    Health challenges and opportunities across stages of migration   370
    Policy and practice responses   374
    Summary   378

Tutorial exercises   378

Further reading   379

References   379

Chapter 21   Understanding health in rural settings   **382**
Alan Crouch, Lisa Bourke and David Pierce

Introduction   383

A framework of rural health   386

Summary   395

Tutorial exercises   396

Further reading   396

References   396

Chapter 22   Drug use in Australia: A public health approach   **399**
Andrew Smirnov and Jake Najman

Introduction   400

Types of drugs   401

The drug-related burden of disease   404

Alcohol and illicit drugs – pleasure and prejudice   409

Why do people use drugs? What types of drugs do they use?   411

Drug policies: A way forward   414

Summary   418

Tutorial exercises   418

Further reading   419

References   419

Index   424

Preface

What is public health? The answer to this question can differ, depending on who provides the answer. One thing that many public health writers tend to agree on is that public health is both a science and an art, and in combination can be used to protect and promote the health of the public (Lin et al., 2014; White et al., 2014). Charles-Edward Amory Winslow, one of the leading figures in the history of public health, stated in 1920 that public health could not be achieved solely through the application of pure science. He saw public health as both the science and art that public health practitioners adopt for the prevention of disease and illness, and for the promotion of health to prolong the life of members of the public. The 'science' that Winslow referred to includes the research, biological, technical and medical knowledge utilised in public health practice. The 'art' is the translation of scientific knowledge into practice in different settings, which can vary according to the situation, circumstances and needs of the people (Lin et al., 2014). This argument is evident in many chapters in this book, which also makes clear that public health deals with health issues of the public as well as with the social, cultural, economic and political issues that influence the health of people. Chapters in the first and second parts of this book point to these issues. More concrete discussions and examples are illustrated in the last part of the book, where chapters discuss public health issues as they affect different groups and communities.

Many changes have occurred in public health over time, including environmental change and social, economic and political developments. For example, human rights and social justice have become central concerns in public health worldwide, yet not many undergraduate texts in public health discuss such important matters. Similarly, the health of some vulnerable groups, including children, adolescents, people living with disability, refugees, migrants, Indigenous peoples and rural people, has been largely neglected in public health texts. These population groups have unique health-related issues that public health practitioners must understand so that sensitive health care can be provided to meet their needs.

The book includes perspectives on public health from both local and global perspectives. Thus, readers will learn about public health issues within local settings as well as about important issues that are occurring globally. The book provides a comprehensive understanding of public health and covers relevant theoretical frameworks, key concepts in public health, the health of special groups and populations, research and policy. The book's authors are from across Australia: public health researchers as well as teachers in public health programs in different Australian universities. All authors are expert in their fields, and their chapters contain information from their own empirical research as well as reviews of literature from local and global perspectives.

The scope of the text is limited to public health as relevant to undergraduate and professional contexts. Although the book is primarily designed for undergraduate students in the public health discipline, it will also be useful for undergraduate students in other disciplines, including nursing, medicine and health social sciences.

Although public health in Australia is the setting, the book also includes public health relevant to other countries and from a global perspective. This provides readers with a comprehensive understanding of public health issues that affect people around the globe. It will help to expand their understanding of public health beyond the Australian context. The text also includes discussion of research methodology and evidence-based practice in public health.

This third edition comprises four parts and 22 chapters. Part one deals with historical and theoretical perspectives. Determinants of health are covered in Part two. Public health and research are discussed in Part three, and public health issues and special populations are covered in Part four.

In bringing this book to life, I owe my gratitude to many people. Like any other publication, this book could not have been possible without assistance from others. First, I wish to express my gratitude to Lucy Russell of Cambridge University Press, who believed in the value of the book and contracted me to edit the third edition. I also thank Jodie Fitzsimmons, who assisted me in bringing this book to the final form. Thank you for your great input into its production. Most importantly, I wish to express my sincere thanks to all the contributors who helped to make this book possible. Most of you worked so hard to meet our timetable and endured our endless emails requesting chapters from you. I hope that this journey has been a positive one for all of you.

This book is dedicated to my parents, who raised their children amidst poverty in Thailand. They believed that only education would improve the lives of their children, and hence worked hard to send us to school. I have made my career thus far because of their beliefs and the opportunities that they both provided for me. I thank them profoundly. I also dedicate this book to my youngest daughter, Emma, who physically left us too soon. You will forever stay in my heart.

Pranee Liamputtong
July 2021

REFERENCES

Lin, V., Smith, J. & Fawkes, S. (Eds.) (2014). *Public health practice in Australia: The organised effort* (2nd ed.). Allen & Unwin.

White, F., Stallones, L., & Last, J. M. (2014). *Global public health: Ecological foundations*. Oxford University Press.

Contributors

Pranee Liamputtong is a medical anthropologist and Professor of Behaviour Sciences at VinUniversity, in Hanoi, Vietnam. Pranee held a personal chair in public health in the School of Psychology and Public Health at La Trobe University, Melbourne until January 2016, and then as Professor of Public Health at the School of Health Sciences at Western Sydney University, until January 2021. She also previously taught in the School of Sociology and Anthropology and worked as a public health research fellow at the Centre for the Study of Mothers' and Children's Health at La Trobe University. Pranee has a particular interest in issues related to cultural and social influences on child-bearing, child-rearing and women's reproductive and sexual health. She works mainly with refugee and migrant women in Melbourne and with women in Asia (mostly in Thailand, Malaysia and Vietnam). She has published several books and many articles in these areas.

Frances Batchelor is a senior principal research fellow, Director of Clinical Gerontology at the National Ageing Research Institute, and honorary Associate Professor at The University of Melbourne. A physiotherapist by background, she has more than 30 years of experience in working with older people.

John Bidewell is a lecturer in the School of Science and Health, Western Sydney University. For many years, John provided technical and inspirational support to academic and student researchers at Western Sydney University's nursing and midwifery school.

Christine Bigby is Professor of Social Work and Director of the multidisciplinary Living with Disability Research Centre at La Trobe University. The focus of her work is policy, programs and frontline practices that support quality-of-life outcomes for people with intellectual disability. She is a national board member of the Australasian Society for Intellectual Disability and founding editor of Research and Practice in Intellectual and Developmental Disabilities (RAPIDD).

Lisa Bourke is a rural sociologist in the Department of Rural Health at The University of Melbourne. She has conducted a range of qualitative and quantitative research projects involving rural communities and health consumers across Australia and the United States. She is particularly interested in power relations and patterns of interaction in rural communities and how these influence health care, access and inclusion.

Lauren Carpenter is a research fellow in the Child and Community Wellbeing Unit in the Melbourne School of Population and Global Health, The University of Melbourne. She is an experienced researcher in the field of child health and wellbeing, using quantitative, qualitative and mixed-methods approaches to research, and has particular interests in child nutrition, oral health and resilience.

Stacy M. Carter is the Founding Director of the Australian Centre for Health Engagement, Evidence and Values (ACHEEV) at The University of Wollongong. She is a chief investigator in the NHMRC-funded collaboration Wiser Healthcare, and works especially on artificial intelligence in health care, overdiagnosis and overtreatment, screening, and vaccine hesitancy and refusal. Twitter handle: @stacymcarter.

Sharon Chirgwin is Associate Dean, Teaching and Learning at Menzies School of Health Research. She is a member of the Aboriginal Ethics Sub-committee, is involved in research in both clinical and community contexts, and has published across a range of areas including ethno-ornithology, nurse education, critical thinking and Indigenous perceptions of work.

Gemma Crawford is the Post Graduate Health Promotion and Public Health Coordinator and a senior lecturer in the Curtin School of Population Health, and a researcher with the Collaboration for Evidence, Research and Impact in Public Health. She is also the national president of the Australian Health Promotion Association. She has a particular interest in working with organisations to evaluate interventions and build public health capacity, and in working with underserved populations and groups across challenging health areas.

Alan Crouch is a retired population health academic holding an honorary senior fellow position with The University of Melbourne's Department of Rural Health. His work includes addressing health disadvantage among communities in remote and rural Australia, with a particular focus on the reduction of burden due to skin cancer disease. Alan has extensive experience and interests in developing country settings and in working with and for Aboriginal and Torres Strait Islander communities in eastern Australia.

Simon Crouch is the lead public health physician at the South East Public Health Unit, based at Monash Health. He is an honorary senior fellow (clinical) at The University of Melbourne. Simon is a public health doctor and the Regional Education Coordinator for Public Health Medicine training in Victoria. He recently served as the Deputy Chief Health Officer for the State of Victoria during the COVID-19 pandemic.

Elizabeth Cyarto is an exercise physiologist and the Lifestyle Program Manager at aged care provider Bolton Clarke. She is also an adjunct associate professor at The University of Queensland. Liz has committed her life and scholarship to developing and evaluating strategies to help older adults flourish, and to translating these strategies into sustainable programs across the aged-care continuum.

Elise Davis is Research and Evaluation Manager at Mind Australia Limited and is an honorary senior research fellow with the Jack Brockhoff Child Health & Wellbeing Program at The University of Melbourne. Her research focuses on the mental health and quality of life of children and families, particularly in relation to children with a disability.

Lisa Gibbs is Director of the Child and Community Wellbeing Unit in the Melbourne School of Population and Global Health at The University of Melbourne. She has been leading public health research for the past 15 years in the fields of child health and wellbeing, and disaster recovery and community resilience. These two fields intersect through her research on child resilience.

Jonathan Hallett is a senior lecturer with the School of Population Health at Curtin University, teaching public health politics and social policy. His research with the Collaboration for Evidence, Research and Impact in Public Health (CERIPH) focuses on community-based evaluation of interventions, evidence-based policy and advocacy methods, and translational research in the areas of sexual health, blood-borne viruses and law reform.

Toni Hannelly is a senior lecturer in health, safety and environment in the School of Population Health at Curtin University. She teaches in the areas of environmental health management and coordinates the Environmental Health Australia-accredited Graduate Diploma in Environmental Health course. Her current research interests include environmental air quality and online learning strategies.

Jessica Heerde is a senior research fellow in the Department of Paediatrics at the Melbourne Medical School. She has been awarded an Emerging Leadership Investigator Grant from the NHMRC (2022–26) and is an inaugural Momentum Research Fellow (2021–23) at The University of Melbourne. Jessica is a recipient of a 2021 Melbourne Medical School Strategic Grant for Outstanding Women. She is an honorary research fellow at the Centre for Adolescent Health (Murdoch Children's Research Institute) and an honorary senior fellow in the Department of Social Work at The University of Melbourne. She is area director of the Homelessness research stream in the International Youth Development Study.

Sheryl Hemphill is a self-employed research writer. She holds honorary positions at The University of Melbourne, Murdoch Children's Research Institute and the School of Education at La Trobe University. Her research interests include school and community contexts, with a focus on the development of marginalised young people.

Teresa Iacono is the Professor of Rural and Regional Allied Health in the La Trobe Rural Health School, Bendigo. She is an experienced clinician and educator, and has gained an international reputation for her research addressing communication supports, accessing health and mental health services and ethical issues in involving people with severe intellectual and developmental disabilities in research.

Jessica Lee is a senior lecturer in health promotion at Griffith University's School of Medicine. Her teaching and research interests are in knowledge translation in health promotion campaigns, public health research methods and community engagement in health promotion.

Patricia Lee is an associate professor in the School of Medicine and Dentistry at Griffith University. She has extensive teaching and working experience in public health, especially in epidemiology and biostatistics. Her research interests include epidemiology, health-risk modelling and analysis, health promotion (specialising in workplace and mental health promotion) and non-communicable disease prevention.

Celia McMichael is an associate professor in the School of Geography, Earth and Atmospheric Sciences at The University of Melbourne. She has conducted research and applied work in international health and development, with particular focus on the health of migrant and mobile populations, including people from refugee backgrounds, populations displaced following disaster, and people moving away from sites of environmental risk. She has a disciplinary background in medical anthropology and health geography.

Kirsty Morgan is a project manager at Frankston Mornington Peninsula Primary Care Partnership and adjunct research associate at Monash University's Addiction Research Centre. She has over 25 years of experience in community and public health sectors, with a focus on addressing social and structural determinants of alcohol and drug-related harms. She previously taught health promotion at Griffith University.

Jake Najman is an emeritus professor in the School of Public Health at the University of Queensland. He has published some 650 research papers, which include a focus on life-course epidemiology and the use of licit and illicit drugs in Australian society.

John Oldroyd is a senior lecturer and Master of Public Health Coordinator at Australian Catholic University. His research includes analyses of real-world datasets, non-communicable diseases in low and middle-income countries, and quality of life in the elderly. He has a particular interest in the effects of migration on health outcomes in ethnic minority populations

Rebecca E. Olson is an associate professor of sociology at the University of Queensland, where she is Program Director of the Bachelor of Social Science and Co-Director of SocioHealthLab, a research collective dedicated to doing health research differently: creatively, collaboratively and with a community focus.

David Pierce is a principal fellow in the Department of Rural Health at The University of Melbourne.

Christina Pollard is an associate professor in public health priorities at Curtin University. She is a dietitian and public health nutritionist who has worked for government for over 30 years. She has planned, implemented and evaluated numerous population-based nutrition interventions, including the Australian Gofor2&5© fruit and vegetable campaign.

Tina Price has worked as a project manager with a nurse-led mobile health clinic and has experience in a range of public health research projects in Australian universities, including at the Curtin School of Population Health. With qualifications in health promotion and business administration, her research interests include social determinants of health, equity, mental health and sexual and reproductive health.

Jennifer Reath is the Foundation Peter Brennan Chair of General Practice at Western Sydney University. She is a general practitioner who has worked for most of her career in Aboriginal Community Controlled Health Services. Her current research interests include Aboriginal ear health and the development and evaluation of innovative models of primary health care.

Zoe Sanipreeya Rice is an independent scholar currently working in London. She graduated from Monash University and The University of Melbourne, and is completing a graduate diploma in psychology at Monash University. She has published several book chapters in health and research methodologies.

Paul Saunders is a Biripi man and a research fellow in the School of Medicine at Western Sydney University. He has a background in medicine and public health, with an interest in Aboriginal and Torres Strait Islander health. His research focuses on cross-cultural capacity building of non-Indigenous health professionals, as well as equitable access to health care for Indigenous Australian populations, with a focus on examining culturally concordant models of care to improve patient outcomes.

Bernadette Sebar is a senior lecturer in the School of Medicine at Griffith University. Her research interests focus on the social determinants of health; in particular, on how the constructions of gender affect people's ability to achieve optimal health.

Marguerite C. Sendall is an associate professor in health promotion in the Department of Public Health, College of Health Sciences, Qatar University. Primarily a methodologist, Marguerite researches in settings-based health promotion; in particular, in workplace health promotion to improve nutrition and increase physical activity for hard-to-reach groups at risk of chronic disease.

Andrew Smirnov is a senior lecturer in the School of Public Health and Deputy Director of the Queensland Alcohol and Drug Research and Education Centre at the University of Queensland. His interests include patterns of substance use over the life course, policies to reduce drug-related harm, hepatitis C treatment and prevention, and the wellbeing of people exposed to the criminal justice system.

Ann Taket is an emeritus professor at Deakin University. She held the Chair in Health and Social Exclusion and was Director of the Centre for Health through Action on Social Exclusion (CHASE) at Deakin University until her retirement at the end of 2019. She has over 30 years' experience in public health-related research, with particular interest in research directed at understanding the complex interactions between social exclusion and health; the design and evaluation of interventions to reduce health inequalities; the use of action research, participatory methods,and experiential learning; and prevention and intervention in violence and abuse. She has a long-term interest in ethics and human rights issues.

Lawrence Tan is a conjoint senior lecturer in general practice in the School of Medicine at Western Sydney University, and a visiting lecturer in the Faculty of Medicine and Health Sciences at the University of Burao, Somaliland. He has extensive experience in practice and teaching family medicine at undergraduate and postgraduate levels in South America and Australia. His research interests lie in understanding how to improve primary care for patients from culturally diverse backgrounds.

Diane Walker is a First Nations Tableland Yidini woman who is a project officer in the Menzies School of Health capacity building unit, Biyamarr ma. She has extensive experience in Indigenous research organisations, including the Cooperative Research Centre for Aboriginal and Torres Strait Islander Health at the Lowitja Institute. In her current role, she assists in the implementation of systems and platforms to maximise opportunities for Aboriginal and Torres Strait Islander people by providing culturally safe spaces to empower Aboriginal and Torres Strait Islander voices and maximise opportunities.

Stuart Wark is the Clinical Academic Coordinator in the School of Rural Medicine at the University of New England, Armidale. His research interests include intellectual disability, ageing, dementia, end-of-life care, mental health and rurality, with a particular focus on effective health services delivery to disadvantaged groups.

Jane Williams is an APPRISE research fellow at Sydney Health Ethics in the School of Public Health at the University of Sydney, specialising in public health ethics. Her research interests include infectious disease emergencies, cancer screening and screening disinvestment, and women's health decision-making. Jane conducts empirical research using qualitative methodologies. Twitter handle: @janewilliams141.

Acknowledgements

The authors and Cambridge University Press would like to thank the following for permission to reproduce material in this book.

Figure 3.1: © World Health Organization. Reproduced from The Ottawa Charter for Health Promotion. Geneva: World Health Organization. Retrieved from https://www.who .int/publications/i/item/ottawa-charter-for-health-promotion; **4.1**: © 2016 Gravity Consulting Services Pty Ltd. Reproduced with permission; **4.2**: © Australian Institute of Health and Welfare 2020. Licensed under Creative Commons BY 3.0 (CC BY 3.0) licence: http://creativecommons.org/licenses/by/3.0/au/; **4.3**: © Springer Nature. Licensed under Creative Commons Attribution 4.0 International (CC BY 4.0) license: https:// creativecommons.org/licenses/by/4.0; **4.4**: Reproduced from World Health Organization, *The top 10 causes of death*, 2020; **6.1**: © 2000, Oxford University Press. S. Carlisle, 'Health Promotion, advocacy and health inequalities: a conceptual framework', *Health Promotion International*, 2000, 15(4), 369–76, by permission of Oxford University Press; **6.2**: © Public Health Advocacy Institute, Curtin University. Reproduced with permission; **7.1**: Reproduced with permission from Dahlgren G, Whitehead M. (1991). *Policies and Strategies to Promote Social Equity in Health*. Institute for Futures Studies; **7.2**: © Office for National Statistics. Contains public sector information licensed under the Open Government Licence v3.0: https://www.nationalarchives.gov.uk/doc/open-government-licence/version/3/; **8.1**: © Australian Institute of Health and Welfare 2014. Licensed under Creative Commons BY 3.0 (CC BY 3.0) license: https://creativecommons.org/licenses/by/3.0/au/; **8.2**: R. Watt (2007). From victim blaming to upstream action: Tackling the determinants of oral health inequalities *Community Dentistry and Epidemiology*, 35. Reproduced with permission of Wiley; **9.2**: Reprinted from I. Ajzen (1991) The theory of planned behavior, *Organizational Behavior and Human Decision Processes*, 50, pp. 179–211, with permission from Elsevier; **9.3**: © Getty Images/John M Lund Photography Inc; **9.4**: © Getty Images/Tara Moore; **13.3**: © Commonwealth of Australia. Reproduced with permission; **13.5**: Reproduced from World Health Organization (2009). *Implementation of the International Health Regulations (2005): Report of the Review Committee on the Functioning of the International Health Regulations (2005) in relation to Pandemic (H1N1)*; **13.6**: © Commonwealth of Australia. Licensed under Creative Commons Attribution 4.0 International licence: http://creativecommons.org/ licenses/by/4.0/; **17.1**: Reproduced from World Health Organization (2015). *World report on ageing and health*.

Extracts from P. Liamputtong (2013). *Women, Motherhood and Living with HIV/AIDS: An Introduction* reprinted by permission from Springer.

Extract from D. Suwankhong & P. Liamputtong (2017). 'I was told not to do it, but ...': Infant feeding practices among HIV-positive women in southern Thailand. *Midwifery*, 48, 69–74. Copyright 2017, with permission from Elsevier.

Extracts adapted from D. Suwankhong & P. Liamputtong (2015). Therapeutic landscapes and living with breast cancer: the lived experiences of Thai women, *Social Science & Medicine*, 128, 263–271, with permission from Elsevier.

Every effort has been made to trace and acknowledge copyright. The publisher apologises for any accidental infringement and welcomes information that would redress the situation.

Public health: An introduction to local and global contexts

1

Pranee Liamputtong

LEARNING OBJECTIVES

After studying this chapter, you should be able to:

1 understand what public health is
2 appreciate the health of Australian people
3 learn about the main public health organisations in Australia
4 understand some global public health concerns
5 learn about the social model of health and the new public health
6 understand health inequality and social justice in health.

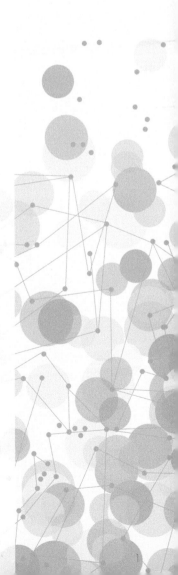

VIGNETTE

Breastfeeding and HIV-positive children: Is it a public health issue?

In 2020, 1.7 million children were living with HIV/AIDS (HIVGov, 2021a; UNAIDS, 2021). In 2019, each day about 880 children became infected with HIV and around 310 children died from AIDS-related causes (UNICEF, 2020). Mostly, this was due to inadequate access to HIV prevention, care and treatment services. Most of children living with HIV/AIDS are born in poor nations, particularly in sub-Saharan Africa, and will die before they reach their fifth birthday. Approximately 40 per cent of HIV-positive children are infected through breastfeeding. This makes breastfeeding the most widespread means of mother-to-child transmission (MTCT) of HIV. For HIV-positive mothers who practice prolonged breast-feeding, the risk of MTCT of HIV spans from 25 to 48 per cent (Blumental et al., 2014).

The transmission of HIV through breast milk has created a dilemma for HIV-positive mothers (Bansaccal et al., 2020). The benefits of breastfeeding and the risks of not breastfeeding have to be weighed against the risk of HIV transmission through breastfeeding. Whereas previously breastfeeding, especially exclusive breastfeeding, was a key child survival strategy, the finding that HIV is present in the breast milk of women living with HIV has led to a re-assessment of the benefits of breastfeeding. Avoiding breastfeeding has been recommended as a means to eliminate breast milk-transmission of HIV (AIDSInfo, 2021; Moseholm & Weis, 2020; HIVGov, 2021b).

Breastfeeding is the most widespread means of mother-to-child transmission of HIV (Moseholm & Weis, 2020; HIVGov, 2021b). As part of the prevention of mother-to-child HIV transmission strategies, there are two options that women with HIV are urged to consider when feeding their infants. These are exclusive breastfeeding with early weaning, or replacement feeding (with breast-milk substitutes). These options may be feasible for women who can afford to do so.

Most HIV-positive mothers follow the advice not to breastfeed their infants (Liamputtong, 2013). However, being unable to connect with their infants through the act of breastfeeding, women may have ambivalent feelings about their motherhood and mothering roles. This may have great ramifica-tions for their emotional wellbeing (Bansaccal et al., 2020). It has been recognised in many societies that breastfeeding is a marked determinant of being a good and responsible mother (Liamputtong, 2011; Suwankhong & Liamputtong, 2017).

Source: Liamputtong 2013 and Suwankhong & Liamputtong 2017.

Introduction

Determinant of health – a factor within and external to the individual that determines their health outcomes; the specific social, economic and political circumstances into which individuals are born and live.

The health of the public is determined by a spectrum of complex individual, social, cultural, economic and environmental factors (White et al., 2013; Turnock, 2016a, b). This has been attributed to **determinants of health** (Marmot, 2004; Commission on Social Determinants of Health, 2014; Liamputtong, 2019; see also the chapters in parts 1 and 2). Determinants of health include genetic and biological factors; sociocultural and socio-economic factors (including social class, gender, ethnicity, education, income and occupation); health behav-iours (such as cigarette smoking, abuse of alcohol and risky lifestyles); and environmental factors (for example, social support, social connection, housing, geographical location and climate). The determinants of health can lead to a change (for better or worse) in the health and wellbeing of individuals, groups and populations (Commission on Social Determinants of Health, 2014; Gleeson & Chong, 2019; Liamputtong, 2019; see also Chapter 7).

Based on the concept of a **new public health**, it is argued that public health practice is situated within the context of broader social issues concerning the underlying social, economic, cultural, environmental and political determinants of health and disease. Thus, this book has its emphasis on the sociocultural environment rather than on the biological and genetic factors associated with health. As illustrated in the opening vignette, the continuing HIV/AIDS epidemic of the past few decades has created a significant challenge for public health practice. It highlights the complex social issues that are fundamental elements of public health (Baum, 2016; Turnock, 2016a, b; Schneider, 2017).

This chapter introduces **public health** and the salient issues relevant to it from local and global perspectives. The definition of public health, its values and major public health organisations are included. The chapter also discusses major public health challenges in Australia and from a global context. The social model of health, health inequalities and social justice are also discussed.

New public health – the concept of public health that moves the focus from behavioural change to healthy public policy, and that focuses on the concept of life-skills enhancement. It also addresses inequalities in health in the population.

Public health – the health of the public, the health profession, health services and the healthcare system, and the knowledge and techniques used to alleviate suffering and disability.

What is public health?

Definition of public health

Public health means different things to different people (White et al., 2013; Lin et al, 2014; Turnock, 2016a, b). Public health may refer to the health of the public, the health profession, health services, the healthcare system and appropriate knowledge and techniques (Turnock, 2016a, b). Regardless of how it is seen, public health aims to promote and improve the health of all people and to prevent injury, disease and premature death. Public health also attempts to alleviate suffering and disability (White et al., 2013). In the Australian context, public health is also about the prevention of illness, disease and injury, as well as the promotion of health, wellbeing and quality of life of people (Fleming, 2019).

It is here that the definition of health needs to be discussed. Health is constructed socially and culturally (Turnock, 2016a, b; Fleming, 2019; Liamputtong & Suwankhong, 2019; Wright & Higgs, 2019). According to the Australian Institute of Health and Welfare (AIHW, 2017), health is seen as a crucial component of wellbeing. Health is also situated within broad social and cultural contexts. The state of the health of populations in society contributes to the social and economic wellbeing of that particular society. Overall, health is perceived as 'a complex outcome' that is influenced by factors including genetic, environmental, economic, social and political circumstances (Baum, 2016).

While medicine has its focus on treating individuals who are ill, public health emphasises the prevention of illness and improvement in the health of people (Schneider, 2017; Parker & Baldwin, 2019). Due to its focus on prevention, the achievements of public health are difficult to recognise. This is why the value of public health tends not to be as highly appreciated as that of medicine. However, most health gains are the result of public health initiatives such as improved nutrition, housing, sanitation and occupational safety (see also Chapter 2 in this book). According to Schneider (2017), effective public health programs save lives and also save money on medical costs. Essentially, public health contributes to the health of people more than medicine is able to do (Turnock, 2016a, b; Schneider, 2017; Fleming, 2019; Parker & Baldwin, 2019). Globally, public health efforts have contributed significantly to improvement in health status of populations. It will continue to play an important role in dealing with new challenges we might face in the future (Turnock, 2016a, b).

Preventive measures in public health can be applied at three levels: primary, secondary and tertiary (Schneider, 2017; Fleming, 2019; Parker & Baldwin, 2019). Primary prevention focuses on the prevention of a disease or injury. Primary prevention includes, for example, anti-smoking campaigns, regulations on the use of seat belts in motor vehicles, prohibition of driving after alcohol consumption (drink-driving campaigns) and nutrition programs. Secondary prevention attempts to reduce the damage caused by the illness through implementation of screening programs (for instance, breast, bowel and prostate cancer screening programs). Secondary prevention also includes the reduction of injury-causing events, such as injuries from competitive sports and motor car racing.

Tertiary prevention aims to minimise any disability that might follow an illness or injury, and is implemented through the provision of medical care and rehabilitation services.

REFLECTION QUESTION

Public health programs have been used to improve the health and wellbeing of people around the world. Since the onset of the COVID-19 pandemic, public health programs have played an essential role in the control of the disease in many parts of the world, including Australia. Why does this happen? How will public health programs help to prevent future pandemics in the world?

Public health disciplines

Commonly, there are five main disciplines under the umbrella of public health. Biostatistics is the application of statistics to the analysis of biological and medical data in public health. Epidemiology refers to the study of the determinants and distribution of health issues within specific groups of the population (see also Chapter 13). Environmental and occupational health sciences deal with a range of environmental determinants of health, including physical, biological, social and behavioural determinants, as well as with diseases that have environmental and occupational origins. Health services administration is concerned with the functioning of public health services in ensuring that they are equitably distributed, work as intended and that policies are implemented as planned. It also plays a crucial role in evaluating the cost-effectiveness of public health programs and medical care (White et al., 2013)

Social and behavioural sciences encompass the application of health education and health promotion to the protection of the health of people (White et al., 2013). Social and behavioural sciences facilitate our understanding of how society and its cultural and belief systems influence health perceptions and the behaviours of individuals and groups (Lin et al., 2014; Liamputtong, 2019). Schneider (2017) points out that social and behavioural sciences have increasingly become major components of public health. More and more people in contemporary societies must deal with illnesses and diseases caused by the social environment and their own behaviour. Some population groups have poorer health overall than others, and the main reasons may be related to social factors. For example, people from low socio-economic groups tend to be less healthy than those with a higher income. People from ethnic minority groups, including indigenous peoples, immigrants and refugees, are at higher risk for many health issues (Schneider, 2017; see also chapters 19 and 20). Additionally, many forms of cancer are caused by smoking; heart disease is linked with exercise patterns and nutrition; drug use and alcohol consumption have been linked with the deaths of many individuals; and violence is a significant cause of death in many societies (see also chapters 7 and 8). These challenges are beyond the questions that biomedical sciences can answer. It is likely that the social and behavioural sciences will make a significant difference to public health policies and practice in the future (Schneider, 2017). Although contemporary public health continues to deal with problems related to sanitation and disease control, increasing attention is now paid to the social determinants of health: 'how the social and behavioural lives of people can affect their health status' (Lin et al., 2014, p. 81). As the complexity of human health patterns increases, the scope of public health interest is widened. This is particularly true in recent times, with the many public health challenges that we have witnessed globally.

The health of Australians

Overall, Australia is doing well in terms of the health of its people. Australia is one of the countries that enjoys the highest levels of life expectancy in the world. From the beginning of the 20th century, the picture of health in Australia changed dramatically. Since 1901, infant and child mortality have decreased significantly, and this has contributed greatly to the increased life expectancy of Australians (AIHW, 2020). Death rates have declined substantially across all age groups. In the past two decades, Australian life expectancy at birth has been located within the top 10 of countries in the Organisation for Economic Co-operation and Development (OECD). According to the AIHW (2020), average life expectancy at birth is 84.9 years for women and 80.7 years for men. Australians also enjoy longer years of living free of disability. Germov (2019a) contends that this health improvement is not due to their biological advantage; instead, it is 'a reflection of our distinctive living and working conditions' (p. 4). Generally, better living conditions, as well as improved public health and safety programs and improved medical care, contribute to the reduction of mortality in Australia (Lin et al., 2014; Fleming, 2015).

However, among some population groups there are several public health issues that need significant improvement. These groups include people from lower socio-economic backgrounds, Indigenous people, people living with disabilities, older people, immigrants and refugees, and people living in rural and remote areas (AIHW, 2020). The health concerns of most of the population groups mentioned here are covered in the chapters of Part 4.

SPOTLIGHT 1.1

Vulnerable people and health in Australia

Even though Australia does well in terms of health and healthcare access, there are certain individuals and groups who do not enjoy the same levels of good health and health care. These individuals and groups have been referred to as 'vulnerable populations' (Lin et al., 2014; AIHW, 2016, 2017). **Vulnerable people** are those individuals or groups who are disadvantaged and susceptible to health adversities (Liamputtong, 2007, 2020). Based on these descriptions, vulnerable people may include children, women, older people, immigrants, refugees, sex workers, homeless people and LGBTIQ+ communities. People living with chronic illness or mental illness and their caregivers are also referred to as vulnerable populations (Liamputtong, 2007, 2020; see also Chapter 7).

In public health, according to Lin, Smith and Fawkes (2014, p. 3660), 'vulnerable people' means 'individuals or populations being at risk of ill-health or other harms, such as injury'. Often, their sociocultural status and living situations have made them vulnerable in various ways. It is suggested that vulnerability is a consequence of inequalities in society. The outcomes of social inequality include ill health and injury. Often, people who are socially disadvantaged are at higher risk of ill health and injury. They tend to have the least social capital and economic resources. Thus, they have reduced capacity to protect themselves from illness and injury. In this sense, vulnerability 'can be thought of in terms of an individual's or group's exposure to a range of psycho-social environmental factors that raise the chances of ill-health' (Lin et al., 2014, p. 366).

QUESTIONS

1   Which other groups would you refer to as 'vulnerable people'?
2   What are the public health issues that these vulnerable people might experience?
3   How can key public health organisations respond to their vulnerability and public health issues?

Key public health organisations in Australia

Public health is closely linked to government, and its processes are intrinsically political. Public health also involves a number of workforces that share a common goal to improve the health of the public (Lin et al., 2014; Wutzke et al., 2018; Fleming, 2019). These characteristics are complex and necessitate the commitments and skills of different professions from different disciplines (Fleming, 2019). This has led Lin, Smith and Fawkes (2014) to refer to public health as an 'organised effort' that requires the contribution of many different parties (see also chapters 2 and 10). Policy, legislative frameworks and resources to support public health services delivery are the responsibility of governments. However, services are provided by specialists and professionals in different locations, including hospitals, general practice, community health centres, non-government organisations (NGOs), schools, media outlets, industry and so on (Lin et al., 2014; Fleming, 2015, 2019).

In Australia, there are several key players in public health (see also Chapter 10). These include organisations both within the government and outside it (Lin et al., 2014; Fleming, 2019). Local and state governments play major roles in public health, whereas the role of the federal government is limited (Lin et al., 2014). Traditionally, local government has a central role in environmental sanitation, food safety and the regulation of building and public accommodation standards. Its role has expanded to include public health activities such as municipal public health plans, which embrace public health strategies to maintain and improve the health of people within a local community. Nowadays, local government is involved in many activities that contribute to the health and wellbeing of the public, including home care, food and nutrition services, child care and transportation (Lin et al., 2014).

State governments are responsible for three key areas in public health: prevention and control of disease; health promotion strategies; and provision of health protection functions (Lin et al., 2014). Each state government has a chief health officer, who gives advice and reassurances to the public when a public health crisis occurs (Lin et al., 2014). The federal government has been responsible mainly for health funding and encouragement to adopt common approaches to health policies and programs by the state and territory governments.

Public health organisations situated outside government comprise a number of key players, including general practitioners (GPs), other health services, NGOs, professional organisations, schools, the media and industry (Lin et al., 2014). GPs play an important role in the provision of health services in the community (Perry & Willis, 2019; Willis et al., 2020; Perry & Sivertsen, 2022). Other public health services are provided mainly through secondary or tertiary prevention strategies. National and state bodies such as the Cancer Council and the National Heart Foundation are strongly involved in public health. They contribute by delivering intervention programs and research (for example, sun protection, women's cancer screening and tobacco control) (Lin et al., 2014; Wutzke et al., 2018).

Public health: Global concerns

Several global public health concerns are prevalent in the 21st century. Some global major public health issues are discussed in this section.

Overweight and obesity

Overweight and obesity are now considered as contributing to the global burden of disease (White et al., 2013; OECD, 2017; World Health Organization (WHO) 2021a). In 2016, a total of 650 million adults and over 340 million children and adolescents (aged 5–19 years) were identified as obese. The prevalence of obesity has tripled in more than 70 nations since 1975, and it continues to increase in most other countries (WHO, 2021a). Overweight and obesity are among the key risk factors for non-communicable diseases, including type 2 diabetes, circulatory disease and musculoskeletal problems (Schneider, 2017). In many developed nations, such as the United States and Australia, a high prevalence of obesity is caused by the combination of eating too much and exercising too little (Schneider, 2017; AIHW, 2020). Rural-to-urban population movements have also contributed to increasing overweight and obesity in many countries (Schneider, 2017). The obesity **pandemic** has become a challenge for both developed and developing nations (White et al., 2013). In Australia, according to the AIHW (2020), between 2017 and 2018, about 12.5 million Australians were overweight or obese. As the prevalence of overweight and obesity has increased so quickly in recent decades, according to Schneider (2017) the health risks of overweight and obesity will reverse many public health improvements achieved in the 20th century (see Chapter 2).

Prevalence rates for overweight and obesity vary in different regions. Countries in Central and Eastern Europe, North America and the Middle East have higher prevalence of these conditions than those northern Europe and Asia (Hou, 2015). This is a major concern for

Pandemic – worldwide spread of a disease.

developing countries with overstretched healthcare systems. They have to deal with the 'double burden' of an 'unfinished agenda' of widespread undernutrition and infectious disease, as well as an emerging burden of disease linked with over-nutrition (White et al., 2013, p. 292). It is estimated that, with the rapid increase in overweight and obesity in developing nations, the number of obese people could double by 2025 (Formiguera & Canton, 2004).

Mental health issues

In developed nations, according to the World Health Organization (WHO), mental health issues constitute greater disability than other illnesses (Schneider, 2017). Among adults, the most common mental health issues are anxiety and mood disorders. One of the most common mental health issues in the general population is major depressive disorder. This illness has a range of symptoms including feelings of sadness and loss of pleasure or interest in things that were once enjoyed. A combination of other symptoms, such as changes in sleep pattern and weight, difficulty concentrating and irritability, may also be experienced by affected individuals (Goldmann & Galea, 2014).

Many mental disorders are the result of environmental impacts. For example, post-traumatic stress disorder is caused by critical, stressful events (Schneider, 2017). This is particularly the case with people who experience disasters such as bushfires and earthquakes, and military workers. There is a clear link between mental disorders and chronic diseases (for example, asthma, diabetes, epilepsy, cardiovascular disease and cancer). Additionally, people with mental health issues are at increased risk of injury (both intentional and unintentional). They tend to use tobacco products and to abuse alcohol and other drugs more than individuals without mental illness (Goldmann & Galea, 2014; Schneider, 2017; Sawyer, 2019).

It is estimated that, like people in most developed countries, about 1 in 5 Australians had a mental or behavioural condition in 2017–18, and females reported more mental health issues than males (AIHW, 2020). In 2015, about 4 million Australian people experienced a common mental health issues (AIHW, 2018). The anxiety and depressive disorders that currently affect Australia and other developed nations are mainly due to the commonplace circumstances and stressors that occur in these societies, including financial strain, unemployment, economic hardship, overwork, pressure to succeed, relationship breakdown and drought (Schneider, 2017; Sawyer, 2019). These stressors are intrinsically connected with salient social and environmental factors such as an increased sense of 'individualism', lack of social support, and anxieties about environmental threats (Sawyer, 2019, p. 249). For some, such as refugees, immigrants, Indigenous people and people with disabilities, this is mainly due to systemic racism and discrimination (Nguyen et al., 2016; Kurban & Liamputtong, 2017; see also chapters 18, 19 and 20).

Migration and health

There are about 1 billion migrants across the world 'whose lives have been shaped by social determinants in their homelands and who face new social, economic, and political conditions in destination countries' (Castaneda et al., 2015, p. 376). Globally, there are approximately 272 million international migrants living outside their countries of origin, and 763 million internal migrants and displaced people living within their countries of birth (WHO, 2018,

2021b). It is projected that, by 2050, there will be 405 million international migrants in the world (International Organization for Migration (IOM), 2020). Migration is a result of several social determinants (for example, poverty, political persecution and occupational and educational opportunities). Many people flee armed conflict, persecution and natural disaster. Economic migrants make up the largest growing portion of the migrating population and, with increases in global economic problems, this is likely to continue and can be associated with human rights issues in the receiving country (Schneider, 2017; Correa-Velez, 2019; WHO, 2021b; see also Chapter 20). This was clearly witnessed in recent years in the number of Rohingya refugees who fled by boat from Myanmar and were denied entry to Thailand, Malaysia and Indonesia, and Syrian refugees who attempted to enter European nations.

Whether voluntary or involuntary, migration affects individuals and communities in many ways. It certainly necessitates a complete change in their daily lives and can have great social, economic and health consequences (Castaneda et al., 2015; IOM, 2020; WHO, 2021b). An important migration issue that has ramifications for public health practice is the increase in the number of women who are migrating (UN Women, 2018). Women generally make up half of the migrating population, and in some countries make up 70–80 per cent. Often, migrant women are forced into low-paid jobs that are unregulated, such as domestic work. They are at high risk of exploitation, violence and abuse, including human trafficking. These can lead to long-term health and social problems for women, including sexually transmitted infection and increased numbers of unplanned pregnancies. Often too, they are rejected by their families when they return home (Schneider, 2017).

Recent global epidemics and pandemics

An epidemic refers to a situation when more cases of a health issue occur than expected in a certain part of the world, but it does not spread further, such as Zika virus. A pandemic is the global spread of a new disease that affects a large number of people; for example, a new influenza virus or the coronavirus, COVID-19 (Madhav at al., 2018). This section outlines some of the recent and serious epidemics and pandemics around the world.

HIV/AIDS epidemic

The HIV/AIDS epidemic has entered its fourth decade and continues to pose a major public health problem worldwide (HIVGov, 2021a). Although earlier in the epidemic it affected mostly intravenous injecting drug users, sex workers and men, it is now also affecting a large number of women and children. According to UNAIDS (2021), in 2020, there were 37.6 million people worldwide living with HIV/AIDS and 1.5 million people became newly infected with it. Around 690 000 people died from AIDS. 34.7 million people have died from AIDS-related illnesses since the beginning of the epidemic. Women and girls made up about 50 per cent of all new HIV infections in 2020 (UNAIDS, 2021). Among young women in developing countries in particular, the rates of infection are increasing rapidly. In sub-Saharan Africa (the region most heavily affected by HIV), women and girls comprised 63 per cent of all new HIV infections. In sub-Saharan Africa, 6 in 7 new HIV infections among young people aged 15–19 years are in girls (UNAIDS 2021). Young women aged 15–24 years are twice as likely to be living with HIV than men in the same age group. Children and young people are also heavily affected by the HIV/AIDS epidemic (UNAIDS, 2021). In 2020, about 1.7 million children and young people aged 0–14 years were living with

HIV/AIDS (UNAIDS, 2021). Women and children tend to suffer from the adverse effects of HIV and AIDS to a greater extent than men (Liamputtong, 2013, 2016). Despite the recent reduction in the number of people infected by HIV/AIDS around the globe, it is suggested that the number of individuals living with HIV/AIDS will continue to grow in sub-Saharan Africa (UNAIDS, 2021).

H1N1 swine 'flu pandemic

The swine 'flu pandemic was brought about by a new strain of H1N1, which emerged in Mexico in the spring of 2009 and then spread to countries all over the world. In one year, the virus affected around 1.4 billion people across the globe. It also killed between 151 700 and 575 400 people in a year (Madhav et al., 2018). The 2009 'flu pandemic infected children and young adults to a greater extent than older people. About 80 per cent of the deaths were in people younger than 65 years. Older people had built up sufficient immunity to the group of viruses to which H1N1 belongs, and thus they were not as affected by the virus as much as young people. Nowadays, there is a vaccine for the H1N1 virus and this is included in the annual 'flu vaccine in most nations.

West African Ebola epidemic

The first known cases of Ebola occurred in the Democratic Republic of Congo and Sudan in 1976. The virus is believed to have its origin in bats. Between 2014 and 2016, Ebola spread across West Africa with 28 646 reported cases and 11 323 deaths (Madhav et al., 2018). In December 2013, the first case was found in Guinea; it then quickly spread to Sierra Leone and Liberia. Most Ebola cases and deaths occurred in those three countries. However, there were also several cases diagnosed in Mali, Senegal, Nigeria, Europe and the United States. Thus far, there is no cure for Ebola, but efforts to develop a vaccine are continuing.

Zika virus epidemic

The Zika virus is dispersed through mosquitoes of the *Aedes* genus. However, in humans, it can also be sexually transmitted. Usually, Zika is not harmful to children or adults, but it can harm infants who are still in the womb, resulting in birth defects. The mosquitoes that transmit Zika multiply well in warm, humid climates. This makes South America, Central America and the southern United States perfect locations for the virus to spread. It has affected 76 countries thus far (Madhav et al., 2018). The effects of the Zika epidemic in South America and Central America will not be known for several years, but scientists have attempted to bring the virus under control.

SARS

Severe Acute Respiratory Syndrome (SARS) is believed to have begun with bats and then spread to humans (Piret & Boivin, 2021). SARS was first detected in humans in China; it was first identified in 2003 after several months of increasing incidence. This was followed by cases in 29 other countries in Asia, Europe, North America and South America, affecting 8437 people, with 774 deaths (Piret & Boivin, 2021). SARS is identified by respiratory problems including fever, dry cough, headaches and body aches. It is transmitted through respiratory droplets from coughs and sneezes. SARS rapidly became a global threat due to its accelerated spread and immense mortality rate (Piret & Boivin, 2021). By July 2003, quarantine efforts contained the transmission of the virus and since then it has not resurfaced. Global health professionals perceived SARS as a forewarning to improve responses to outbreaks. Lessons from the pandemic were employed to keep global diseases like H1N1, Ebola and Zika under control.

COVID-19

In late December 2019, SARS-CoV-2, a new strain of coronavirus that had not been previously detected in humans, was first reported in Wuhan, China (Chatterjee, 2021; Piret & Boivin, 2021). This virus created a cluster of cases of an acute respiratory disease, referred to as coronavirus disease 2019, or COVID-19. Symptoms include respiratory problems, cough and fever, which can lead to pneumonia and death. Similar to SARS, it is spread through short-range aerosol transmission.

At present, the virus has spread to almost all countries around the world, with unanticipated repercussions for the health and wellbeing of millions of people (Zoumpourlis et al., 2020; Béland et al., 2021; Chatterjee, 2021). COVID-19 has created fear among people and uncertainty at all economic and socio-political levels. It markedly complicates people's daily life, travel and trade, and local and global economies (Béland et al., 2021; Chatterjee, 2021; Moreira & Hick, 2021; Thoradeniya & Jayasinghe, 2021). Due to restriction strategies, such as lockdowns restricting people to their homes, which have been taken to stop the spread of the virus, mental health problems (particularly depression) have resulted in many individuals around the globe (Zoumpourlis et al., 2020).

The WHO declared the spread of COVID-19 as a pandemic on 11 March 2020. This marks the first global pandemic since the 2009 swine 'flu. More than 200 nations have now been affected by the virus. Major outbreaks first appeared in India, Mexico, Peru, Brazil, South Africa, Western Europe, Russia and the United States. By December 2020, it had affected more than 74 million people and led to more than 1.6 million deaths worldwide (WHO, 2020a). The number of new cases grew quickly, with more than 500 000 reported each day, on average.

As of July 2021, the number of people affected with COVID-19 reached 182 319 261 worldwide, and the death toll reached 3 954 323 (WHO, 2021c). However, it is suggested that these figures are underestimated as testing did not start at the beginning of the outbreak, and many people may not have been tested because they had no symptoms, or only mild symptoms. At the time of writing (July 2021), several vaccines have been approved, and are being rolled out in many countries. However, we have also witnessed new and more serious strains of the virus emerging in different parts of the world (Béland et al., 2021).

COVID-19 is unlikely to be the last pandemic that we witness. Carrol and colleagues (2021) suggest that epidemics and pandemics will continue to increase as they will be 'driven mainly by demographic trends, such as urbanisation, environmental degradation, climate change, persistent social and economic inequalities, and globalised trade and travel' (p. 2). This has prompted serious discussions among scholars about the future of global public health. Zoumpourlis and colleagues (2020), for example, contend that COVID-19 'should ring like a very loud bell to the ears of the global financial elite and of every single consumer. If global environmental, health and development issues are not addressed holistically, new pandemics will continue to emerge' (p. 3046).

SPOTLIGHT 1.2

Urbanisation and public health

Where we live influences our health and our chances of thriving. Even though people living in urban areas do better in terms of health and healthcare access in Australia, globally we witness a somewhat different pattern. Urbanisation creates major environmental challenges, particularly climate change, for many nations (Hanna, 2019). It is a significant impact in many low-income countries and among vulnerable people (McMichael et al., 2008). They are not only vulnerable to health hazards from climate change, but also need to deal with increasing problems associated with rapid development (Commission on Social Determinants of Health, 2014). Urbanisation has reshaped the health problems of individuals and groups with increasing alcohol and substance abuse, injuries and non-communicable diseases, and from ecological disasters. This is particularly so among the urban poor (Campbell & Campbell, 2007).

Increasingly, in the cities of high-income countries (including Australia), violence and crime have become significant problems in urban neighbourhoods. This is particularly noticeable in the large-scale suburban housing estates of large cities. Mental health problems contribute to approximately 14 per cent of the global urban burden of disease (Prince et al., 2007). Common mental disorders include depression, psychoses and alcohol and substance abuse disorders (Prince et al., 2007; AIHW, 2017, 2020). It is thought that by 2030 the burden of major depression will create a major urban health challenge, and it is expected to become the second-highest cause of loss of disability-adjusted life years among urban populations (Commission on Social Determinants of Health, 2014). Urban populations will also get older. In low-income and middle-income nations, the numbers of older people in urban areas are expected to swell to more than 16 times the current levels, from about 56 million in 1998 to more than 908 million in 2050. There will also be more people living in poverty, slums and squatter settlements in these nations (Campbell & Campbell, 2007). People living with disability in urban areas are also vulnerable to health threats. This is due to a high population density, crowding, unsuitable living design and lack of social support (Frumkin et al., 2004; Commission on Social Determinants of Health, 2014).

QUESTION

What challenges might highly urbanised countries encounter, and how can they go about ensuring that their urban populations have better health and quality of life?

Social model of health and the new public health

Since the 1970s, there has been a shift in the public health sector to try to understand why some individuals and groups of people become sicker and have a lower life expectancy than others (Lin et al., 2014; Baum 2016; Germov, 2019a; Liamputtong, 2019). There has been increasing awareness that medicine alone cannot adequately improve health overall or decrease health inequalities without examining where and how people live (Braveman et al., 2011; Turnock, 2016a, b; Germov, 2019a).

The 'old public health' model focuses on behavioural change. Causes of disease are analysed in terms of lifestyle 'factors' within the individual, as well as in the social and physical environments. Health education, service provision and legislation are used as strategies to interrupt the 'chain of causation' for a disease (Fleming, 2019). The 'new public health' approach moves the focus from behavioural change to **healthy public policy** (see Chapter 3), and supersedes the lifestyle approach with the concept of life-skills enhancement (Fleming, 2015, 2019). The new public health approach underscores the importance of addressing inequalities in health among populations. This can be done through effective public policies including education, employment and economic policies so that adequate standards of living, and thus, better health for all, can be achieved (Fleming, 2019; Liamputtong, 2019).

In health sociology, the new public health approach is referred to as the **social model of health**. The social model of health endeavours to ascertain the societal factors that hinder the health of individuals and groups (Germov, 2019a; Wright & Higgs, 2019). The model attempts to tackle **health inequity** by emphasising the prevention of illness through social reforms that have their focus on the living conditions of people (Henderson-Wilson, 2012). According to Germov (2019a), the social model of health places an emphasis on health determinants and health intervention at the societal level. It draws attention to the fact that health and illness take place within a social context (Wright & Higgs, 2019). As such, for health interventions and preventive efforts to be effective, they must move away from emphasis on the medical treatment of an individual. Within the social model of health, Germov (2019a) suggests that 'health is a social responsibility' (p. 15) and the social determinants of an individual's health status and health-related behaviour must be carefully examined. Importantly, the social model of health underscores societal factors that impose risks and induce illnesses (for example, racism, discrimination, poverty, homelessness, unemployment and stressful work). In particular, it emphasises the **health inequalities** that individuals who are located within some social groups (based on their social class, gender, ethnicity, age, sexual orientation and occupational experience). The model also suggests that any attempts to improve the overall health of the individuals and groups must tackle both living and working conditions, including poverty, possibilities for employment, and health and safety in the workplace. Additionally, Germov (2019a) argues that these attempts must also cater for cultural differences within the population. This is crucial for a multicultural society like Australia, where people come from many cultural backgrounds (including refugees, immigrants and Indigenous peoples; see chapters 19 and 20). In sum, the priority of the social model is the prevention of illness (along with the treatment of illness), and it endeavours to lessen health inequality within the population.

As the social model examines health and illness beyond the medical model, it enables us also to understand how people perceive health and illness (Henderson-Wilson, 2012; Wright & Higgs, 2019). The perspectives of lay individuals, including those experiencing ill health, can be drawn upon in public health prevention and health service provision (Liamputtong, 2019). By moving the focus away from a biomedical framework towards the social model, health and illness can be perceived within a framework of individuals and society (Henderson-Wilson, 2012; Fleming, 2015; Wright & Higgs, 2019). The social model of health, according to Henderson-Wilson (2012), 'allows for a comprehensive understanding of health, illness and well-being, by exploring the range of influential social and cultural contexts within an individual's environment' (p. 200).

Healthy public policy – an explicit concern for health and equity in all areas of policy, and characterised by an accountability for health effects.

Social model of health – an approach to health that views health as influenced by social structures and attempts to identify the factors within society that hinder the health of individuals, groups and populations.

Health inequity – the disparity between health resources and outcomes across populations.

Health inequality – the disparities in the health achievements of some individuals and groups. Inequality disproportionately affects the health of the most disadvantaged members of society, particularly in resource-poor nations.

SPOTLIGHT 1.3

Social factors and tobacco use

Globally, 1.1 billion people currently smoke cigarettes or use other tobacco products. Most smokers live in low-income and middle-income nations (WHO, 2020b). It was estimated that in 2020 more than 9 million annual tobacco-related deaths would occur. Seven million were expected to take place in developing countries. To address this pandemic of tobacco-related diseases, the WHO launched the Framework Convention on Tobacco Control in 2005 (White et al., 2013). Tobacco control aims to prevent tobacco-related disease and premature death. Thus, programs are devised to prevent the start of tobacco use, and to help current smokers to stop smoking. The reduction of exposure to second-hand smoke is included in control programs. The most successful attempt to date has been the prohibition of smoking in public places. Worldwide, tobacco control efforts also include labelling tobacco products as hazardous, increasing their prices and taxation, prohibiting the advertising of tobacco and sponsorship of entertainment events by tobacco companies, and scrutinising the illicit trade of tobacco (White et al., 2013).

However, the social and cultural contexts of the involved populations have been recognised as crucial elements of successful control programs (White et al., 2013). Creating tobacco prevention programs for specific populations necessitates an appreciation that the prevalence and patterns of tobacco use differ across gender, social class, race, ethnicity and age groups (WHO, 2020b). One important aspect of an attempt to develop appropriate programs is to focus on the functional use of cigarettes within different groups of populations. Tobacco may be used for socialisation in a few ways. Peers may have a significant role in modelling tobacco use and thus play a crucial role in tobacco control for some groups. For example, in the United States, peers have been reported as having a strong role in the initiation of smoking among whites and Hispanics, compared with African-Americans. Thus, while using peers as a way to influence smoking behaviour may be effective among white and Hispanic young people, it may not work effectively with African-Americans. Working closely with adult role models and/or parents may be more effective when tailoring intervention programs for African-American young people (White et al., 2013; WHO, 2020b).

QUESTION
What does this Spotlight tell you about the importance of social factors for understanding public health challenges?

Health inequality and social justice

A number of circumstances and conditions have created basic inequalities that contribute to the ill health of people within the current sociocultural, economic and political contexts around the globe, including in Australia (Germov, 2019a; Liamputtong, 2019). Therefore, health inequalities exist among populations (Bleich et al., 2012; Commission on Social Determinants of Health, 2014; Gleeson & Chong, 2019; see also Chapter 7). 'Health inequality' is a term that is employed 'to designate the differences, variations, and disparities in the health achievements of individuals and groups' (Kawachi et al., 2002, p. 647).

In the past three decades, we have witnessed the steady growth of economic inequality across the globe (Wilkinson & Pickett, 2006; OECD, 2011; Gleeson & Chong, 2019). This has crucial implications for population health because of the clear evidence of the negative effects of income inequality on the morbidity and mortality of populations. This inequality disproportionately affects the health of the most disadvantaged members of society, particularly in poorer nations (Turnock, 2016a, b). However, it is detrimental for everyone. Inequality has contributed to the psychosocial burden of many people (Kawachi & Kennedy, 2006; Cushing et al., 2015). Importantly, a growing body of research is revealing that polluted and degraded environments tend to occur more often in unequal societies (Cushing et al., 2015). This helps to explain 'why more unequal societies are often less healthy' (Cushing et al., 2015, p. 193).

Social inequalities intersect in a way that can create further inequalities in health among some individuals and groups (Broom et al., 2019). For example, men from ethnic minority groups and lower social classes are also likely to be disadvantaged in terms of health and wellbeing, when compared to white Anglo-Celtic men with higher incomes (Germov, 2019b; Julian, 2019). Among migrant populations, those from refugee backgrounds are more likely to fare worse in all aspects (including health status and health needs) than economic migrants from higher social classes and those who have higher educational attainments. Even among these populations, women are more disadvantaged than men (see also Chapter 20). Within the Australian context, we have witnessed many examples of these interrelationships within Indigenous populations. Indigenous Australians fare worse in health issues than non-Indigenous Australians, and often women and children and those who live in remote areas fare worse than Indigenous men who live in urban settings (AIHW, 2020; see also Chapter 19).

Since inequalities are the consequence of inequitable societies, they are addressed through the concept of **social justice** (Bleich et al., 2012; Commission on Social Determinants of Health, 2014; Miles, 2019). It has been suggested that social justice approaches to health are crucial for public health because all individuals have the right to achieve good health outcomes (Wilkinson, 2005; Wilkinson & Pickett, 2006; Commission on Social Determinants of Health, 2014; Keleher & MacDougall 2016; Miles, 2019; see chapters 7 and 11). According to Turnock (2016a), social justice is 'the foundation of public health' (p. 19). This concept was born around 1848, a time considered to be the 'birth of modern public health' (Turnock, 2016a, p. 19). Social justice suggests that public health is essentially 'a public matter'. The consequences of social injustice by means of disease, ill health and death are the reflection of 'the decisions and actions that a society makes, for good or for ill' (Turnock, 2016a, p. 19). Justice means that there is an equitable distribution of benefits and burdens among populations. Injustices happen when an unwarranted burden is placed on some individuals and groups, and they lack access to a benefit to which they are entitled. Turnock (2016a) contends that 'if access to health services, or even health itself, is considered to be a societal benefit (or if poor health is considered to be a burden), the links between the concepts of justice and public health become clear' (p. 19; see also Chapter 11).

Social justice – the equitable distribution of benefits and burdens among populations.

SPOTLIGHT 1.4

Gender inequality and women living with HIV/AIDS

Gender inequality is widespread in all societies. It damages the health of millions of girls and women. Both within and outside the health sector, gender inequity means women's voices, authority, decision-making power and recognition are diminished (Commission on Social Determinants of Health, 2014).

Gender inequality can be seen clearly in the area of HIV/AIDS (Liamputtong, 2013; Paudel & Baral, 2015; Cuca & Rose 2016; Malik & Dixit 2017). When a woman is labelled as having HIV, she is treated with suspicion, her morality is questioned, and blame is often placed on her. Because of their HIV status, many women are subjected to violence from their partners or family members. Perceived gender differences, delay in diagnosis, inferior access to healthcare services, internalised stigma and poor utilisation of health services can affect women living with HIV/AIDS. This makes it extremely difficult for women to take care of their own health needs. Women who are living with HIV/AIDS and who are mothers carry the triple burden of being HIV-infected: they are mothers of children who may or may not be positive themselves and often are also caregivers to their HIV-positive partners.

Men living with HIV/AIDS have to deal with the stigma associated with the illness, but that stigma can have particularly painful consequences for women and mothers living with HIV (Liamputtong, 2013; Paudel & Baral, 2015; Suwankhong & Liamputtong, 2017). For example, if their HIV status becomes known in the community, their children may be stigmatised and their family members may see them as 'unfit' mothers (Davies et al., 2009, p. 553). Hence, these mothers may decide not to disclose their HIV status to anyone (including their children) for fear of experiencing negative consequences such as feelings of shame, social ostracism, violence or expulsion from home. Women may even isolate themselves from their social networks and hide their illness so that their families can be protected from the stigma associated with it (Paudel & Baral, 2015; Suwankhong & Liamputtong, 2017). Not surprisingly, we witness many mothers with HIV/AIDS living 'in social isolation to avoid stigmatization', and frequently experiencing 'anxiety and depression in confronting their seropositive status' (Davies et al., 2009, p. 552).

QUESTIONS

1   How is this Spotlight related to the concept of social justice discussed above?
2   What can be done to eradicate gender inequality in public health?

REFLECTION QUESTION

We know now that health inequalities exist among populations everywhere around the world, even in Australia. Why do these inequalities persist around the globe? What will be the implications of these inequalities for some vulnerable groups, in particular Indigenous peoples? In your view, how can we reduce or even eradicate these inequalities?

SUMMARY

This chapter has provided an overview of the central issues that have shaped public health locally and globally. By now you should have a good understanding of the nature, value and scope of public health, both in Australia and within the global context.

Learning objective 1: Understand what public health is
Public health is grounded in science and focuses on preventive strategies. Public health is concerned with the prevention of disease and disability, and the promotion of the health of the public.

Learning objective 2: Appreciate the health of Australian people
Australia enjoys good health in comparison with other nations. However, there are some population groups whose health continues to be disadvantaged, and these are considered vulnerable populations.

Learning objective 3: Learn about the main public health organisations in Australia
There are several public health disciplines and organisations. Each has its own focus and roles, but all share the goals of prevention of injury and ill health, and improvement in good health. Public health organisations include local and state/territory governments, which legislate on public health and allocate resources and services provided by specialists and professionals in different locations, including hospitals, general practices, community health centres, NGOs, schools, media outlets, industry and so on.

Learning objective 4: Understand some global public health concerns
There are several major public health concerns around the globe, and these have been discussed in this chapter, including HIV/AIDS, overweight and obesity, migration and mental health.

Learning objective 5: Learn about the social model of health and the new public health
This chapter has discussed the importance of the social model of health, which is situated within the new public health paradigm. Within this model, it is the responsibility of society to ensure that the living and working conditions of individuals and groups are equitable in all areas, including health prevention, health promotion and the provision of health care. These are crucial if improvement in the health of the public is to be achieved.

Learning objective 6: Understand health inequality and social justice in health.
Public health is based on the principles of social justice, and often deals with continuing health issues and emerging health challenges. Disparities in health, wellbeing and illness are all products of inequality in society. These inequalities render some individuals and groups vulnerable to ill health and are closely linked with the concept of social justice.

TUTORIAL EXERCISES

1   Find articles in a daily newspaper or news site (on any day) that reference public health issues.
   a   What are the main public health issues covered?
   b   Why have they become public health concerns?
   c   Are there articles that do not make it clear that the issues discussed are related to public health?
   d   What could be the reason for this unclear message?
2   It has been suggested that the prevalence of infectious diseases such as HIV/AIDS and tuberculosis among migrants, who are confronted with structural disadvantage, including poor nutrition, inadequate housing, lack of sufficient education and limited access to health care, has led to migrants being considered a 'risk group'. In some nations, this characterisation of migrants as 'carriers of disease' has

been used to justify restrictive immigration policies that ignore the effects of political and economic determinants on the prevalence of infectious diseases among this population.

From the social model of health and the new public health perspectives, what does this case tell us? Discuss.

FURTHER READING

Baum, F. (2016). *The new public health: An Australian perspective* (4th ed.). Oxford University Press.

Chatterjee, S. (2021). *COVID-19: Tackling global pandemics through scientific and social tools.* Academic Press.

Germov, J. (Ed.) (2019). *Second opinion: An introduction to health sociology* (6th ed.). Oxford University Press.

Liamputtong, P. (Ed.) (2019). *Social determinants of health: Individuals, community and healthcare.* Oxford University Press.

Turnock, B. J. (2016). *Public health: What it is and how it works* (6th ed.). Jones & Bartlett Learning.

REFERENCES

AIDSInfo (2021). Panel on treatment of pregnant women with HIV infection and prevention of perinatal transmission. Recommendations for use of antiretroviral drugs in transmission in the United States, 2018: Counseling and management of women living with HIV who breastfeed perinatal [Internet]. AIDSinfo. [cited 2019 Jan 24]. Retrieved: https://aidsinfo.nih.gov/guidelines/html/3/perinatal/513/counseling-and-management-of-women-living-with-hiv-who-breastfeed.

Australian Institute of Health and Welfare (AIHW) (2016). *Australia's health 2016 – In brief.* AIHW.

——(2017). *Australia's welfare, 2017.* AIHW.

——(2018). *Mental health services in Australia.* AIHW. Retrieved https://www.aihw.gov.au/reports/mental-health-services/mental-health-services-in-australia/report-contents/summary

——(2020). *Australia's health 2020 – In brief.* AIHW. Retrieved https://www.aihw.gov.au/getmedia/2aa9f51b-dbd6-4d56-8dd4-06a10ba7cae8/aihw-aus-232.pdf.aspx?inline=true

Bansaccal, N., Van der Linden, D., Marot, J-C., & Belkhir, L. (2020). HIV-infected mothers who decide to breastfeed their infants under close supervision in Belgium: About two cases. *Frontiers in Pediatrics*, 8, article 248.

Baum, F. (2016). *The new public health: An Australian perspective* (4th ed.). Oxford University Press.

Béland, D., Cantillon, B., Hick, R., & Moreira, A. (2021). Social policy in the face of a global pandemic: Policy responses to the COVID-19 crisis. *Social Policy & Administration*, 55, 249–60.

Bleich, S. N., Jarlenski, M. P., Bell, C. N., & LaVeist, T. A. (2012). Health inequalities: Trends, progress, and policy. *Annual Review of Public Health*, *33*, 7–40.

Blumental, S., Ferster, A., Van den Wijngaert, S., & Lepage, P. (2014). HIV transmission through breastfeeding: Still possible in developed countries. *Pediatrics*, *134*(3), e875–9.

Braveman, P., Egerter, S., & Williams, D. R. (2011). The social determinants of health: Coming of age. *Annual Review of Public Health*, *32*, 381–98.

Broom, D., Freij, M., & Germov, J. (2019). Gendered health. In J. Germov (Ed.), *Second opinion: An introduction to health sociology* (6th ed.) (pp. 133–160). Oxford University Press.

Campbell, T., & Campbell, A. (2007). Emerging disease burdens and the poor in cities of the developing world. *Journal of Urban Health*, *84*, i54–i64.

Carroll, D., Morzaria, S., Sylvie, B., Johnson, C. K., Morens, D., Sumption, K., Tomori, O., & Wacharphaueasadee, S. (2021). Preventing the next pandemic: The power of a global viral surveillance network. *British Medical Journal (Online)*, 372(485).

Castaneda, H., Holmes, S. M., Madrigal, D. S., DeTrinidad Young, M-E., Beyeler, N., & Quesada, J. (2015). Immigration as a social determinant of health. *Annual Review of Public Health*, *36*, 375–92.

Chatterjee, S. (2021). *COVID-19: Tackling global pandemics through scientific and social tools*. Academic Press.

Commission on Social Determinants of Health (2014). *Closing the gap in a generation: Health equity through action on the social determinants of health. Final report of the Commission on Social Determinants of Health*. World Health Organization.

Correa-Velez, I. (2019). Global health. In M.L. Fleming (ed.), *Introduction to public health*, 4th edn (pp. 197–212). Elsevier.

Cuca, P. V., & Rose, C. D. (2016). Social stigma and childbearing for women living with HIV/AIS. *Qualitative Health Research*, *26*(11), 1508–18.

Cushing, L., Morello-Frosch, R., Wander, M., & Pasto, M. (2015). The haves, the have-nots, and the health of everyone: The relationship between social inequality and environmental quality. *Annual Review of Public Health*, *36*, 193–209.

Davies, S. L., Horton, T. V., Williams, A. G., Martin, M. Y., & Stewart, L. E. (2009). MOMS: Formative evaluation and subsequent intervention for mothers living with HIV. *AIDS Care*, *21*(5), 552–60.

Fleming, M. L. (2015). Social and emotional determinants of health. In M. L. Fleming, & E. Parker (Eds.), *Introduction to public health* (3rd ed.) (pp. 140–59). Churchill Livingstone.

——(2019). Defining health and public health. In M. L. Fleming (Ed.), *Introduction to public health* (4th ed.) (pp. 3–15). Elsevier.

Formiguera, X., & Canton, A. (2004). Obesity: Epidemiology and clinical aspects. *Best Practice in Research & Clinical Gastroenterology*, *18*, 1125–46.

Frumkin, H., Frank, L., & Jackson, R. (Eds.) (2004). *Urban sprawl and public health: Designing, planning and building for healthy communities*. Island Press.

Germov, J. (2019a). Imagining health problems as social issues. In J. Germov (Ed.), *Second opinion: An introduction to health sociology* (6th ed.) (pp. 2–23). Oxford University Press.

——(2019b). The class origins of health inequality. In J. Germov (Ed.), *Second opinion: An introduction to health sociology* (6th ed.) (pp. 88–110). Oxford University Press.

Gleeson, D., & Chong, S. (2019). Social determinants of health on a global scale. In P. Liamputtong (Ed.), *Social determinants of health: Individuals, community and healthcare* (pp. 353–81). Oxford University Press.

Goldmann, E., & Galea, S. (2014). Mental health consequences of disasters. *Annual Review of Public Health*, *35*, 169–83.

Hanna, L. (2019). Health and the living environment. In P. Liamputtong (Ed.), *Social determinants of health: Individuals, community and healthcare* (pp. 265–97). Oxford University Press.

Henderson-Wilson, C. (2012). Health as a social construct. In P. Liamputtong, R. Fanany & G. Verrinder (Eds). *Health, illness and well-being: Perspectives and social determinants* (pp. 197–212). Oxford University Press.

HIVGov (2021a). *The global HIV/AIDS epidemic*. Retrieved https://www.hiv.gov/hiv-basics/overview/data-and-trends/global-statistics

——(2021b). Counseling and management of women living with HIV who breastfeed perinatal. Retrieved https://aidsinfo.nih.gov/guidelines/html/3/perinatal/513/counseling-and-management-of-women-living-with-hiv-who-breastfeed

Hou, X-U. (2015). The impact of globalisation on health. In M. L. Fleming, & E. Parker (Eds.), *Introduction to public health* (2nd ed.) (pp. 332–54). Churchill Livingstone.

International Organization for Migration (IOM) (2020). *World migration report 2020*. IOM. Retrieved https://publications.iom.int/books/world-migration-report-2020

Julian, R. (2019). Ethnicity, health and multiculturalism. In J. Germov (Ed.), *Second opinion: An introduction to health sociology* (6th ed.) (pp. 180–204). Oxford University Press.

Kawachi, I., & Kennedy, B. P. (2006). *The health of nations: Why inequality is harmful to your health.* New Press.

Kawachi, I., Subramanian, S. & Almeida-Filho, N. (2002). A glossary for health inequalities. *Journal of Epidemiology and Community Health (Glossary), 56*(9), 647–52.

Keleher, H., & MacDougall, C. (2016). Determinants of health. In H. Keleher, & C. MacDougall (Eds.), *Understanding health: A determinants approach* (4th ed.) (pp. 19–34). Oxford University Press.

Kurban, H., & Liamputtong, P. (2017). Stigma, social attitudes and social connections: The lived experience of young Middle-Eastern refugees in Melbourne. *Youth Voice Journal, 7.* Retrieved https://www.rj4allpublications.com/yvj-2017-vol-7/

Liamputtong, P. (2007). *Researching the vulnerable: A guide to sensitive research methods.* Sage Publications.

——(Ed.) (2011). *Infant feeding practices: A cross-cultural perspective.* Springer.

——(Ed.) (2013). *Women, motherhood and living with HIV/AIDS: A cross-cultural perspective.* Springer.

——(Ed.) (2016). *Children, young people and living with HIV/AIDS: A cross-cultural perspective.* Springer.

——(Ed.) (2019). Health, illness and well-being: An introduction to social determinants of health. In P. Liamputtong (Ed.), *Social determinants of health: Individuals, community and healthcare* (pp. 1-27). Oxford University Press.

——(2020). *Qualitative research methods* (5th ed.). Oxford University Press.

Liamputtong, P., & Suwankhong, D. (2019). Culture as a social determinant of health. In P. Liamputtong (Ed.), *Social determinants of health: Individuals, community and healthcare* (pp. 51–82). Oxford University Press.

Lin, V., Smith, J., & Fawkes, S. (2014). *Public health practice in Australia: The organised effort* (2nd ed.). Allen & Unwin.

Madhav, N., Oppenheim, B., Gallivan, M., Mulembakani, P., Rubin, E., & Wolfe, N. (2018). Pandemics: Risks, impacts, and mitigation. In D.T. Jamieson, H. Gelband, S. Horton, P. Jha, R. Laxminarayan, C.N. Mock, & R Nugent (Eds.), *Disease control priorities: Improving health and reducing poverty* (pp. 315–46). The World Bank.

Malik, A. & Dixit, S. (2017). Women living with HIV/AIDS: Psychosocial challenges in the Indian context. *Journal of Health Management, 19*(3), 474–94.

Marmot, M. (2004). *Status syndrome: How your social standing directly affects your health and life expectancy.* Bloomsbury Press.

McMichael, A. J., Friel, S., Nyong, A., & Corvalan, C. (2008). Global environmental change and health: Impacts, inequalities, and the health sector. *British Medical Journal, 336*(7637), 191–94.

Miles, D. (2019). Social justice, human rights and social determinants of health. In P. Liamputtong (Ed.), *Social determinants of health: Individuals, community and healthcare* (pp. 107–30). Oxford University Press.

Moreira, A., & Hick, R. (2021). COVID-19, the great recession and social policy: Is this time different? *Social Policy and Administration,* 1–19.

Moseholm, E., & Weis, N. (2020). Women living with HIV in high-income settings and breastfeeding. *Journal of Internal Medicine, 287*(1), 19–31.

Nguyen, A. T., Liamputtong, P., & Monfries, M. (2016). Reproductive and sexual health of people living with physical disabilities: A meta-synthesis. *Sexuality and Disability, 34,* 3–26.

Organisation for Economic Co-operation and Development (OECD). (2011). *Divided we stand: Why inequality keeps rising.* OECD.

——(2017). *Obesity update 2017.* Retrieved https://www.oecd.org/els/health-systems/Obesity-Update-2017.pdf

Parker, E., & Baldwin, L. (2019). Refocusing public health: Emphasising health promotion and protection. In M.L. Fleming (ed.), *Introduction to public health* (4th ed.) (pp. 172–83). Elsevier.

Paudel, V., & Baral, K. P. (2015). Women living with HIV/AIDS (WLHA), battling stigma, discrimination and denial and the role of support group as a coping strategy: A review of literature. *Reproductive Health*, *12*(53).

Perry, Y., & Sivertsen, N. (2022). Social inclusion and the role of health care system. In P. Liamputtong (Ed.), *Handbook of social inclusion, research and practices in the health and social sciences* (Chapter 111). Springer.

Perry, Y., & Willis, E. (2019). Social determinants and the health care system. In P. Liamputtong (Ed.), *Social determinants of health: Individuals, community and healthcare* (pp. 330–52). Oxford University Press.

Piret, J., & Boivin, G. (2021). Pandemics throughout history. *Frontiers in Microbiology*, 11, 631736.

Prince, M., Patel, V., Saxena, S., Maj, M., Marselko, J., Phillips, M. R., & Rahman, A. (2007). No health without mental health. *Lancet*, *370*(9590), 859–77.

Sawyer, A-M. (2019). Mental illness: Understanding, experience, and service provision. In J. Germov (Ed.), *Second opinion: An introduction to health sociology* (6th ed.) (pp. 307–24). Oxford University Press.

Schneider, M-J. (2017). *Introduction to public health* (5th ed.). Jones & Bartlett.

Suwankhong, D., & Liamputtong, P. (2017). 'I was told not to do it, but . . .': Infant feeding practices among HIV-positive women in southern Thailand. *Midwifery*, *48*, 69–74.

Thoradeniya, T., & Jayasinghe, S. (2021). COVID-19 and future pandemics: A global systems approach and relevance to SDGs. *Globalization and Health*, 17, 59.

Turnock, B. J. (2016a). *Public health: What it is and how it works* (6th ed.). Jones & Bartlett Learning.

——(2016b). *Essentials of public health* (3rd ed.). Jones & Bartlett Learning.

UN Women (2018). *Women refugees and migrants*. Retrieved http://www.unwomen.org/en/news/in-focus/women-refugees-and-migrants

UNAIDS (2021). *Global HIV statistics — Fact sheet 2021*. Retrieved https://www.unaids.org/en/resources/fact-sheet

UNICEF (2020). *HIV/AIDS: Global and reginal trends*. Retrieved https://data.unicef.org/topic/hivaids/global-regional-trends/

White, F. M. M., Stallones, L., & Last, J. M. (2013). *Global public health: Ecological foundations*. Oxford University Press.

Wilkinson, R. G. (2005). *The impact of inequality: How to make sick societies healthier*. New Press.

Wilkinson, R. G. & Pickett, K. E. (2006). Income inequality and population health: A review and explanation of the evidence. *Social Science & Medicine*, *62*(7), 1768–84.

Willis, E., Reynolds, L., & Rudge, T. (eds.) (2020). *Understanding the Australian health care system*, 4th edn. Elsevier.

World Health Organization (WHO). (2018). *Refugee and migrant health*. WHO.

——(2020a). WHO Coronavirus Disease (COVID-19) Dashboard. Retrieved https://covid19.who.int/

——(2020b). *Tobacco – Fact sheet*. Retrieved http://www.who.int/en/news-room/fact-sheets/detail/tobacco

——(2021a) *Obesity and overweight*. Retrieved https://www.who.int/news-room/fact-sheets/detail/obesity-and-overweight

——(2021b). *Refugee and migrant health*. Retrieved https://www.who.int/health-topics/refugee-and-migrant-health#tab=tab_1

——(2021c). *WHO Coronavirus (COVID-19) dashboard*. Retrieved https://covid19.who.int/

Wright, C., & Higgs, P. (2019). Health as a social construct. In P. Liamputtong (Ed.), *Social determinants of health: Individuals, communities and healthcare* (pp. 31–50). Oxford University Press.

Wutzke, S., Morrice, E., Benton, M., Milat, A., Russell, L., & Wilson, A. (2018). Australia's National Partnership Agreement on preventive health: Critical reflections from States and Territories. *Health Promotion Journal of Australia*, 29, 228–35.

Zoumpourlis, V., Goulielmaki, M., Rizoz, E., Baliou, S., & Spandidos, D.A. (2020). The COVID-19 pandemic as a scientific and social challenge in the 21st century. *Molecular Medicine Reports*, 22, 3035–48.

PART 1

Historical and theoretical perspectives

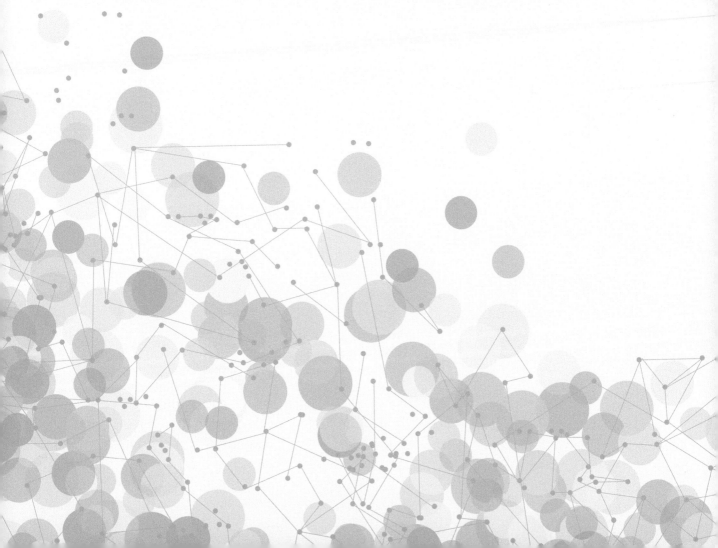

Historical and contemporary principles and practices of public health

2

Rebecca E. Olson and Paul Saunders

LEARNING OBJECTIVES

After studying this chapter, you should be able to:

1   identify stages in public health's history, drawing examples from ancient and modern history
2   identify individual, social, environmental, cultural and political factors shaping health outcomes and public health action
3   understand the significance of politics and policy to effective public health interventions
4   explain the effects of traditional and contemporary definitions of health on public health practice
5   explain the tension between individual and collective perspectives within public health
6   understand the influence of social, economic and political ideologies on public health throughout Europe's, Australia's and Aotearoa New Zealand's recent histories.

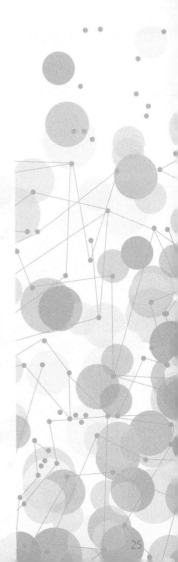

VIGNETTE

Health: Who is responsible?

Who is responsible for health? Consider your own health status. Is it due to your genetics or your personal choices? Perhaps you are an accomplished swimmer – from a long line of athletes – who watches what you eat, gets adequate sleep and drives with care. Or perhaps your health is a reflection of your upbringing? Maybe you grew up in a family that could not afford regular visits to the dentist, and you now have gum disease and tooth decay. To what extent is your health a reflection of government policy? Perhaps you required treatment in a hospital and, despite being on a low student income, you gained access to treatment through your country's universal health insurance. This tension between individual and collective responsibility for health is a common thread in the history of public health. As you read this chapter, ask yourself: how has this tension developed over time, and why does it persist?

Introduction

This chapter explores the assumptions and struggles that have occurred over the long history of public health. It provides an opportunity to question what public health is and where it is going, based on where it has been. A comprehensive history is outside the scope of a single chapter; instead, the chapter takes a critical overview. Following the social philosopher Michel Foucault (1926–84), the public health knowledge presented is considered a product of its time, culture and context, rather than the result of 'progress': a linear path of discovery (Foucault, [1969] 2002). Accordingly, the chapter examines contemporary public health principles and practices that have resulted from the actions of historic heroes and innovators as much as from chance or folly.

With a critical examination of its history, this chapter shows that public health is more than a health discipline. It is a scientific profession, a social science and a political endeavour to empower individuals and improve health through organised collective intervention (see also chapters 1, 5, 10 and 14). This chapter introduces readers to the different lenses through which public health has been viewed and practised, from individualist, behaviourist and biomedical perspectives through to cultural and socio-environmental; from ancient Greece to 19th-century Prussia. Australia's and Aotearoa New Zealand's histories are also explored, to show how different approaches to public health have (de)emphasised the importance of collective action. The chapter concludes with an examination of this tension in contemporary public health through the example of tobacco control.

This chapter's central theme – reflected in the above vignette – is the tension between the concepts of individual choice and collective action. In one view, individuals are seen to be responsible for their own health and hygiene (see Chapter 9). In the other, individuals are considered the products of their social, economic and historical circumstances: what the World Health Organization (WHO, 2008) refers to as health being socially determined (see Chapter 7).

This tension between individual and collective responsibility is also found in politics (see Chapter 10). The major political parties in Australia and Aotearoa New Zealand value individual liberties and economic stability, but view the government as playing different roles in achieving those goals. Neo-liberalism is an overarching term for political ideologies that support free market trading, privitisation and the achievement of (individualistic) self-interest, such as consumer choice that is unhampered by collectivist interventions (Venugopal, 2015). By and large, neo-liberalism is the political philosophy underpinning the Liberal Party of Australia and the National Party in Australia and in Aotearoa New Zealand. Social democracy, a political philosophy central to the Australian Labor Party and the New Zealand Labour Party (Rōpū Reipa o Aotearoa), and also important to the Australian Greens, is committed to ensuring the right to equal treatment through (collective) government interventions that aim to counter existing systems of privilege and the ill-effects of capitalism and neo-liberalism (Jackson, 2013). Our exploration of public health's history and politics begins in the birthplace of democracy: ancient Greece.

> **Neo-liberalism** – a political ideology that values limited government involvement in capitalist markets, viewing regulation as an encroachment on free-market principles and individual consumer choice.
>
> **Social democracy** – a political philosophy committed to ensuring the individual's right to equal treatment through collective interventions that aim to counter inequality in capitalist systems.

Ancient to medieval Europe: Sports, swamps and citizens

Throughout its history, as far back as ancient Greek and Roman societies, public health has emphasised competing approaches: empowering individuals to make healthy choices and pursuing collective efforts to improve population health.

Ancient Greece

The ancient Greeks (1000 to 27 BCE) treated health as an individual accomplishment. Their history is characterised by war, sporting competition and religious belief. During times of peace, young (male) warriors channelled their energies into the sporting arena. Athletic competitions served two religious purposes. First, wreaths won during sporting events could be offered to the gods, signifying the winner's 'worthiness to approach the gods' (Curtius, 1899, p. 33). Second, sport helped Greek athletes to sculpt their bodies in ways that were considered pleasing to the gods. Unlike the gods of their enemies, who cherished sacrifice, Hellenic gods were believed to favour 'healthful, vigorous, and strong' bodies (Curtius, 1899, p. 32). These characteristics, along with cleanliness, are epitomised in the Greek goddess Hygeia – from whom the term 'hygiene' originates (Taylor, 2017). The ancient Greeks were not alone in entangling individual health and religion. Many religions throughout history have directed followers in which foods to avoid (e.g. pork or beef), how to prepare foods safely and respectfully, and in hygiene and sexual practices.

Ancient Greece's sporting and religious cultures encouraged a view of health as due to rigorous individual training and diet. The practices of ancient Greek physicians reflected this individual focus. Following the legacy of the famous physician Hippocrates (460–370 BCE), doctors considered each person to be different, and thus tailored treatment and advice to each individual's circumstances (Cuartas, 2018). Their advice was often centred on dietary changes rather than pharmaceutical or surgical intervention. The word for 'diet' (*diaita*) in ancient Greek, however, encompassed one's lifestyle, including everything from food, drink and exercise through to bathing and sexual activity (Tsiompanou & Marketos, 2013).

SPOTLIGHT 2.1

Hippocrates

While the ancient Greeks saw health as achieved largely through individual lifestyle, the environment was also important. For example, in Hippocrates' (400 BCE) book, *On Airs, Waters, and Places*, we can clearly see consideration of both lifestyle and environment:

> Whoever wishes to investigate medicine properly, should proceed thus: in the first place to consider the seasons of the year, and what effects each of them produces … Then the winds, the hot and the cold … We must also consider the qualities of the waters … whether they be marshy and soft, or hard, and running from elevated and rocky situations … and the ground, whether it be naked and deficient in water, or wooded and well watered … and the mode in which the inhabitants live … whether they are fond of drinking and eating to excess, and given to indolence, or are fond of exercise and labor, and not given to excess in eating and drinking. (Hippocrates, 400 BCE, part 1)

Hippocrates considered health to be an individual accomplishment and a reflection of available natural resources. Thus, he was probably one of the first advocates for a behaviourist (focused on individual behavioural change) and socio-environmental (focused on the social and environmental circumstances) understanding of health.

QUESTION
How does the environment (indoors and outdoors, across seasons and settings) shape your health?

Ancient Rome to medieval Venice

Epidemic – the occurrence of a disease or a health-related event in a community that exceeds the usual expected occurrence.

Ancient Greek conceptualisations of health included the environment (see Spotlight 2.1), but it featured even more prominently in ancient Rome (27 BCE to 476 CE). **Epidemics** were said to be caused by the location of cities and camps. Misty, swampy and foggy environments were deemed unhealthy. What would come to be known as 'miasmas' – malodorous and contaminated air particles – were thought to proliferate in these conditions, causing sickness (Narins, 2020). This theory of miasma was replaced by germ theory more than a century ago; we now know that smells from the swamps were not to blame. Nonetheless, moving settlements away from those swamp locations was probably sound advice; mosquitos breed in stagnant water. Epidemics in these swampy locations were most likely the result of the **vector-borne disease** malaria, which is spread by mosquitos (Sallares, 2002).

Vector-borne disease – an infectious disease spread through a 'vector', such as a mosquito or tick.

Like the ancient Greeks, the ancient Romans, especially their most famous physician, Galen (129–216 CE), promoted good hygiene, diet and exercise such as gymnastics and wrestling (Nutton, 2020). The ancient Romans, however, took an organised approach to improving their citizens' health (they did not prioritise the health of their slaves). With the rise of the imperial state, an elaborate system of aqueducts was established to carry fresh water into the more than 800 public baths within the city, and to carry wastewater and sewage out ('The baths of ancient Rome', 1877). The ancient Romans also regulated the supply of water, street cleaning, burial of the dead, containment of dangerous animals, sex work (prostitution) and the sale of contaminated food, which illustrates a collective approach to what we would now call 'public health' (Baum, 2015).

While the Roman Empire's concern for its citizens may seem benevolent, it was most likely preservationist. Plagues had the potential to decimate a population, threaten commerce and challenge the legitimacy of those in power (Hamlin, 2013).

A concern for order and health was epitomised by the response to the bubonic plague (1347–52) in Europe during the Middle Ages. In 1377, citizens of Dubrovnik, Croatia were the first to cordon off the sick from the well. The merchant city Venice followed suit, ordering infected people to reside in 'plague hospitals' located away from the city for 40 (*quaranta*) days. From these practices, the idea of quarantine (isolation) was born (Narins, 2020; Tognotti, 2013). Avoiding the threats to health, wealth and authority posed by epidemics provided a strong incentive for collective public health measures such as quarantine.

REFLECTION QUESTION

What legacies of ancient Greece and Rome can be found in contemporary public health practices?

Modern European history part one: Statistics, socialism and science

Concern for individual hygiene and collective health continued in 19th-century Europe as a concern for the wealth of nations. The Industrial Revolution (mid-18th to mid-19th century) was a time of great change. Many people moved from farms to cities. Work hours shifted from following the rhythms of the seasons to following the foreman's watch. Instead of outdoor work, industrial labourers now toiled in factories blanketed by the smoke and dust of machines. Overcrowding became problematic. Many working-class families lived in cellars no larger than a single room, in close proximity to their neighbours and factories emitting pollutants (see Spotlight 2.2). Middle-class families preferred to reside in suburbs beyond the city, thereby escaping the smog, din and disease. Communicable diseases, such as typhoid, and sexually transmissible infections, such as syphilis, proliferated in cities, where overworked and malnourished labourers lived side by side (Hamlin, 2013).

Communicable disease – a contagious illness usually caused by a virus or bacterium that is spread from one person to another.

Sexually transmissible infection – a communicable disease spread from one person to another through sexual contact.

Public health's story, as it is often told, begins in this bleak urban landscape. Its narrative is one of statistics, politics and science. Its key players include medical officers and medical police, the socialist physician Dr Rudolph Virchow in Prussia and the founder of epidemiology, Dr John Snow. Their stories illustrate the push and pull between individual and collective action: the intersecting relationship between state power, politics and scientific discovery.

Medical police and medical officers

During the Industrial Revolution, European monarchies continued to expand their empires and amass wealth through manufacturing, trade and discovery or invasion. Illness could threaten these pursuits, so monitoring the nation's health was prioritised. Offices were established to collect statistical information on births, deaths and marriages (Narins, 2020). To improve the health of their citizens, European nation-states took a twofold approach.

First, a medical police force was instituted to monitor health and hygiene, and to regulate all manner of human life, from child-rearing, nutrition and clothing to sanitation and exercise (Dew, 2012). Second, 'medical officers' were introduced, reflecting a simultaneous collective effort. These medical officers monitored population health and inspected living quarters to report to government officials. One such officer, Dr William Henry Duncan (1805–63), campaigned for collective action to establish the *Liverpool Building Act 1842* (Engl.) on basic housing standards (Battersby, 2017). The appointment of medical police officers and medical officers is significant to public health's history as it marks the beginning of the use of statistical data and government offices for individual and collective health reform.

Dr Rudolph Virchow

Duncan's continental counterpart, Dr Rudolph Virchow (1821–1902) took a more radical approach to his post. The Prussian government hired this Berlin-based physician to study the cause of a severe typhus outbreak in 1848 in Upper Silesia (now Poland). In accepting his post, Virchow, an accomplished linguist and medical researcher, lived among the labourers of Upper Silesia (Scarani, 2003). Rather than making a medical assessment, Virchow concluded that social conditions were responsible for the epidemic (Dew, 2012). Victims of exploitation, the labourers were poor, uneducated and malnourished. Virchow prescribed democracy, education, higher wages, tax reform and safer working conditions, famously stating that 'medicine is a social science, and politics is nothing but medicine on a grand scale' (Reilly & McKee, 2012, p. 303). Virchow's recommendations are significant to public health's history, as an early acknowledgement of the social determinants of health (Baum, 2015; see also Chapter 7). His socialist recommendations, however, were largely disregarded by the conservative Prussian government (Scarani, 2003).

Dr John Snow

While Virchow contributed the social determinants of health to public health's modern history, Dr John Snow (1813–58) contributed epidemiology (see also Chapter 13). In 1854, Snow took leave from his practice as an anaesthetist to assess a serious cholera outbreak in London. Snow found it strange that some houses were unaffected, despite neighbours in all adjacent houses being stricken with the illness. Snow concluded that the drinking water was at fault. Nearly all residents of houses with water sourced through the Southwark and Vauxhall water company fell ill, while very few residents of houses serviced by the Lambeth company showed symptoms of cholera. Snow hypothesised that this was because the former water company sourced water from a part of the Thames River into which sewage was drained. Using mortality reports from the General Registrar Office and a map, Snow plotted the residences of the deceased and their water sources to show a cluster localised around one pump (Narins, 2020; Thomas, 2017). At a public meeting to discuss the epidemic, Snow urged the removal of the water pump handle to contain the outbreak.

Water-borne disease – an infectious illness spread by the consumption of pathogenic micro-organisms in contaminated water.

Snow published a book in 1849 on the causes of cholera, asserting it was a **water-borne disease** spread by drinking water contaminated with faeces from infected people. Despite Snow's convincing evidence, his findings were largely ignored – mostly due to the continuing popularity of miasma theory (Narins, 2020; Dew, 2012).

Snow's story shows the significance of scientific observation to understanding disease, and the significance of action to public health improvement. It also offers a lesson for public health practitioners: that policy is important to effective collective action. Based on contemporaneous understandings of infectious disease, Snow's conclusions were ahead of their time – germ theory did not gain traction until after Snow's death (Ekelund & Price, 2012; Thomas, 2017). Snow's message was largely ignored because of a failure to consider political ramifications. If germs, spread from person to person through air and water, were to blame, this would necessitate the enactment of quarantine measures. Quarantine, however, would interrupt trade and profits (Baum, 2015). Miasma theory may have been more palatable to 19th-century elites, posing a lesser threat to profits. The latter theory was employed by Sir Edwin Chadwick, whose achievements are explored next.

SPOTLIGHT 2.2

The living and labouring conditions of the working class

Friedrich Engels, the son of a German manufacturer, spent two years observing the labouring classes in England. In the following excerpt from Engels' book, *The Condition of the Working Class in England in 1844* ([1845] 1950), their woeful living conditions are described.

> The filth and tottering ruin surpass all description. Scarcely a whole window-pane can be found, the walls are crumbling, doorposts and window-frames loose and broken, doors of old boards nailed together . . . Heaps of garbage and ashes lie in all directions, and the foul liquids emptied before the doors gather in stinking pools. Here live the poorest of the poor, the worst paid workers . . . (Engels, [1845] 1950, p. 27)

> Over 50 years later, Dr Alice Hamilton told a story about pathogenic working conditions in Chicago's factories. 'Living in the working-class quarter . . . I could not fail to hear tales of dangers that workingmen faced . . . carbon-monoxide gassing in the great steel mills . . . painters disabled by lead palsy' (Hamilton, 1943, p. 114). Hamilton later became known as the 'mother' of occupational health, for pioneering investigations – using inspections and interviews – into the medical effects of industrialisation, which led to the implementation of laws on occupational disease (Fee & Greene, 1989; Baron & Brown, 2009; Narins, 2020).

QUESTION

Engels and Hamilton, along with Duncan, Virchow and Snow, all showed that social patterns underpinned disease. In what other ways are diseases socially patterned or determined by social factors?

Modern European history part two: Economics and excretory ducts

More so than Duncan, Virchow and Snow, Sir Edwin Chadwick's (1800–90) story is about employing political savvy to enable public health reform. Chadwick was a lawyer, politician, economist and author of the influential government report, *The Sanitary Conditions of the Labouring Population of Great Britain* (1843). Using basic statistical tables, Chadwick argued that differences in life expectancy were primarily due to miasmas and the environment: 'inadequate supplies of fresh water, excess ground moisture … inadequate waste removal' and poisonous smells from decomposing waste (Ekelund & Price, 2012, p. 189). Chadwick asserted that this harmful atmosphere posed an economic threat. Unsanitary conditions allowed miasmas to proliferate, leading to high mortality among labourers, and subsequently a growing number of widows and orphans reliant on government poorhouses.

Chadwick's solution: plumbing. Chadwick advocated for 'the installation of a complete water and sewer system with extensions to every household' (Ekelund & Price, 2012, p. 193). As a means of improving population health, the city's atmosphere and economic growth, Chadwick promoted this solution to parliamentarians. 'Night soil' (human excrement) was often deposited in basement cesspools and, according to miasma theory, was a significant contributor to London's pathogenic environment (Angus, 2018). This night soil could be sold as a fertiliser to farmers, thereby increasing their yields. The cost of transporting the fertiliser to outlying farms posed a barrier, but Chadwick's system of excretory ducts provided a lower-cost solution. Thus, Chadwick convinced those in power of the benefits of improving London's water supply, and thereby lowering death rates from the numerous epidemics flourishing among the working class, as good for profit, productivity and the public purse. These efforts formed the basis for development of a plumbing system to evacuate of human waste; one that would eventually supply clean drinking water to London residences. Chadwick's story illustrates the effectiveness of shrewd political argument. Rather than revolutionary science (as used by Snow) or radical socialism (Virchow), Chadwick framed reform in terms that were relevant to the concerns of the elite: savings on government spending and increased profits for private business.

At first glance, 19th-century European public health was largely about reform in the areas of sanitation, housing, working conditions and waterworks. Upon reflection, it was also a story of science and politics: the tensions between commercial interests, individual freedoms and government regulation (Dew, 2012), and the imperative of countering, working within or, at minimum, acknowledging the importance of politics to effective public health decision-making.

Early Antipodean health

With poorhouses and jails overflowing, King George III (1738–1820) was eager to expand the British Empire. With the American colonies challenging British authority, Australia became the new destination for Britain's convicts. The first Europeans to disembark on the land that would later become known as Australia commented on the health of the people they found there. Aboriginal people were described as tall, lean, athletic and free from disease (Moodie, 1973). Many argue that the first Australians were healthier than the British arrivals (Franklin & White, 1991), many of whom had been living in overcrowded and unsanitary urban slums (see Spotlight 2.2). This section provides an overview of how health was conceptualised by the First Peoples of Australia and Aotearoa New Zealand during the many eras before British settlement/invasion: as a collective, cultural, social, environmental and individual phenomenon.

Traditional Aboriginal conceptualisations of health

Archaeological evidence suggests that the First Peoples of Australia arrived approximately 65 000 years ago (Clarkson et al., 2017). Prior to the arrival of the British, Aboriginal and Torres Strait Islander conceptualisations of health were similar in many ways to those of the ancient Greeks and Romans; all linked health with diet and environment. In other ways, Aboriginal and Torres Strait Islander conceptions of health differed, reflecting the continent's isolation, a spiritual connection to land and ancestry, a reciprocal social construct, and a mixed hunter–gatherer and agricultural way of life (Butler et al., 2019; Keen, 2021; Sherwood, 2021). While the ancient Greeks and Romans endured repeated waves of plagues, the extended isolation and mix of settled and nomadic existence of Australia's Indigenous peoples (dependent on seasonal variations) meant there was a relative dearth of vector-borne and communicable diseases (Moodie, 1973; Sherwood, 2013; Sherwood, 2021). Mapping illness in Aboriginal and Torres Strait Islander peoples prior to European settlement is difficult, but skin irritations, influenza, snake bites and injuries were probably the most common health complaints (Saggers & Gray, 1991; Dowling, 1997). These were thought to result from physical, social and spiritual causes. For example, illness might be considered a consequence of violating a taboo and a lack of dietary variety, prompting a healer to prescribe a visit to relatives in a location where different foods were available (Saggers & Gray, 1991).

A spiritual connection between land and people is a defining feature of traditional Aboriginal and Torres Strait Islander cultures. This connection reflects traditional stories about ancestors who lived in, ate from and hunted the land as an extended kinship network over millennia (Saggers & Gray, 1991). Although largely undocumented, Aboriginal and Torres Strait Islander communities have assessed their environments to develop public health responses for their communities over millennia. Practices such as the strategic burning of flora to locate food sources and prevent inhalation of thick smoke and catastrophic wild-fires is an Aboriginal practice pre-dating ancient European civilisation (Johnston et al., 2007). Given the importance of family, community and land to their cultures, it is perhaps not surprising that traditional Indigenous concepts of health encompass 'the social, emotional and cultural well-being of the whole Community' (National Aboriginal Community Controlled Health Organisation, 2001, p. 5; see also Chapter 19).

Traditional Māori conceptualisations of health

The First Peoples of Aotearoa New Zealand, the Māori, shared a similar connection to land and sky through their creation story. Traditional Māori conceptualisations of health can be summarised in the concept of *te whare tapa wha*, which 'compares health to a four-sided house in which there is a balance between spiritual, physical, intellectual/emotional, and family domains' (Durie, 2004, p. 818; Warbick et al., 2016). Spirituality encompasses a connection with, and humility towards, one's tribal lands. Physical health incorporates important hygienic rituals; food preparation and consumption, and bathing and bodily functions are activities that should take place in separate spaces. Mental health is an holistic concept, incorporating the individual's thoughts, emotions and integration with their community. Family and a person's extended kinship are also implicated in health, with identity derived from tribal affiliation (Durie, 1985; Warbick et al., 2016). Thus, the collective – family, community, environment and spirituality – is central to traditional Māori and Aboriginal and

Torres Strait Islander conceptualisations of health. Public health practices that work within culturally appropriate conceptualisations of health enjoy wider success – a finding demonstrated by the actions of the first Māori health officer, Dr Maui Pomare (see Spotlight 2.3)

SPOTLIGHT 2.3

Dr Maui Pomare

Dr Maui Pomare is an important figure in Aotearoa New Zealand's public health history. Pomare was the first Māori person to graduate from medical school and the first Māori health officer, appointed in 1901 by the then-new Department of Public Health (Durie, 2000). Some of Pomare's decisions as Māori health officer were controversial, such as prohibiting the practising of traditional Māori medicine (*tohunga*). But, overall, Pomare's record in Māori health improvement is unmatched. The success of Pomare's efforts can be attributed to embracing a Māori view of health as more than an individual phenomenon: as a collective state reflecting the health of a person's community and following the directions of community leaders. With this conceptualisation of health in mind, Pomare worked closely with Māori tribal leaders to implement sanitary, legal and economic reforms, thereby improving the health, social infrastructure and social standing of Aotearoa New Zealand's early 20th-century Māori population (Durie, 2000; Riches & Palmowski, 2016).

QUESTIONS

1   In what ways does the Māori concept of *te whare tapa wha* and the Aboriginal and Torres Strait Islander concept of health and wellbeing challenge medical definitions of health and public health practices?
2   How do these differences affect the ability of Indigenous peoples to achieve and maintain their health? Provide examples.

The Antipodean public health story: 'Old public health'

Like their European contemporaries (and the indigenous peoples they displaced), 19th-century Australian and Aotearoa New Zealand settlers experienced high rates of infant mortality and infectious diseases associated with overcrowded urban housing and under-developed sanitation systems (Dew, 2012). Extending into the first two decades of the 20th century, Australian cities faced outbreaks of the plague, measles, tuberculosis, smallpox and influenza (Saggers & Gray, 1991; Lawson & Bauman, 2001; Webster, 2020). This section outlines public health responses in Australia and Aotearoa New Zealand in the first half of the 20th century. It includes a shameful history of scapegoating Indigenous and minority groups, as well as nation-building, biomedical interventions and individual responsibility.

Scapegoating

In Aotearoa New Zealand, Indian vendors' working-class living conditions were blamed for spreading disease (Dew, 2012). In Australia, Chinese immigrants and Aboriginal and Torres

Strait Islander peoples were treated as scapegoats (Baum, 2015). Having endured warfare, dispossession, displacement and debilitation from new communicable diseases, poor health in Māori and Aboriginal and Torres Strait Islander communities was seen as a threat to the wider population (Carson et al., 2020; Durie, 2000). Between 1911 and the 1930s, several Australian states passed legislation to implement compulsory medical examinations of First Australians to 'protect' the health of non-Indigenous Australians (Saggers & Gray, 1991). Other than implementing a Māori health officer in Aotearoa New Zealand (see Spotlight 2.3), the overarching response to the dwindling numbers of indigenous peoples there and in Australia was to do nothing (Durie, 2000), based on a belief that these populations were unlikely to survive. This belief – social Darwinism – emerged from an erroneous adaption of Darwin's concept of the 'survival of the fittest' in seeking to understand different racial groups (Hofstader, [1944] 2016; O'Connell & Ruse, 2021). Thus, Australia's and Aotearoa New Zealand's first public health interventions as young nations were shamefully xenophobic.

Nation-building

Building the nation in number and resilience was another public health response to the continuing threat of infectious disease in both countries. With the aim of growing, strengthening and 'promoting the health of (white) [non-Indigenous] populations from the early years of the 20th century,' (Madsen, 2016, p. 149) new organisations and curricula were introduced to encourage physical fitness and individual responsibility for health. Both countries established departments of public health to oversee hygiene and health services for mothers and infants, among other responsibilities (Dow, 1995; Baum, 2015; Madsen, 2016). In schools, child health was fostered through physical fitness programs and regular medical examinations (Lawson & Bauman, 2001; Madsen, 2016). The tension between national and individual responsibility can be seen clearly during the nation-building era. Although in Australia the emerging states organised services for collective health improvement, health was largely depicted as an individual responsibility.

Medicine

The years preceding and following World War II (1939–45) are credited with extraordinary medical advances for population health, including the increased availability of antibiotics and vaccinations (Dew, 2012; Baum, 2015). A significant gap, however, remained in the health and social outcomes between Indigenous and non-Indigenous populations in Australia, due to the continuing effects of colonial government policies and biomedical approaches to health based on Eurocentric interpretations (Moodie, 1973; Paradies, 2016).

With better control of infectious diseases and improvements in maternal and child health, overall population infant mortality decreased and life expectancy improved substantially in Australia. Many declared the work of public health done. These biomedical and population health advances, however, perpetuated an individualistic approach to public health, encouraging individual vigilance on hygiene and fitness standards, and compliance with advice from medical practitioners, that is arguably still present today (Kriznik et al., 2018). Research from McKeown would challenge this biomedicine-centric perception of health (see Spotlight 2.4), but as we conclude this overview of this period of public health's history, an emphasis on the individual rather than social determinants of health is clear.

SPOTLIGHT 2.4

Dr Thomas McKeown

In 1979, British academic Dr Thomas McKeown published his statistical analysis of life-expectancy improvements in the 20th century. His findings challenged the dominant perception that medical advances, namely vaccination, were responsible for the significant decreases in mortality witnessed in developed countries. McKeown, and later McKeown's students McKinlay and McKinlay, showed that mortality rates from many infectious diseases began declining *before* vaccinations became available (Kindig, 2020; McKeown, 1979). Medical interventions had only minor effects, making a mere '3.5% contribution to the decline in total mortality' in the United States between 1900 and 1973 (Kindig, 2020). Instead, McKeown attributed significant advances in health to improvements in affluence, nutrition and hygiene, thereby (unintentionally) reinforcing a picture of health as an individual accomplishment. McKeown's argument was happily used by conservative (neo-liberal) politicians to support arguments for unrestricted growth and limited government services, ushering in the closure of services and widening income and health disparities in many countries (Szreter, 2002). More recently, these arguments have been adopted by anti-coronavirus vaccine advocates (Kindig, 2020).

Questioning the use of McKeown's thesis to support the contraction of public health efforts, in 1988, American academic Simon Szreter re-examined and challenged McKeown's work, showing that organised efforts of public health movements and local interventions, coordinated by the federal government, were also important to health outcomes (Szreter, 2002; Baum, 2015). McKeown's story illustrates that public health is socio-political (see Part 2). In addition to generating and analysing scientific findings, practitioners must always consider their work's political implications.

QUESTION

McKeown's story shows that scientific research is never neutral. How does this story undermine perceptions of science as unbiased, objective and absolute?

The Antipodean public health story: 'New public health'

Mid-20th century dreams that public health's work was done were soon dashed. As people lived longer, chronic disease became more prevalent. By the 1970s, the post-war boom had ended; a recession saw widespread unemployment and poverty return. Along with them came new health concerns: HIV/AIDS, cancer, diabetes and cardiovascular disease (Baum, 2015). With the exception of HIV/AIDS, the infectious disease eradication focus of the mid-20th century was replaced with a focus on 'lifestyle' diseases by the 1970s to 1980s. In response, many public health practitioners began re-thinking individualistic and biomedical approaches, returning to more collective approaches to addressing social and environmental determinants of health (de Camargo, 2017). It was amid this public suffering that a so-called 'new public health' was born, taking a more holistic approach to public health by acknowledging the importance of individual *and* collective action situated within social, cultural, political and ecological environments (Baum, 2015).

REFLECTION QUESTION

How do recent epidemics and pandemics (SARS, Ebola, COVID-19) illustrate the continuing tension between the individual and the collective in public health's history?

Nonetheless, the tension between individual and collective responsibility persists. Many contemporary public health campaigns take a behaviourist approach, urging citizens to take responsibility for their health. Though often underpinned by altruism, such interventions have repeatedly hindered particular groups, namely indigenous and other minority populations in which a cultural and lifestyle conflict exists, and thereby perpetuating social disadvantage correlated with poor health outcomes over the life-course. Tobacco control efforts (see Spotlight 2.5) offer a primary example. While at times it may seem appropriate, an individualistic approach risks compounding health inequities through **victim blaming**: 'attributing to a person the cause of their own misfortune' (White, 2006, p. 24). As one of the leaders of the WHO's Commission on the Social Determinants of Health, Professor Michael Marmot (2004), explained: when we focus on individual behaviours, 'we may miss the big picture' (p. 33). That is, we 'miss out on the major influences on health of the way we live our lives in society. The circumstances in which people live and work are intimately related to risk of illness and length of life' (Marmot, 2004, p. 14). Thus, while threats to health have changed over time, the individual–collective tension remains.

Victim blaming – ignoring the social determinants of health and placing responsibility for poor health solely with the individual.

SPOTLIGHT 2.5

Tobacco control

How we define health problems shapes how public health practitioners respond. Take cigarette smoking. As nicotine addiction, smoking becomes a medical problem warranting a medical intervention, such as nicotine patches. Defined as a lifestyle disease, many tobacco-control campaigns depict smoking as an individual choice and respond by encouraging individuals to quit (Adams et al., 2019). But such conceptualisations are narrow and do not always go to plan. Many people feel **stigmatised** by such messaging and continue to smoke in resistance (Occhipinti et al., 2018; Bond et al., 2012). Furthermore, such messaging is based on understandings of people in isolation, but we are all interdependent.

Stigma – the shame of having a tarnished identity as someone who is deviant, often due to one's moral social standing.

If, however, we define smoking as a social determinant of health (Marmot, 2004), smoking becomes a response to the stresses of poverty and parenting in working-class communities (Graham et al., 2014). Subsequently, we are more likely to respond with social support and collective interventions, such as government policies to subsidise child care or to ameliorate insecurities associated with precarious labour. This approach avoids blaming or stigmatising.

QUESTION

Are current tobacco-control initiatives working? In addition to improving childcare support and job security, what other public health and government interventions could be introduced to address smoking as a collective concern?

SUMMARY

More than a story of progress, the critical examination of public health's history presented in this chapter reveals the continuing tension within social, cultural and political contexts and their contribution to our understanding of health, disease and the interrelated principles and practices of public health.

Learning objective 1: Identify stages in public health's history, drawing examples from ancient and modern history.

From a religious concern for individual diet and physique in ancient Greece to a collective concern for social order in the Roman Empire, we see the early stages of public health. During the Industrial Revolution, public health matured; medical officers and key figures, such as Snow and Virchow, combined statistics and observation to draw links between environmental conditions, social policy, civil infrastructure and individual health outcomes. It is here that practices emerge that we now recognise as public health: collective action to improve living and working conditions, using a combination of science and advocacy.

Learning objective 2: Identify individual, social, environmental, cultural and political factors shaping health outcomes and public health action.

Changes in diet and exercise have long been the focus of individualistic approaches to public health – from ancient Greece to Australia's nation-building and lifestyle-diseases eras in the 20th century. However, Engels' and Virchow's exposés of the abysmal living and working conditions of the Industrial Revolution brought attention to the environmental factors shaping health and the socio-political interventions necessary to address them.

Learning objective 3: Understand the significance of politics and policy to effective public health interventions.

Chadwick's story aptly illustrates the political 'savvy' necessary to enacting public health interventions that address the social and environmental determinants of health. McKeown's story serves as a further warning: failure to take politics into account may see public health research used for purposes counter to those intended. The context in Australia and Aotearoa New Zealand provides an important example of entire populations inaccurately perceived as threats to public health; accusers harboured an array of infectious diseases on arrival, facilitating the emergence of many of the health problems that the nation currently faces.

Learning objective 4: Explain the effects of traditional and contemporary definitions of health on public health practice.

Our metaphorical voyage to the Antipodes showed that reflecting on cultural and historical circumstances is important to understanding and addressing health. Definitions of health vary across peoples and time. But, as Pomare's work exemplifies, public health interventions only reach their full potential if they are based on culturally appropriate conceptualisations of health. Furthermore, considering all aspects of people's lives in the contexts of social, cultural and physical environments is vital to understanding health risk and public health responses. This relatively new and comprehensive approach to public health is heavily influenced by traditional Indigenous conceptualisations, encompassing environment, socio-political community dynamics and the broader population.

Learning objective 5: Explain the tension between individuals and collective perspectives within public health.

Reflecting historical religious and cultural influences, health has to some extent always been seen as an individual achievement. If we only acknowledge the individual contributions, however, we risk overlooking social and environmental determinants of health, and blaming victims of these circumstances. Many indigenous populations, in contrast, have traditionally perceived health as a communal responsibility and, equally, as something that generates communal effects. Such a collectivist approach avoids victim-blaming.

Learning objective 6: Understand the influence of social, economic and political ideologies on public health throughout Europe's, Australia's and Aotearoa New Zealand's recent histories.

From the Industrial Revolution era through to the present, economic and political concerns have influenced our understanding of health (as a social or individual responsibility) and our responses to health. Today, conservative political parties frame health as an individual responsibility, shifting much of the perceived responsibility for health onto individuals, thus partially obscuring health's social determinants. The continuing social exclusion and colonisation of indigenous populations – in Australia, Aotearoa New Zealand and elsewhere – through the application of Eurocentric political, economic and social systems maintains a state of disadvantage that continues to have strong effects on health outcomes at both individual and population levels, further perpetuating differences in population outcomes, such as life expectancy between indigenous and non-indigenous groups.

In sum, it should be clear from this overview of public health's history that it is by no means linear or complete. Public health continues to wax and wane in response to political, economic, social and scientific trends. The challenges of the 21st century – the return of certain highly infectious diseases, the ageing of populations, global inequality – demand an organised, collective strategy that recognises the lessons and triumphs of public health's rich history.

TUTORIAL EXERCISES

1   List everything you have purchased over the past two days. What prompted you to purchase these items? Do these purchases reflect individual choices or social circumstances and obligations? What would need to change for you to stop purchasing these items? Now, answer these questions about your health choices over the past two days.
2   Based on the history presented in this chapter, what key principles define public health?
3   Review media coverage of a recent public health issue. What responses are suggested? What political ideologies underpin these recommendations?
4   In addition to Dr Alice Hamilton, which other women have contributed to public health's history?

FURTHER READING

Baum, F. (2015). *The new public health* (4th ed.). Oxford University Press.

Dew, K. (2012). *The cult and science of public health: A sociological investigation*. Berghahn Books, Inc.

Engels, F. ([1845] 1950). *The condition of the working class in England in 1844* (F. K. Wischnewetzky, Trans.). Allen & Unwin.

Stewart, J. (Ed.) (2017). *Pioneers in public health: Lessons from history*. Routledge.

REFERENCES

Adams, G., Estrada-Villalta, S., Sullivan, D., & Markus, H. (2019). The psychology of neoliberalism and the neoliberalism of psychology. *Journal of Social Issues*, *75*(1), 189–216.

Angus, I. (2018). Cesspools, sewage, and social murder: Environmental crisis and metabolic rift in nineteenth-century London. *Monthly Review*, *70*(3), 32–68.

Baron, S., & Brown, T. (2009). Alice Hamilton (1869–1970): Mother of US occupational medicine. *American Journal of Public Health*, *99*(S3), S548.

Battersby, S. (2017). Duncan of Liverpool: The first medical officer of health. In J. Stewart (Ed.), *Pioneers in public health: Lessons from history* (pp. 56–65). Routledge.

Baum, F. (2015). *The new public health* (4th ed.). Oxford University Press.

Bond, C., Brough, M., Spurling, G., & Hayman, N. (2012). 'It had to be my choice' – Indigenous smoking cessation and negotiations of risk, resistance and resilience. *Health, Risk & Society*, *14*(6), 565–81.

Butler, T. L., Anderson, K., Garvey, G., Cunningham, J., Ratcliffe, J., Tong, A., Whop, L., Cass, A., Dickson, M., & Howard, K. (2019). Aboriginal and Torres Strait Islander people's domains of wellbeing: A comprehensive literature review. *Social Science & Medicine*, 233, 138–57.

Carson, B., Dunbar, T., Chenhall, R. D., & Bailie, R. (Eds.). (2020). *Social determinants of Indigenous health. Protection, exploitation and activism: Indigenous health in the interwar years.* Routledge.

Clarkson, C., Jacobs, Z., Marwick, B., Fullagar, R., Wallis, L., Smith, M. . . . Pardoe, C. (2017). Human occupation of northern Australia by 65,000 years ago. *Nature*, *547*(7663), 306–310.

Cuartas, J. R. (2018). Challenges of health education in the 21st century. *Revista Cuidarte*, *9*(3), 2291–3.

Curtius, E. (1899). *The history of Greece* (A. W. Ward, Trans.). Charles Scribner & Co.

de Camargo, K. (2017). Democratic policy, social movements, and public health: A new theme for AJPH Public Health Forum. *American Journal of Public Health*, *107*(12), 1855.

Dew, K. (2012). *The cult and science of public health: A sociological investigation.* Berghahn Books, Inc.

Dow, D. A. (1995). *Safeguarding the public health: A history of the New Zealand Department of Health.* Victoria University Press.

Dowling, P. (1997). *'A great deal of sickness': Introduced diseases among the Aboriginal people of colonial southeast Australia 1788–1900* [Doctoral thesis, Australian National University]. Retrieved from Proquest Database.

Durie, M. (1985). A Māori perspective of health. *Social Science & Medicine*, *20*(5), 483–6.

——(2000). Public health strategies for Māori. *Health Education & Behavior*, *27*(3), 288–95.

——(2004). Māori. In C. R. Ember & M. Ember (Eds.), *Encyclopedia of medical anthropology: Health and illness in the world's cultures* (pp. 815–22). Kluwer Academic Publishers.

Ekelund, R., & Price, E. (2012). *The economics of Edwin Chadwick: Incentives matter.* Edward Elgar Publishing.

Engels, F. ([1845] 1950). *The condition of the working class in England in 1844* (F. K. Wischnewetzky, Trans.). Allen & Unwin.

Fee, E., & Greene, B. (1989). Science and social reform: Women in public health. *Journal of Public Health Policy*, *10*(2), 161–77.

Foucault, M. ([1969] 2002). *The archaeology of knowledge* (A. M. Sheridan Smith, Trans.). Routledge.

Franklin, M.-A., & White, I. (1991). The history and politics of Aboriginal health. In J. Reid, & P. Trompf (Eds.), *The health of Aboriginal Australia* (pp. 1–36). Harcourt Brace Jovanovich Publishers.

Graham, H., Flemming, K., Fox, D., Heirs, M., & Sowden, A. (2014). Cutting down: Insights from qualitative studies of smoking in pregnancy. *Health & Social Care in the Community*, *22*(3), 259–67.

Hamilton, A. (1943). *Exploring the dangerous trades: The autobiography of Alice Hamilton, M.D.* Little, Brown and Company.

Hamlin, C. (2013). The history and development of public health in developed countries. In R. Detels, R. Beaglehole, M. A. Lansang, & M. Gulliford (Eds.), *Oxford textbook of public health* (5th ed.) (pp. 20–38). Oxford University Press.

Hippocrates. (400 BCE). *On airs, waters, and places* (F. Adams, Trans.).

Hofstadter, R. ([1944] 2016). *Social Darwinism in American thought, 1860–1915*. University of Pennsylvania Press.

Jackson, B. (2013). Social democracy. In M. Freeden, & M. Stears (Eds.), *The Oxford handbook of political ideologies* (pp. 348–63). Oxford University Press.

Johnston, F. H., Jacups, S. P., Vickery, A. J., & Bowman, D. M. (2007). Ecohealth and Aboriginal testimony of the nexus between human health and place. *EcoHealth, 4*(4), 489–99.

Keen, I. (2021). Foragers or farmers: Dark Emu and the controversy over Aboriginal agriculture. *Anthropological Forum* (pp. 1–23). Routledge.

Kindig, D.A. (2020). The (still) limited contribution of medical measures to declines in mortality. *The Milbank Quarterly, 98*(4), 1053–7.

Kriznik, N. M., Kinmouth, A. L., Ling, T., & Kelly, M. P. (2018). Moving beyond individual choice in policies to reduce health inequalities: The integration of dynamic with individual explanations. *Journal of Public Health, 40*(4), 764–75.

Lawson, J. S., & Bauman, A. E. (2001). *Public health Australia: An introduction*. McGraw-Hill.

Madsen, W. (2016). Partnerships and the past: Reflections on 1940s community centre endeavours of the National Fitness Council. *Health Promotion Journal of Australia, 27*, 148–52.

Marmot, M. (2004). *Status syndrome: How your social standing directly affects your health and life expectancy*. Bloomsbury Publishing.

McKeown, T. (1979). *The role of medicine: Dream, mirage or nemesis?* Blackwell.

Moodie, P. M. (1973). *Aboriginal health*. Australian National University Press.

Narins, B. (ed.) (2020). *The Gale Encyclopedia of Public Health*. Gale.

National Aboriginal Community Controlled Health Organisation (NACCHO). (2001). *Constitution for the National Aboriginal Community Controlled Health Organisation*. NACCHO.

Nutton, V. (2020). *Galen: A thinking doctor in imperial Rome*. Routledge.

Occhipinti, S., Dunn, J., O'Connell, D., Garvey, G., Valery, P.C., Ball, D., . . . Chambers, S. (2018). Lung cancer stigma across the social network: Patient and caregiver perspectives. *Journal of Thoracic Oncology, 13* (10), 1443–53.

O'Connell, J., & Ruse, M. (2021). *Social Darwinism*. Cambridge University Press.

Paradies, Y. (2016). Colonisation, racism and indigenous health. *Journal of Population Research, 33*, 83–96.

Reilly, R. G., & McKee, M. (2012). 'Decipio': Examining Virchow in the context of modern 'democracy'. *Public Health, 126*, 303–7.

Riches, C., & Palmowski, J. (2016). *A dictionary of contemporary world history* (4th ed.). Oxford University Press.

Saggers, S., & Gray, D. (1991). *Aboriginal health and society: The traditional and contemporary Aboriginal struggle for better health*. Allen & Unwin.

Sallares, R. (2002). *Malaria and Rome: A history of malaria in ancient Italy*. Oxford University Press.

Scarani, P. (2003). Rudolf Virchow (1821–1902). *Virchows archives, 442*, 95–8.

Sherwood, J. (2013). Colonisation – It's bad for your health: The context of Aboriginal health. *Contemporary Nurse, 46*(1), 28–40.

——(2021). Historical and current perspectives on the health of Aboriginal and Torres Strait Islander people. In O. Best, & B. Fredericks (Eds.), *Yatdjuligin: Aboriginal and Torres Strait Islander Nursing and Midwifery Care* (pp. 6–33). Cambridge University Press.

Szreter, S. (2002). Rethinking McKeown: The relationship between public health and social change. *American Journal of Public Health, 92*(5), 722–5.

Taylor, R. (2017). *The amazing language of medicine*. Springer.

The baths of ancient Rome (1877). *The British Architect and Northern Engineer, 7*(14), 205–6.

Thomas, H. (2017). John Snow: A pioneer in epidemiology. In J. Stewart (Ed.), *Pioneers in public health: Lessons from history* (pp. 33–9). Routledge.

Tognotti, E. (2013). Lessons from the history of quarantine, from plague to influenza A. *Emerging Infectious Diseases, 19*(2), 254–9.

Tsiompanou, E., & Marketos, S. G. (2013). Hippocrates: Timeless still. *Journal of the Royal Society of Medicine, 106*(7), 288–92.

Venugopal, R. (2015). Neoliberalism as concept. *Economy and Society*, *44*(2), 165–87.

Warbick, I., Dickson, A., Prince, R., & Heke, I. (2016). The biopolitics of Māori biomass: Towards a new epistemology for Māori health in Aotearoa/New Zealand. *Critical Public Health*, *26*(4), 394–404.

Webster, E. (2020). Tubercular landscape: Land use change and Mycobacterium in Melbourne, Australia, 1837-1900. *Journal of Historical Geography*, *67*, 48–60.

White, K. (2006). *Sage dictionary of health and society*. Sage Publications.

World Health Organization (WHO). (2008). *Closing the gap in a generation: Health equity through action on the social determinants of health*. WHO.

Health promotion principles and practice: Addressing complex public health issues using the Ottawa Charter

3

Bernadette Sebar, Kirsty Morgan and Jessica Lee

LEARNING OBJECTIVES

After studying this chapter, you should be able to:

1 discuss the role of governments in promoting health through healthy public policy
2 discuss how physical and social environments can be health-promoting
3 discuss the role communities can play in promoting health
4 explain how individual, health-compromising behaviours can be addressed
5 discuss the role of health services in promoting health.

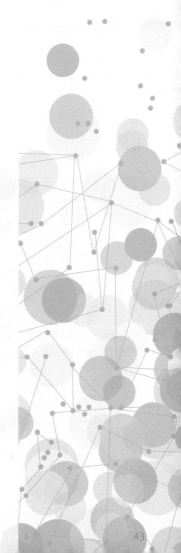

VIGNETTE

'Big Tobacco' and public health

Reducing tobacco use is a priority action area in the National Preventive Health Strategy 2021–2030, and one of its targets is the protection of public health policy, including tobacco-control policies, from interference by the tobacco industry (Commonwealth of Australia, 2021). The Australian Institute of Health and Welfare (AIHW) has reported a decline in daily smoking rates among people aged 18 years and older, from 28 per cent in 1989–90 to 14.5 per cent in 2014–15 and 11.6 per cent in 2019 (AIHW, 2020a). This decline is attributed to Australia's strong tobacco-control regulations, which limit tobacco promotions, place high taxes on tobacco products and restrict smoking areas (AIHW, 2020a). Despite significant progress in combatting smoking in high-income countries, smoking is still at pandemic proportions in low-income and middle-income countries. Smoking prevalence remains particularly high in South East Asia and the Balkans region in Europe (World Population Review, 2021). For example, in Indonesia, the prevalence of daily cigarette smoking among males is 64.3 per cent (WHO, 2019). The WHO (2003) has responded to the globalisation of the tobacco epidemic with its Framework Convention on Tobacco Control, which is an evidence-based treaty to provide countries with a legal basis from which to implement regulatory measures that reduce the demand for, and exposure to, tobacco.

Despite the global effort, the tobacco industry continues to aggressively promote tobacco products in South East Asia, which provide them with less regulated environments compared to high-income countries. Tobacco giant Phillip Morris has rebranded to increase their products' appeal to their target markets. The company launched a new cigarette brand in Indonesia at the same time as their 'Unsmoke Your World' campaign in the United Kingdom, and positioned itself as 'part of the solution' by announcing a pledge to stop selling cigarettes (Campaign for Tobacco-Free Kids, 2021). Big Tobacco has also been focusing its efforts on creating new markets in wealthier nations, with alternative nicotine-delivery systems (ANDS) and by increasing investment in e-cigarettes and vaping products (Bauld et al., 2016). Switching from selling tobacco products to ANDS is a means of shoring up declining profit margins and improving Big Tobacco's corporate image by associating with less-harmful products that are more socially acceptable to younger people (Dewhurst, 2020). Between 2011 and 2015, there was a 900 per cent increase in e-cigarette use by high school students in the United States, with 1.7 million using them in the previous 30 days (US Surgeon General Report, cited in Binns & Low, 2018). With emerging evidence linking e-cigarettes and lung disease, Australia has chosen to take a precautionary approach to the marketing and sale of e-cigarettes, preventing the proliferation of their use through regulations that prohibit the importation of e-cigarettes containing nicotine, and the requirement of a doctor's prescription to possess liquid nicotine (Department of Health, 2021). While applauded by the Australian Cancer Council, Australian and WHO policies on vaping have been criticised by some addiction medicine specialists, who argue that access to e-cigarettes is needed to support smoking cessation; they are calling for the inclusion of tobacco harm reduction into the Framework Convention on Tobacco Control (Abad et al., 2021). However, there is consensus that protecting public health from Big Tobacco will require both stronger tobacco regulatory measures in developing countries – similar to what has been implemented in Australia – and counter-measures globally to combat the tobacco industries' tenacious efforts to escalate e-cigarette use among nicotine-naïve adolescents. Cunning marketing techniques such as producing flavoured e-cigarettes and targeting promotions by using 'influencers' on social media are contributing to creation of a new generation addicted to nicotine while ensuring that transnational tobacco companies continue to rake in big profits.

Introduction

We live in a world in which we are faced with a myriad of health issues, including communicable and non-communicable diseases such as COVID-19, HIV/AIDS, obesity, malnutrition, heart disease, occupational injuries and drug and alcohol misuse. Addressing our most pressing concerns is a complex task that requires action on several levels, from global to local, and from prevention through to treatment. At the global level, the World Health Organization (WHO) is a United Nations (UN) agency whose primary role is to lead and coordinate global health efforts. This chapter introduces readers to the discipline of **health promotion**, a core function of the WHO. The WHO defines health promotion as 'the process of enabling people to increase control over their health and its determinants, and thereby improve their health … and contributes to the work of tackling communicable and non-communicable diseases and other threats to health' (WHO, 1986, para. 3). This definition encompasses two important aspects. First, it is based on the WHO's holistic, positive definition of health and second, it necessitates an understanding of health that goes beyond the physical and/or psychological body to an understanding that there are many factors that influence a person's ability to be healthy (see chapters 1 and 7).

Health promotion – the practice of working with individuals and communities to enable them to improve their health by addressing the multiple determinants of health.

Using the opening vignette of tobacco use, readers can explore how Australia has attempted to curb the uptake of tobacco smoking and to encourage those who already smoke to quit. This has been undertaken by implementing public health interventions that target both individuals' smoking behaviours and the social and economic conditions surrounding tobacco use. The *Ottawa Charter for Health Promotion* ('Ottawa Charter') is used to frame the discussion.

The **Ottawa Charter** is the guiding framework used by health promotion practitioners to address the multiple determinants of health through multi-sectoral and multi-level approaches. While conceived in 1986, the Ottawa Charter continues to be considered the 'gold standard' for those attempting to promote health and reduce inequalities in health (Thompson, Watson & Tilford, 2018). The Ottawa Charter (Figure 3.1) is guided by three main principles: advocate, enable, and mediate. The aim of the advocate principle is to create favourable conditions for health by championing the case for action. The enable principle focuses on achieving equitable opportunities and resources. It also recognises that all sectors have a role to play and that health promotion professionals have a responsibility to mediate between various stakeholders in the pursuit of health. The three guiding principles facilitate implementation of the Ottawa Charter's five action areas: building healthy public policy, creating supportive environments, strengthening community action, developing individual skills and re-orienting health services. Each of the action areas is explored in the rest of the chapter.

Ottawa Charter – the *Ottawa Charter for Health Promotion* is a strategic framework for action in health promotion, recognising the need for multi-level, multi-sectoral action to address the determinants of health.

Addressing the multiple determinants of health is not an easy task. It requires input from all sectors of society. To successfully and sustainably promote health, governments, communities and organisations need to appreciate the long-term effort required to address complex health issues, rather than depending solely on non-integrated policy change and behavioural change, as is the current trend.

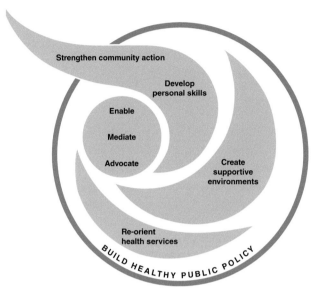

Figure 3.1   The Ottawa Charter.
Source: WHO (1986).

Building healthy public policy

Healthy public policy – a viewpoint that requires policy (not just health policy) to be cognisant of, and accountable for, any health effects influenced by policy.

Healthy public policy is created to address the structural and environmental determinants of health. Its main aim is to create a supportive environment in which healthy choices are the easier choices or, in the case of legislated policy, the only choice (WHO, n.d.-c). There is an abundance of evidence that healthy public policy has a profound and positive effect on the health status of populations. We have witnessed a decrease in the burden of disease following the implementation of several policies, such as seat-belt legislation, free and compulsory education, smoking legislation (see Spotlight 3.1), regulations on workplace health and safety, and environmental protection, to name a few. Health policies can be implemented in organisations (e.g. healthy tuckshop initiatives and healthy canteens in workplaces), but this section focuses on the government's responsibility, as set out in the Ottawa Charter (WHO, 1986), to create the conditions that support health by putting it on the agenda of all policymakers in all sectors. This requires governments to consider the health implications of all their decisions.

SPOTLIGHT 3.1

Tobacco legislation in Australia

Australia is a world leader in using healthy public policy approaches such as legislation and taxation to address tobacco consumption. Daily adult (18 years and older) smoking rates in Australia have declined from 28 per cent in 1989–90 to 11.6 per cent in 2019 (AIHW, 2020a). Since the 1990s, the federal, state and territorial governments have introduced legislation restricting tobacco advertising and access to tobacco products and places where tobacco can be consumed. Despite smoking behaviour still being inversely related to socio-economic status, with disadvantaged groups more likely to initiate and continue smoking (Greenhalgh et al., 2021), policy measures have led to significant declines in smoking across all socio-economic groups and age groups. Importantly, although smoking has continued to steadily decline since the 1990s, it has not always declined at the same rate across all age groups. According to the AIHW's National Drug Strategy Household Survey Report, the prevalence of regular smokers aged 25–39 years declined more sharply between 2007 and 2013, dropping from 25.5 per cent to 17 per cent (AIHW, 2020b) and coinciding with the introduction of several strong tobacco-control policy measures, including:

- graphic health warnings required on packaging of most tobacco products from 2006
- a 25 per cent increase in tobacco control excise in 2010, followed by 12.5 per cent tobacco excise increases implemented each year from 2013 to 2020 inclusive
- bans on point-of-sale tobacco product displays between 2010 and 2012
- legislation introduced in 2012 that makes it an offence to publish tobacco advertising on the internet or other electronic media
- plain packaging legislation and expanded graphic health warnings introduced in 2012
- complete bans on smoking in all enclosed public places, including pubs and licensed premises, between 2006 and 2010 (Commonwealth of Australia, 2018).

Increased taxes on tobacco products has been shown to have an effect on trends in tobacco consumption and prevalence. According to the 2019 National Drug Strategy Household Survey, the most frequently nominated reasons for quitting were health concerns and the cost of tobacco (AIHW, 2020b). An evaluation assessing the effects of plain packaging with large and graphic health warnings indicates that the legislation has been effective in achieving its objectives to reduce the appeal of tobacco, increase the effectiveness of health warnings and reduce the ability of packaging to mislead consumers about smoking harms (Wakefield et al., 2015). For examples of plain packaging, see Department of Health (n.d.).

QUESTION

A contemporary challenge facing policymakers in Australia is an increase in the use of e-cigarettes. There is conflicting evidence about the harms and benefits of e-cigarettes, from both the tobacco industry and health practitioners. Australia is taking a precautionary approach to vaping. Do you agree with the Australian government's approach to addressing this issue?

REFLECTION QUESTION

The taxes on tobacco have seen major increases in recent years. Has this resulted in a significant decrease in tobacco use in all groups? If yes, in which groups and why? If not, why do you think people continue to smoke or take up smoking?

Creating the 'nanny state'?

What level of responsibility should the government take in intervening in a population's behavioural choices, and where do we draw the line and enable adults to make their own — even if health-compromising — choices? These questions are usually couched in terms of whether government interference is creating a 'nanny state' in which basic human rights are being taken away from individuals or curtailing their freedom. Hoek (2015) argues that we need government intervention because citizens are not provided with clear, rational information about the potential harms to their health, particularly from the tobacco industry, and are bombarded with advertising that distorts rather than informs. Furthermore, there is evidence to suggest that implementing healthy policies that may be initially resisted can sway public opinion in the long run. This is clearly demonstrated in the case of tobacco legislation: smoking used to be highly acceptable, even desirable, but in recent years it has become a far less acceptable behaviour. History has also shown that those who stand to lose most from legislating for health, such as multinational tobacco, soda and fast-food industries, are the most vocal 'nanny state' dissenters.

Challenges in creating healthy public policy

Researchers in public health policy (e.g. Brownson et al., 2009; Eyler et al., 2016) suggest that there is a variety of scientific, social, economic and political forces that influence healthy public policy at local, state and national government levels. These include a lack of value placed on prevention (see also 'Re-orienting health services'), insufficient evidence of the effectiveness of government interventions, election cycles that are out of sync with the time required for interventions to be effective, and the disproportionate power and influence of vested interests such as the tobacco industry. Furthermore, researchers argue that there is a gap between the understandings of policymakers and research – a gap that results in a lack of evidence-based policymaking and, instead, a reliance on a 'business-as-usual approach' based on habit, stereotypes and cultural norms (see also Baker et al., 2017).

REFLECTION QUESTION

What would be the public health implications of criminalising tobacco use? Think about this in relation to the debates on legalising the use of recreational drugs. Should only certain recreational drugs be legalised, or all of them? Why or why not?

Creating supportive environments

Creating supportive environments is the area of health promotion that is concerned with generating 'living and working conditions that are safe, stimulating, satisfying and enjoyable' (WHO, 1986, para. 13). Creating environments that support health refers to their natural, physical and social aspects (WHO, 2009; Taylor et al., 2021). We need to conserve the natural environment in order to minimise the effects of environmental degradation, such as climate change and declining water, land and air quality (WHO, n.d.-c). In the built environment, we need environments for living, work and leisure that create and promote health. These conditions are most successfully produced through establishing healthy public policy such as the provision of subsidies, restrictions on purchasing and limits on advertising (Agide & Shakibazadeh, 2018) (see Spotlight 3.2). Changing health policies to create supportive environments not only restricts unhealthy individual behaviour but can also contribute to changes in social perceptions of unhealthy behaviours. For example, a Queensland campaign associated with the introduction of laws restricting smoking in certain environments (such as eating areas and enclosed liquor premises) adopted the slogan, 'Nobody smokes here anymore'. This message initiated a positive change in what is considered acceptable in a social environment. The ways in which health issues are framed in terms of policy can create healthy social environments as well as healthy natural and built environments.

SPOTLIGHT 3.2

Creating smoke-free work environments

Smoking policies were implemented in most Australian workplaces from the mid-1990s to the early 2000s before legislation to ban smoking in indoor workplaces was introduced. Most employers recognised that failure to protect their employees from exposure to environmental tobacco smoke would breach their duty-of-care obligations under occupational health and safety legislation, which requires employers to provide employees with a safe and healthy work environment.

Across Australia, Cancer Councils have developed resources to guide employers on how to best implement smoke-free policies to create safer, healthier work environments. Cancer Councils advised employers that the development of a smoke-free workplace policy should involve active participation from smoking and non-smoking employees, should specify where smoking is prohibited and the time frame for implementation, and should state the consequences for non-compliance. In addition to restricting smoking in the workplace, Cancer Councils emphasised the importance of providing information and support for smoking employees to quit and suggested that smokers be allowed to attend 'quit smoking' courses during work time (Cancer Council NSW, 2020). However, some work environments, such as prisons, were not made smoke-free until 2013–15. Prisons are both workplaces and the homes of those incarcerated, which poses a different set of complexities. Prior to the introduction of smoking bans in prisons, some argued that it would infringe on the human rights of a disenfranchised group, while prison guards raised concerns about the potential for increased tensions and violence within the prison. Although workplace smoking bans primarily aim to protect non-smokers from secondhand smoke, studies have shown that they also provide an environment that encourages smokers to quit. A systematic review of the effectiveness of smoke-free policies found that there was a median increase in cessation of 6.4 per cent among smokers exposed to a smoke-free policy, compared to smokers who were not (Hopkins et al., 2010). A high proportion of both prisoners and prison staff smoke, and therefore smoking contributes to substantial mortality in prisons (Binswanger, 2014). Spaulding and colleagues (2018) estimate that globally nearly 15 million smokers pass through prisons annually, and thus policies and legislation that ban smoking in prisons, accompanied by evidence-based interventions for smoking cessation, have potential to make a significant contribution to global health.

QUESTION
In proposing to make prisons smoke-free, how can we respond to the argument that a prison is home to many people with associated rights while balancing the rights of workers to a smoke-free workplace?

The settings-based approach

Settings approach to health promotion – an approach based on the understanding that health is created where people live, love, work and play. Using settings to promote health enables intersectoral collaboration and promotes working relationships between the health sector and other sectors to address health issues close to the source.

Creating supportive environments is often achieved by addressing determinants, using a **settings approach to health promotion**. The 'setting' is considered 'the place or social context in which people engage in daily activities in which environmental, organizational, and personal factors interact to affect health and wellbeing.' (WHO, n.d.-a, para. 5). Typical settings for health promotion are schools, workplaces and hospitals. An example of the settings approach that creates a supportive environment is that of health-promoting schools (see Langford et al., 2015). The health-promoting school is an environment 'that constantly strengthens its capacity as a healthy setting for living, learning and working' (WHO, n.d.-b, para. 1). Through an integrated focus, healthy school policies (e.g., on tuckshop menus, sun safety), school ethos and culture, along with the development of individual skills, can create conditions that are conducive to health. Not only are children required to engage in healthy behaviours according to school policies such as wearing a hat and sunscreen, but they are also provided with appropriate knowledge and resources and are supported through cultural understandings and expectations.

Challenges to creating supportive environments

Creating supportive environments relies on an integrated approach involving governments, businesses, organisations, communities and individuals. Collaborating across multiple levels can be time-consuming and expensive. Furthermore, the policies that help to create supportive environments are susceptible to change under different government agendas and budgetary restrictions. Not least, people – in general – can be resistant to change, particularly in the most significant environments in which they live their lives, such as school and work.

Strengthening community action

Health promotion is most effective and sustainable when it is achieved through community action on setting priorities, making decisions, planning strategies and implementing them to achieve better health (WHO, 1986). That is, the role of the health practitioner shifts to being facilitative – to enable community members to be more directly involved in identifying health needs and implementing solutions (Taylor et al., 2021). Indeed, the active role of community members is considered central to the settings approach, by which changes are made by people in their own communities to address local issues of health and wellbeing (Taylor et al., 2021). Strengthening community action focuses on community empowerment by recognising that community members themselves are the experts in their own settings (Taylor et al., 2021; see also Chapter 4). As such, community members are afforded greater power and control over health promotion action and, in so doing, the social environment becomes the focus for action rather than the individual (Taylor et al., 2021). By working *with* communities rather than *for* communities in a way that community members feel they have control over strategies and outcomes is health promoting in itself, since it promotes self-esteem, a sense of worth and social capital (Kickbusch, 2003). Furthermore, it is likely that changes will be sustained once health promotion experts have completed their project or funding has run out.

The WHO has identified social media as an important tool in strengthening community action; not only for risk communication (Tambo et al., 2021), but in engaging community volunteer action. One example is Syria's 'Volunteers against Corona' campaign (Ekzayez et al., 2020), which utilises the social media platforms Facebook and WhatsApp to mobilise community volunteers to raise awareness and promote campaigns and community-based referrals.

Community development

Community development is one approach through which community action on health can be achieved. Community development places communities as central to the identification of priorities and decision-making, and is recognised as a 'bottom-up' approach (Taylor et al., 2021). Engaging communities in forging their own health futures has the potential to address some of the social and economic determinants of health, particularly at the local level. As such, community development is necessarily political, since it means working for change to create social justice (Taylor et al., 2021).

Often, health promoters can become acutely aware of inequalities and obvious health needs within the communities in which they work (see Part 4). While communities can be empowered to set priorities, plan and implement strategies, it is more difficult for them to influence policies that may be compromising to their health. As such, health promoters may become advocates for change in lobbying governments for health policy reform. Spotlight 3.3 details the example of BUGA UP, one of the earliest examples of community-based advocacy for public policy to ban tobacco advertising. Other community initiatives led by health promotion organisations seek to upskill community members to join in health advocacy activities on their own behalf, such the Campaign for Tobacco-Free Kids and the Tobacco-Free Kids Action Fund (see Spotlight 3.3).

SPOTLIGHT 3.3

Community action in tobacco control

Australia has a long history of community action on tobacco control. One of the most noted early examples of community-based advocacy for public policy to ban tobacco advertising is that of BUGA UP (Billboard Utilising Graffitists against Unhealthy Promotions). BUGA UP was formed in 1978 by an environmentalist, an artist and a health educator. The group graffitied tens of thousands of billboards across Australia, and their actions are credited as being key in the campaign to end tobacco advertising, which was finally banned in 1994 (Chapman, 1996). Youth activists and civil society organisations continue to play a key role in strengthening community action on tobacco control. The Campaign for Tobacco-Free Kids and the Tobacco-Free Kids Action Fund are two organisations based in the United

States, with a national and international focus, who are leading global community advocacy efforts (www.tobaccofreekids.org). Through strategic communications and policy advocacy campaigns, they work to change public attitudes about tobacco and call on governments to reform policy and strengthen regulations on all tobacco products, including e-cigarettes. In addition to global online campaigns, they have developed advocacy action guide toolkits to build community capacity and support civil organisations to undertake advocacy campaigns that target policymakers in their local region.

QUESTION

We know that vaping is a problem in different population groups, including culturally and linguistically diverse (CALD) communities, young people and Aboriginal and Torres Strait Islander communities. What kind of community action would you be interested in promoting, and how would you like to be engaged in decision-making and policy development about vaping?

Challenges to facilitating community action

Health promoters who are facilitating community action need to be aware of the extent of participation of community members, to avoid their input being tokenistic (Taylor et al., 2021) – that is, gathering community input but not acting on it. Assumptions about communities can also hinder progress on health action. A thorough understanding of how the community defines itself (this may be different for different factions within the community), and the strengths and weaknesses within current practices and resources, is required. Community members themselves may be reluctant to participate in community action because they may feel they lack the knowledge and skills required, and that this task should be undertaken by the health promotion 'experts'. Strategies and theories as part of the community development framework can help to overcome these potential challenges.

Developing personal skills

KAB (Knowledge, Attitude, Behaviour) – a behavioural-change theory arguing that an increase in knowledge will encourage a change in attitude and a subsequent change in behaviour. While on the surface this appears logical and forms the basis of many campaigns, it is an outdated and contentious behavioural-change theory that fails to consider the influence of the broader determinants of health.

While the Ottawa Charter was in large part a response to the failure of behavioural-change interventions to encourage people to change their behaviours and subsequently to reduce the burden of non-communicable diseases, it recognised the role that behaviour and lifestyle play in promoting health. Developing personal skills, as framed within the Ottawa Charter, includes not only distributing health information but also understanding the structural and cultural factors that influence health and behaviours. This contrasts with the theory that if knowledge is increased attitudes will change and, consequently, there will be a change in behaviour (**KAB**). Furthermore, the Charter calls for skills to be extended to community organisations, lobbying and advocacy (Baum, 2016a).

Behavioural-change interventions

There are several ways that we can encourage the uptake of health information through behavioural-change interventions. These include direct efforts, such as teaching cooking skills and delivering weight-loss programs, quit-smoking programs and screening of at-risk, asymptomatic people for such conditions as breast or bowel cancer. A common behavioural-change intervention in Australia is social marketing. **Social marketing** in the public health context is defined as the application of commercial marketing techniques to influence the voluntary or involuntary behaviour of target audiences to improve health and wellbeing (Andreasen, 1995). Contemporary social marketing commentators argue that to achieve this social good, societal structures need to be targeted and that a move away from individual approaches to a systems approach is needed (Flaherty et al 2020; Rundle-Thiele et al 2019). However, most campaigns continue to focus on individual risk behaviours, and ignore the social and physical environments in which the behaviours are embedded.

Social marketing – the application of commercial marketing techniques to influence the voluntary behaviour of target audiences to achieve a social good.

Limitations of behavioural-change approaches

Behavioural-change interventions are very limited in their effect if they are not conducted in conjunction with structural change to provide the target group with the opportunity to modify their behaviour (see Spotlight 3.4). Furthermore, ignoring the social and economic circumstances may lead to victim-blaming for poor health. Research has shown that people who have greater access to society's resources are more likely to change their behaviours than those who have limited access (Baum, 2016a). That is, if you have a good job and good social networks and are free of disease, the benefits you accrue from changing your physical activity behaviour, for example, will be much greater than for someone who does not have the same social and economic advantages.

SPOTLIGHT 3.4

Social marketing campaigns

Social marketing campaigns against smoking have been used extensively since the 1990s in Australia, with the aim of increasing individuals' knowledge of tobacco-related risks and improving quitting behaviours. The first National Tobacco Campaign was launched in 1997, and subsequently state Cancer Councils produced many mass media campaigns, such as 'Sponge', 'Bubblewrap', 'Cough' and 'Who will you leave behind?' (Carroll, Cotter & Purcell, 2012). The 2013–15 campaign 'Breathless' shows a man being buried alive and struggling to breathe, and likens this to the experience of smoking-induced emphysema. Durkin, Brennan and Wakefield's (2012) review of mass-media anti-smoking campaigns suggests that messages conveying negative health effects such as 'Breathless' may be more effective in increasing knowledge and changing quitting behaviours at the population level. More recent mass-media campaigns have targeted specific population groups focusing on pregnant women and Indigenous smokers. For example, the 2017–18 'Don't make smokes your story', features an Indigenous man describing his experiences with smoking and quitting. However, mass-media smoking campaigns are costly, and critics have suggested that investment towards more cost-efficient tobacco control measures would be more effective. Atusingwize and colleagues' (2015) systematic review of economic evaluations of tobacco control mass-media campaigns concluded that they offer good value for money. Yet, there is consensus in the literature that social marketing is unlikely to provide the same return on investment as priced-based (tobacco taxes) and non-priced-based smoking cessation legislative interventions (such as smoking restrictions in public places). A major review of the evidence on the economic effects of tobacco (Ekpu & Brown, 2015) found that the cost-effectiveness ratio of implementing non-price-based smoking cessation legislation ranged from US $2 to US $112 per life year gained, and Vos and colleagues (2010) concluded that a 30 per cent tobacco tax in Australia would be the most cost-effective intervention with the greatest public health benefits. Globally, with the advent of the digital age, the public's exposure to media has significantly changed since mass-media TV campaigns were launched in Australia in the 1990s, and there is emerging evidence suggesting that online campaigns may be substantially more cost effective than other media campaigns (Eku & Brown, 2015). Social media campaigns integrated with smartphone apps to promote smoking cessation to younger adult smokers are being used in Canada. One such example is the Break It Off (BIO) campaign. The evaluation of BIO found that users of the campaign materials had significantly higher 7-day and 30-day quit rates when compared to users of telephone quitlines of the same age (Baskerville et al., 2015). Regardless of the type of media or platform used in social marketing for smoking cessation, evidence suggests that for such campaigns to be optimally effective in reducing smoking prevalence they need to be sustained, since campaign effectiveness is 'dose-dependent' (Wakefield et al., 2011) and they are most effective when conducted in conjunction with other tobacco-control measures, as part of suite of tobacco-control interventions.

QUESTION

How sustainable are the effects of the social marketing campaigns highlighted in Spotlight 3.4, and do they address the social and environmental determinants of health?

Re-orienting health services

Determinant of health – a factor within and external to the individual that determines their health; the specific social, economic and political circumstances into which individuals are born and live.

The healthcare sector is a powerful **determinant of health** (Baum, 2016b). According to the Ottawa Charter (WHO, 1986), the main purposes of re-orienting health services are three-fold. First, we must recognise that the responsibility for health promotion needs to be shared among individuals, community groups, health professionals, health service institutions and governments. Second, there needs to be a move away from healthcare services focusing primarily on clinical and curative services and an increase in investment in population health initiatives, prevention and health promotion. Finally, health services need to be culturally sensitive and support the needs of individuals and communities. This includes recognising the broader social, political, economic and environmental components of health that affect different populations. This has the potential to empower individuals and communities to take control of the determinants of their health (see the definition of 'health promotion') and enables them to actively participate in the development of interventions that are appropriate and relevant to their population.

Challenges of re-orienting health services

Of all the Ottawa Charter strategies, there has been little progress in re-orienting health services, except at the local level with individual health services or community organisations (Wilberg et al., 2019; see Spotlight 3.5). This is despite mounting evidence that even a modest increase in investment in public health services can produce improved health in populations

(Leider et al., 2018). That is, a modest change from investment in curative services to investment in health promotion services will see lives saved, illnesses and injuries prevented, and associated cost benefits to societies. Furthermore, there is ample evidence that improved life expectancy is linked to improved living and working conditions, rather than to improvements in healthcare services per se (Baum, 2016a).

This raises the question of why governments do not heed the evidence and invest more in prevention. In Australia, as in most countries, the health budget primarily funds curative services, particularly hospital services. The most recent available figures indicate that Australia's total government expenditure on public health activities was 1.6 per cent of the total health expenditure (AIHW, 2018). This proportion is lower than in many other OECD (Organisation for Economic Co-operation and Development) countries, including Aotearoa New Zealand, Canada and the United Kingdom (Jackson & Shiell, 2017) and lower than reported in the previous period (AIHW, 2011). Baum and colleagues (2009) argue that the emphasis on curative medicine reflects the 'dominance of the medical imagination' (p. 1969). That is, as powerful actors, medical professionals can set the agenda and influence policy decisions on how best to address and fund health.

SPOTLIGHT 3.5

Re-orienting health services at the local level

In Melbourne, Australia, the Dandenong and District Aborigines Co-operative (DDAC), incorporating the Bunurong Health Service and the Bunurong Healthy Lifestyle Team, delivers programs ranging from medical services to youth and women's community development projects that strengthen social supports and connectedness to improve health and wellbeing. Developing and delivering community-based interventions that reduce tobacco consumption is a key priority action area for the service, because tobacco is the leading preventable cause of disease and death among the local Indigenous population (AIHW, 2020a).

In 2012, the service developed the 'Kick the Butt' initiative, using funding from the Department of Health and Ageing. A steering committee was established comprising health experts of 50 per cent Indigenous and 50 per cent non-Indigenous origin. The committee decided it would target its efforts on reducing the uptake of smoking among the youth population (12–25 years of age) in the southern region of Melbourne. The primary aim of the project was to change young people's perception of smoking as a social norm within Indigenous communities. Therefore, a social marketing approach was employed. The project team partnered with agencies including Quitline, the Cancer Council of Victoria, OxyGen and the Hawthorn Football Club. A media consultant was contracted to support the project, and focus groups were held with local Indigenous young people to inform the development of social marketing content and determine the best communication channels for reaching the target group. Initially, the project developed a series of four advertisements broadcast on SBS and National Indigenous TV, and the campaign was promoted through radio broadcasts and billboards on buses. Feedback from the target group indicated that the billboards were particularly useful in increasing campaign exposure.

Mainstream tobacco-control advertising has predominantly emphasised the negative health effects of smoking by using 'scare tactics' to prompt behavioural change. The view of the project steering committee was that this negative, directive approach was less likely to be effective among their community members. Therefore, they chose to frame their tobacco-prevention messages with a positive approach that highlighted the importance of living longer for the sake of kin. They also leveraged the significance of Australian Rules football to Indigenous young people and featured a prominent player from the Australian Football League (AFL) in the advertisements as a means of motivating young people to avoid smoking. DDAC received further funding for its Tackling Indigenous Smoking (TIS) program, and has developed more resources in the Kick the Butt campaign to reduce tobacco use. This includes online resources such as interactive games and the stories of campaign ambassadors who have successfully quit smoking. Online resources also link to several social media channels, including Facebook and Instagram (see Quit Victoria 2021 and Tobacco Cessation (vaccho. org.au)).

We thank Chris Tsagaris from DDAC and the Bunurong Health Service for his time and for sharing his knowledge to inform this case example.

QUESTION

The WHO is calling for health services to be more preventative in focus. How can healthcare services work in a more integrated way with the community and other sectors to achieve this?

SUMMARY

This chapter has discussed the principles and practices of health promotion in public health. Salient issues are summarised below.

Learning objective 1: Discuss the role of governments in promoting health through healthy public policy.
History has shown that policy and legislation have positive effects on the status of our health, as demonstrated by the tobacco legislation in Australia. The Ottawa Charter requires governments to consider the health implications of all their decisions. However, governments face several scientific, social, economic and political challenges when creating public health policy.

Learning objective 2: Discuss how physical and social environments can be health-promoting.
Creating environments that support healthy living involves social, natural and built environments. This is most often achieved by establishing strong public health policy. Positive changes in policy for natural and built environments can promote the creation of healthy social environments by influencing public perceptions of healthy norms.

Learning objective 3: Discuss the role communities can play in promoting health.
Health promotion is most effective and sustainable when it is achieved through community action on setting priorities, making decisions, planning strategies and implementing them to achieve better public health outcomes. It is difficult, however, for communities to influence policies that may be compromising their health. As such, health promoters may become advocates for change in lobbying governments for health policy reform.

Learning objective 4: Explain how individual health-compromising behaviours can be addressed.
There are several ways in which health-compromising behaviours can be addressed at the individual level. These include direct behavioural-change efforts such as teaching cooking skills and implementing weight-loss and 'quit smoking' programs. The major limitations of behavioural-change programs include the lack of recognition of the social and economic environments in which behaviours are embedded, and that can lead to victim-blaming and program failure.

Learning objective 5: Discuss the role of health services in promoting health.
Traditionally, the role of health services has been to provide clinical and curative treatment. Re-orienting health services shifts this focus to include investment in population health initiatives, prevention and health promotion. It recognises that the responsibility for health lies both within and outside the healthcare sector.

TUTORIAL EXERCISES

1   Despite the positive effects of legislation and policy on smoking prevalence in most of the population, smoking rates are persistently high among our most disadvantaged groups, including people who are homeless, illicit substance users, people living with a mental illness and Indigenous peoples. The challenge in Australia is to reduce this disparity. Discuss a possible way forward for the Australian government.
2   Based on your understanding of the Ottawa Charter and using each action area, what recommendations would you suggest to address malnutrition in a high-income country (over-nutrition) and a low-income country (under-nutrition).

3   Discuss the barriers and enablers of implementing each of the interventions in the countries you have identified in question 2 (including political, sociocultural, economic, multi-sectoral action, behavioural change and community action).

4   How would you respond if your university banned the sale and consumption of sugary drinks on your campus to help make 'the healthier choice the easier choice' for students? This would include energy drinks, soft drinks, sports drinks and some juices. Discuss notions of free choice versus 'the nanny state' (as discussed in this chapter). Do the benefits outweigh the costs? For example, does improved student health trump lost revenue from sales?

FURTHER READING

Almestahiri, R., Rundle-Thiele, S., Parkinson, J., & Arli, D. (2017). The use of the major components of social marketing: A systematic review of tobacco cessation programs. *Social Marketing Quarterly*, *23*(3), 232–48.

Bodkin, A., & Hakimi, S. (2020). Sustainable by design: a systematic review of factors for health promotion program sustainability. *BMC Public Health*, *20* (964).

Department of Health Victoria. (2012). *Integrated health promotion resource kit*. Retrieved https://content. health.vic.gov.au/sites/default/files/migrated/files/collections/policies-and-guidelines/i/integrated_health_promo--pdf.pdf

Mercado, S. P. (2020). COVID-19, the WHO Ottawa charter and the Red Cross-Red Crescent Movement. *Global Social Policy*, *20*(3), 406–11.

Moodie C, Hoek J, Scheffels J, Gallopel-Morvan, K., & Lindorff, K. (2019). Plain packaging: Legislative differences in Australia, France, the UK, New Zealand and Norway, and options for strengthening regulations. *Tobacco Control*, *28*(5), 485–92.

REFERENCES

Abad, M. L. et al. (2021). One hundred specialists call for WHO to change its hostile stance on tobacco harm reduction – new letter to FCTC delegates published. Retrieved https://clivebates.com/documents/WHOCOP9LetterOct2021-EN.pdf

Agide, F. D., & Shakibazadeh, E. (2018). Contextualising Ottawa Charter frameworks for type 2 diabetes prevention: A professional perspective as a review. *Ethiopian Journal of Health*, *28*(3), 355–64.

Andreasen, A. (1995). *Marketing social change: Changing behavior to promote health, social development, and the environment*. Josey-Bass.

Atusingwize, E., Lewis, S., & Langley, T. (2015). Economic evaluations of tobacco control mass media campaigns: a systematic review. *Tobacco Control*, *24*(4), 320–7.

Australian Institute of Health and Welfare (AIHW). (2011). Public health expenditure in Australia 2008–09. Health and welfare expenditure series No. 43. (Cat. No. HWE 52). AIHW. Retrieved http://www.aihw.gov.au

——(2018). Health expenditure Australia 2016–17. Health and welfare expenditure series No. 64. (Cat. No. HWE 74). AIHW. Retrieved http://www.aihw.gov.au

——(2020a). Australia's health 2020. AIHW. Retrieved https://www.aihw.gov.au/reports-data/australias-health

——(2020b). *National Drug Strategy Household Survey 2019*. AIHW. Retrieved https://www.aihw.gov.au/reports/illicit-use-of-drugs/national-drug-strategy-household-survey-2019/contents/summary

Baker, P. Gill, T., Friel, S., Carey, G., & Kay, A. (2017). Generating political priority for regulatory interventions targeting obesity prevention: An Australian case study. *Social Science & Medicine*, 177, 141–9.

Baskerville, N.B. Azagba, S., Norman, C., McKeown, K., & Brown, K.S. (2015). Effect of a digital social media campaign on young adult smoking cessation. *Nicotine & Tobacco Research*, *18*(3), 351–60.

Bauld, L., Angus, K., de Andrade, M., & Ford A. (2016). *Current research and policy*. Cancer Research UK. Retrieved https://www.cancerresearchuk.org/sites/default/files/electronic_cigarette_marketing_report_final.pdf.

Baum, F. (2016a). *The new public health* (4th ed.). Oxford University Press.

——(2016b) Health systems: How much difference can they make to health inequities? *Journal of Epidemiology and Community Health*, *70*(7), 635–6.

Baum, F., Bégin, M., Houweling, T., & Taylor, S. (2009). Changes not for the fainthearted: Reorienting health care systems toward health equity through action on the social determinants of health. *American Journal of Public Health*, *99*(11), 1967–74.

Binns, C., & Low, M. K. (2018). Big tobacco finds a new way to make profits: And still kill people. *Asia Pacific Journal of Public Health*, *30*(4), 312–14.

Binswanger, I. A., Carson, A. E., Krueger, P. M., Mueller, S. R., Steiner, J. F., & Sabol, W. J. (2014). Prison tobacco control policies and deaths from smoking in United States prisons: population based retrospective analysis. *British Medical Journal 349*. Retrieved https://doi.org/10.1136/bmj.g4542

Brownson, R., Chriqui, J., & Stamatakis, K. (2009). Understanding evidence-based public health policy. *American Journal of Public Health*, *99*(9), 1576–83.

Campaign for Tobacco-Free Kids. (2021). Philip Morris international's massive public relations push: The Foundation for a Smoke-Free World. Retrieved https://www.tobaccofreekids.org/what-we-do/industry-watch/pmi-foundation

Cancer Council NSW. (2020). Comprehensive smoking policies. Retrieved https://www.cancercouncil.com.au/cancer-prevention/smoking/tackling-tobacco/how-the-program-works/comprehensive-smoking-policies/

Carroll, T., Cotter, T., & Purcell, K. (2012). Tobacco-control campaigns in Australia: Experience. In M. M. Scollo & M. H. Winstanley (Eds.), *Tobacco in Australia: Facts and issues* (4th ed.). Cancer Council Victoria. Retrieved http://www.tobaccoinaustralia.org.au

Chapman, S. (1996). Civil disobedience and tobacco control: The case of BUGA UP. *Tobacco Control*, *5*, 179–85.

Commonwealth of Australia. (2018). Tobacco control timeline. Retrieved https://www1.health.gov.au/internet/publications/publishing.nsf/Content/tobacco-control-toc~timeline

——(2021). *Draft National Preventative Health Strategy 2021–2030*. Retrieved https://consultations.health.gov.au/national-preventive-health-taskforce/draft-national-preventive-health-strategy/

Department of Health. (n.d.). Tobacco plain packaging resources. Retrieved https://www.health.gov.au/resources/collections/tobacco-plain-packaging-resources

——(2021). About e-cigarettes. Retrieved https://www.health.gov.au/health-topics/smoking-and-tobacco/about-smoking-and-tobacco/about-e-cigarettes

Dewhurst, T. (2020). Co-optation of harm reduction by Big Tobacco (Editorial). *Tobacco Control*, 30(e1). doi:10.1136/ tobaccocontrol-2020-056059

Durkin, S., Brennan, E., & Wakefield, M. (2012). Mass media campaigns to promote smoking cessation among adults: An integrative review. *Tobacco Control*, *21*, 127–38.

Ekpu, V.U & Brown, A.K. (2015). The economic impact of smoking and of reducing smoking prevalence: Review of evidence. *Top Use Insights*, *8*, 1–35.

Ekzayez, A., Al-Khalil, M., Jasiem, M., Al Saleh, R., Alzoubi, Z., Meagher, K., & Patel, P. (2020). COVID-19 response in northwest Syria: Innovation and community engagement in a complex conflict. *Journal of Public Health*, *42*(3), 504–9.

Eyler, A. A., Chriqui, J. F., Moreland-Russell, S., & Brownson, C. (Eds.). (2016). *Prevention, policy, and public health*. Oxford University Press.

Flaherty, T., Domegan, C., Duane, S., & Anand (2020). Systems social marketing and macro-social marketing: A systematic review. *Social Marketing Quarterly*, *26*(2), 146–66.

Greenhalgh, E.M., Bayly, M., & Scollo, M. (2021). 1.7 Trends in the prevalence of smoking by socio-economic status. In Greenhalgh, E.M., Scollo, M.M., & Winstanley, M.H. (Eds.), *Tobacco in Australia: Facts and issues*. Cancer Council Victoria. Retrieved http://www.tobaccoinaustralia.org.au

Hoek, J. (2015). Informed choice and the nanny state: Learning from the tobacco industry. *Public Health*, *129*(8), 1038–45.

Hopkins, D. P., Razi, S., Leeks, K., Geetika, P. K., Chattopadhyay, S. K., & Soler, R. E. (2010). Smokefree policies to reduce tobacco use: A systematic review. *American Journal of Preventative medicine*, *38*(2), 275–89.

Jackson, H. & Shiell, A. (2017). *Preventive health: How much does Australia spend and is it enough?* Foundation for Alcohol Research and Education.

Kickbusch, I. (2003). The contribution of the World Health Organization to a new public health and health promotion. *American Journal of Public Health*, *93*(3), 383–8.

Langford, R., Bonell, C., Jones, H., Pouliou, T., Murphy, S., Waters, E., ... Campbell, R. (2015). The World Health Organization's Health Promoting School's framework: A Cochrane systematic review and meta-analysis. *BMC Public Health*, *15*, 130.

Leider, J. P., Alfonso, N., Resnick, B., Brady, E., McCullough, J. M., & Bishai, D., (2018). Assessing the value of 40 years of local public expenditures on health. *Health Affairs; Chevy Chase 37*(4), 560–9.

Quit Victoria. (2021). Tackling Indigenous smoking. Retrieved https://www.quit.org.au/resources/aboriginal-communities/tackling-indigenous-smoking/

Rundle-Thiele., David, P., Willmott, T., Pang, B., Eagle, L., & Hay, R. (2019). Social marketing theory development goals: An agenda to drive change. *Journal of Marketing Management*, *35*(1-2), 160–81.

Spaulding, A. C., Eldridge, G. D., Chico, C. E., Morisseau, N., Drobeniuc, A., Fils-Aime, R., Day, C., Hopkins, R., Jin, X., Chen, J., & Dolan, K. A. (2018). Smoking in correctional settings worldwide: Prevalence, bans, and interventions. *Epidemiologic Reviews*, *40*(1), 82–95.

Tambo, E., Djuikoue, I. C., Tazemda, G. K., Fotsing, M. F., & Zhou, X. N. (2021). Early stage risk communication and community engagement (RCCE) strategies and measures against the coronavirus disease 2019 (COVID-19) pandemic crisis. *Global Health Journal*, *5*(1), 44–50.

Taylor, J., O'Hara, L., Talbot, L., & Verrinder, G. (2021). *Promoting health: The primary health care approach*. (7th ed.). Elsevier.

Thompson, S. R., Watson, M. C., & Tilford, S. (2018). The Ottawa Charter 30 years on: Still an important standard for health promotion. *International Journal of Health Promotion and Education, 56*(2), 73–84.

Vos, T., Carter, R., Barendregt, J., Mihalopoulos, C., Veerman, L., Magnus, A., Cobiac, L., Bertram, M. & Wallace, A. (2010). *Assessing cost-effectiveness in prevention. (ACE–prevention): Final report*. University of Queensland and Deakin University.

Wakefield, M., Coomber, K., Zacher, M., Durkin, S., Brennan, E., & Scollo, M. (2015). Australian adult smokers' responses to plain packaging with larger graphic health warnings 1 year after implementation: Results from a national cross-sectional tracking survey. *Tobacco Control*, *24*, ii17–ii25.

Wakefield, M. A., Spittal, M. J., Yong, H-H., & Borland, R. (2011). Effects of mass media campaign exposure intensity and durability on quit attempts in a population-based cohort study. *Health Education Research, 26*(6), 988–97.

Wilberg, A., Saboga-Nunes, L., & Stock, C. (2019). Are we there yet? Use of the Ottawa Charter action areas in the perspective of European health promotion professionals. *Journal of Public Health: From Theory to Practice 29*, 1–7.

World Health Organization (WHO). (1986). *The Ottawa Charter for Health Promotion*. WHO. Retrieved https://www.who.int/publications/i/item/ottawa-charter-for-health-promotion

——(2003). *WHO Framework Convention on Tobacco Control*. Retrieved https://www.who.int/fctc/text_download/en/

——(2009). *Milestones in health promotion: Statements from global conferences*. Retrieved http://www.who.int/healthpromotion/Milestones_Health_Promotion_05022010.pdf

——(2019). *WHO report on the global tobacco epidemic*. Country Profile Report: Indonesia. Retrieved https://www.who.int/tobacco/surveillance/policy/country_profile/

——(n.d.-a). *Health promoting schools.* Retrieved https://www.who.int/health-topics/health-promoting-schools#tab=tab_1

——(n.d.-b). *Healthy settings*. Retrieved https://www.who.int/teams/health-promotion/enhanced-wellbeing/healthy-settings

——(n.d.-c). *Health promotion action means*. Retrieved https://www.who.int/teams/health-promotion/enhanced-wellbeing/healthy-settings

World Population Review. (2021). (Website). Retrieved https://worldpopulationreview.com/country-rankings/smoking-rates-by-country

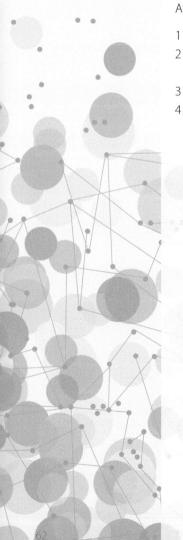

4

Primary health care and community health

Lawrence Tan and Jennifer Reath

With acknowledgements to Irene Blackberry for her contribution to the chapter in the second edition of this book

LEARNING OBJECTIVES

After studying this chapter, you will be able to:

1 define primary health care, primary care and community health
2 describe the contexts of primary health care and community health in Australian and global healthcare systems
3 discuss effective models of care within primary health care and community health
4 identify challenges and future directions in primary health care.

VIGNETTE

Carmen encounters the health system

Carmen, aged 56, immigrated to Australia with her family six years ago. She speaks some English but prefers to use her first language, Spanish. When she needs health care, Carmen first goes to her pharmacist, dentist or general practitioner (GP). Her regular GP can speak Spanish, also. Carmen's main health concerns have been overweight, high blood pressure and prevention of diabetes, since her mother is on insulin medication. Carmen's GP has discussed with her options for healthy eating and increasing her physical activity. The GP also ensures Carmen has regular screening for bowel and cervical cancer. One morning Carmen's GP receives the results of Carmen's screening from the government-funded BreastScreen unit. The mammography indicates that Carmen has a suspicious lesion, and on biopsy it is found to be malignant. The GP makes an appointment for Carmen to come in to discuss the report. When she walks into the consultation room, Carmen bursts into tears. Together they work out the next steps, including referral to a breast surgeon at the local public hospital, who organises further investigation and surgery. Following discharge, Carmen is visited at home by the McGrath community breast cancer nurse for additional care, education and support. Her GP uses a GP Management Plan to organise Medicare-funded referrals for physiotherapy to treat her lymphedema, a dietitian for weight loss and an exercise physiologist. The hospital oncologist phones the GP, asking them to clarify instructions for ongoing chemotherapy with Carmen, as she seems confused despite the assistance of an interpreter. The GP also directs Carmen to a Spanish-speaking community cancer support group, and to multilingual resources on the Cancer Council website. Carmen's friends and family become enthusiastic supporters of the Pink Ribbon campaign, which raises community aware-ness about breast cancer, and funds for breast cancer research. Carmen is now in remission but has developed diabetes. Her GP refers her to a diabetes educator and to a community pharmacist, who completes a home medication review to help Carmen understand her new medications. The GP continues to work with Carmen and her allied health providers on her health goals, monitors the diabetes and organises surveillance for cancer recurrence.

Introduction

This chapter introduces readers to **primary health care (PHC)** and **community health** in Australia. PHC is an integral part of health care provision and the first point of contact with the country's health system. In this chapter, definitions of PHC and its rationale are described. Then an overview of current PHC in both Australian and global healthcare systems is provided, including discussion of health reforms that have shaped PHC develop-ment and funding models. Finally, effective models of care within PHC and community health are examined using a range of examples in Australia and elsewhere. The final section of the chapter provides insights into some of the current challenges and future directions in PHC to respond to rising healthcare expenditure resulting from increasing costs of investi-gations, medications and health services and an epidemic of chronic diseases in a rapidly ageing population.

Primary health care (PHC) – is a whole-of-society approach, aiming to provide people with equitable access within their communities, to the highest level of health and wellbeing (WHO & UNICEF, 2018).

Community health – integrated health and social services provided by public and private partnerships to meet the health and welfare needs of individuals and their families in the community.

Definition and concept of PHC and community health

Confusingly, the term 'PHC' is often used interchangeably with '**primary care**' and 'community health'. In this section, working definitions of PHC and how it relates to primary care and community health are discussed.

The origin of PHC and community health

In 1978, the WHO hosted the International Conference on Primary Health Care in Alma-Ata (now Almaty), Kazakhstan (WHO, 1978) to introduce 'primary health care' and to declare 'health care for all by the year 2000'. The commitment was strengthened with the launch of the *Ottawa Charter for Health Promotion* (WHO, 1986; see also Chapter 3).

The movement towards PHC was a reaction to the emphasis at the time on highly technological healthcare provided in hospitals that was unaffordable for many. PHC is about universal access to fundamental health care for individuals and their families in the community, within the health system, in order to maintain health and wellbeing (WHO, 1978). PHC is a key strategy enabling individuals and their families to access affordable and equitable health care in their communities (Talbot & Verrinder, 2017). To achieve this goal, government, communities and individuals need to work in partnerships within their sociocultural, economic, political, biomedical and public health contexts. The Declaration of Alma-Ata specified the core elements of PHC as:

- education concerning health literacy
- promotion of food supply and proper nutrition
- an adequate supply of safe water and basic sanitation
- maternal and child health care, including family planning
- immunisation against major infectious diseases
- prevention and control of locally endemic diseases
- appropriate treatment of common diseases and injuries
- provision of essential drugs (WHO, 1978).

Community health is one of the ways in which PHC is implemented, focusing on working with communities to improve upstream determinants of health such as social and welfare issues. Communities are groups of individuals who have geographical or cultural aspects in common, or who share common interests such as sport, religion or leisure activities. While public health protects and improves the health of whole populations, PHC and community health focus on individuals, families and communities.

From Alma Ata to Astana

A common criticism of the Declaration of Alma-Ata was that it was too idealistic to be practical (Rifkin, 2018). There was a move to simplify PHC by promoting vertical interventions to target prevention and the cure of specific diseases such as tuberculosis and malaria. This selective PHC approach attracted funding from entities such as the World Bank and the Bill and Melinda Gates Foundation, and was successful in improving outcomes for those targeted conditions. However, it did not address the broader issues of health inequity, nor did it facilitate the multi-sectoral involvement espoused by the comprehensive PHC approach envisioned by the Alma-Ata Declaration (Hall & Taylor, 2003). WHO responded by championing Universal Health Coverage (UHC), whereby all people would have access to the services they need without causing financial hardship. UHC became incorporated as target 3.8 of the United Nation's Sustainable Development Goals:

> Achieve universal health coverage, including financial risk protection, access to quality essential health-care services and access to safe, effective, quality and affordable essential medicines and vaccines for all (United Nations, 2015).

In 2018, world leaders from health, finance, education and social welfare sectors, as well as patient advocates and youth representatives, committed to the Declaration of Astana (WHO, 2018a). This global conference on PHC returned to Kazakhstan to reaffirm the Declaration of Alma-Ata, this time with a broader scope. The Declaration of Astana prioritised three key components of PHC:

- Empowering individuals and communities as advocates and architects of their health
- Using evidence-based, multi-sectoral policies to address determinants of health
- Strengthening primary care and public health as integral to service delivery.

REFLECTION QUESTION

Think about Carmen and her encounters with the health system. In what ways did the three key components of the Declaration of Astana come into play in the PHC-based prevention, diagnosis, management and continuing care of her health problems?

PHC and community health in Australia

Definition of PHC in Australia

Australian PHC is 'socially appropriate, universally accessible, scientifically sound first level care provided by health services and systems with a suitably trained workforce comprised of multi-disciplinary teams' (Lunnay, McIntyre, Oliver-Baxter, 2014, p. 1). It coordinates with the rest of the health system through referral pathways in order to address health inequalities, increase individual and community self-reliance and collaborate with other sectors to improve public health.

In contrast to primary care, PHC goes beyond the biomedical model of health care using a social model of care that addresses the various determinants of health described in Part 2 of this book.

Definitions of 'primary care' and 'community health' in Australia

Primary care (PC) is part of PHC and the first point of entry for individuals into the healthcare system. Australia and Aotearoa New Zealand, among other nations, have a 'gatekeeper' system whereby access to secondary and tertiary levels of health care requires referral from the PC level (apart from emergency services). PC covers services that individuals can gain

General practitioners (GPs)
– provide person-centred, continuing, comprehensive and coordinated whole-person medical care to individuals and families in their communities (Royal Australian College of General Practitioners, n.d.).

access to directly, such as general practice, allied health services, dentistry, Aboriginal health, community health and pharmacy. **General practitioners (GPs)** are medical specialists trained in PC. They have an important role in maintaining continuity and coordinating care for individuals and communities within an often-fragmented healthcare system.

While general practice in Australia has a medical and biological focus, community health operates under social, environmental and economic models. As such, community health services develop strong partnerships with their local stakeholders and target disadvantaged population groups, including:

* Aboriginal and Torres Strait Islander peoples
* people with an intellectual disability
* refugees and people seeking asylum
* homeless people and people at risk of homelessness
* people living with a serious mental illness.

Community health offers a comprehensive PHC, with funding usually from state or local governments, or community organisations. The range of services varies between states and territories, and between communities, and these may include:

* rural primary health services to remote and very remote communities
* maternal and child community health services
* women's health
* men's health
* community rehabilitation
* mental health
* aged care.

Community health services are delivered in a variety of settings, including community health centres, health services, public venues, local councils, schools and in the individual's home. An example of community health services in Australia is provided by Aboriginal Community Controlled Health Organisations (ACCHO) (see Spotlight 4.1).

SPOTLIGHT 4.1

Aboriginal Community Controlled Health Services

The first Aboriginal Community Controlled Health Service (ACCHS) was established in Sydney in 1971, in response to failure of the health system to meet the needs of Aboriginal and Torres Strait Islander peoples. Since then, the sector has come a long way, and continues from strength to strength, consolidating its unique place in Australia's health system by establishing models of care and achieving outcomes that others seek to emulate.

There are more than 140 ACCHSs across Australia. The National Aboriginal Community Controlled Health Organisation (NACCHO) is the peak organisation, participating in national health policy development on behalf of the ACCHSs and eight state and territory affiliates supporting the services. ACCHS funding includes government block grants, Medicare billings, targeted program funding, other grants and contracts. The ACCHS sector is one of the largest employers of Aboriginal and Torres Strait Islander peoples nationally.

Health inequities result from maldistribution of money, power and resources and, uniquely in Australia for Aboriginal and Torres Strait Islander peoples, from the history of colonisation and continuing unreconciled effects of institutionalised racism and structural disempowerment. In a critical act of self-determination, the ACCHSs have developed a comprehensive, holistic, person-centred model of PHC, grounded in cultural understandings of relationships across the individual, country, kin, community and spirituality contexts. Though pre-dating Alma-Ata, the ACCHS model is consistent with this approach. Each ACCHS, governed by a community-elected board, enables local communities to identify needs and decide best approaches to health issues. These include management of illnesses as well as preventive medicine, health promotion, environmental health, and provision of medications, counselling and rehabilitation.

Through needs-based, community controlled, comprehensive primary health care, as well as employment, engagement, empowerment and social action, the ACCHSs enable Aboriginal and Torres Strait Islander people to take responsibility for their health.

Source: based on NACCHO, 2021. With acknowledgement to Dr Dawn Casey, Deputy Chief Executive Officer, NACCHO.

QUESTION

Many would see the ACCHOs as models of high-quality primary health organisations. How do these organisations exemplify the key features of PHC described by Lunnay and colleagues (2014)?

Understanding the context of PHC and community health within Australian and global healthcare systems

This section describes the context of PHC within the Australian healthcare system and elsewhere. Development of PHC through various health reforms and funding models in the Australian healthcare system is also discussed.

Overview of PHC within the Australian healthcare system

According to the Australian Medical Association (2020), '[t]he primary health care system is designed to provide the right care at the right time, at the right place, ensuring a healthier population' (p. 6). PHC ranges from health promotion and prevention to early detection and treatment of acute and chronic conditions by various health professionals, including Aboriginal health workers, allied health professionals, nurses, dentists and GPs (AIHW, 2020a). The Australian health system, including PC, was rated by the Commonwealth Fund as the second-best performing health system of 11 high-income OECD countries in 2017 (Schneider et al., 2017). An overview of PHC within the Australian healthcare system and other health services is provided here.

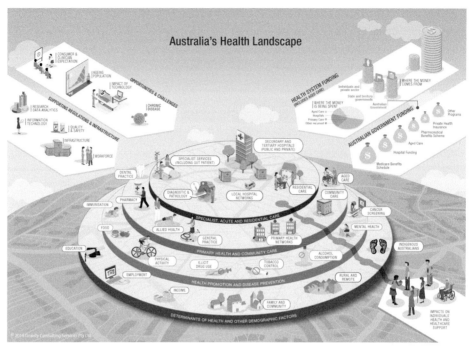

Figure 4.1   Australia's health landscape.
Source: Department of Health (2017).

PHC reforms in Australia

Rising costs and expectations of health care, along with Australia's ageing population and the epidemic of chronic diseases, present significant challenges to the healthcare system (Duckett & McGannon, 2013). PHC meets these challenges by providing a holistic, preventive and patient-centred care approach (Harris, Islam et al., 2013). Barriers to this approach identified by the Standing Council on Health (2013) include:

- fragmentation between federally funded services (such as general practice) and state-funded services (such as hospitals and community health centres)
- funding, governance and reporting complexities
- poor coordination of service planning and delivery across different sectors
- workforce shortages and maldistribution.

PHC organisations

The early 1990s saw the formation of Divisions of General Practice, the first national network of regional PHC organisations in Australia. In 2011, they were replaced by Medicare Locals and then superseded by Primary Health Networks (PHNs). PHNs aim to reduce fragmentation of care, commission primary care services for patients, increase coordination between local hospitals and PC services and improve the overall operational efficiency within their networks. Freeman, Baum and colleagues (2021) noted considerable variation in PHN collaboration with state health systems and appealed for greater resourcing and less ambiguity in state versus federal responsibilities to support a well-integrated PHC system.

Funding for PHC in Australia

Funding for PHC services in Australia, illustrated in Figure 4.2, is derived from multiple sources (AIHW, 2020b):

- Australian government programs such as Medicare, the Pharmaceutical Benefits Scheme (PBS), specific funding for Aboriginal and Torres Strait Islander health organisations, and preventive health and quality improvement programs
- state and territory government programs, including health and community services
- other government-funded programs, such as immunisation
- patient out-of-pocket payments
- private health insurers and workers' compensation insurers
- non-government funding sources such as private charities focused on specific issues.

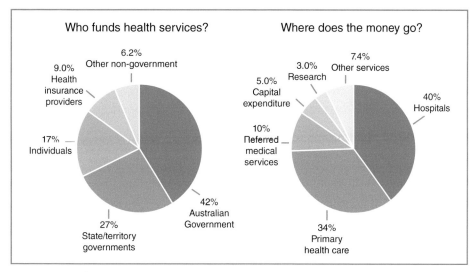

Figure 4.2   Funding for PHC services in Australia.
Source: AIHW (2020b).

Medicare, a universal public health insurance scheme, was introduced by the Australian government in 1984 (Biggs, 2003). It aims to provide affordable, accessible and high-quality care for all Australians. Medicare reimburses a proportion of patient costs related to:

- out-of-hospital medical services, including GP, diagnostic and other specialist services
- dental care for children (in limited circumstances)
- eye checks by optometrists
- allied health services for patients with a GP management plan
- medical services for private patients in public and private hospitals (Boxall & Gillespie, 2013).

PHC services represent the second-largest health expenditure (Figure 4.2), comprising GP services, dental services, allied health services, community and public health initiatives, and the cost of many medications through the PBS (AIHW, 2020b), and is one of the most cost-efficient sectors of the health system. For example, a Category 5 (non-urgent) visit to an emergency department costs the health system $533 (Hendry, 2019), while a 20–40-minute complex GP consultation currently costs the system $75.75 (Australian Government Department of Health, 2021a). Despite the efficiencies of investing in PHC, successive Australian governments have reduced PHC funding, including by imposing a Medicare rebate freeze for GP consultations from 2013 to 2020, and ceased funding for key PHC research and training programs. The continuing devaluing of PHC has contributed to PC workforce shortages and maldistribution. More promisingly, a $45-million federal government investment in a new PHC research initiative was announced in 2019 (Australian Government Department of Health, 2021b). This initiative aimed to support research relevant to PC over its nine-year duration.

Global PHC

While all signatories to the Declaration of Astana embraced PHC as fundamental to improving the health of their populations, the ways in which care is delivered vary as they are dependent upon the health system, funding mechanisms and workforce skills in each country. Bitton and others (2017) have developed a Primary Health Care Performance Initiative framework with key 'vital signs' (indicators) that can be used to compare the progress of PHC in low and middle-income countries (LMIC) – see Figure 4.3. Rasanathan and Evans (2020) suggest that the COVID-19 pandemic revealed a problematic emphasis on secondary and tertiary care facilities rather than on PHC in many countries. Reports following the peak of the COVID-19 pandemic in Australia suggested an increase in emergency department (ED) attendance and ambulance callouts was possibly due to people deferring regular primary care visits during this crisis. Rasanathan and Evans (2020) proposed five priority actions to support PHC efforts globally:

- Assist countries to clarify and monitor their priorities and implementation of PHC
- Provide essential technical assistance for PHC tailored to each country's requirements
- Support countries to overcome political resistance to investment and implementation of PHC
- Genuinely aligned partnerships
- Mobilise funding within countries to support PHC.

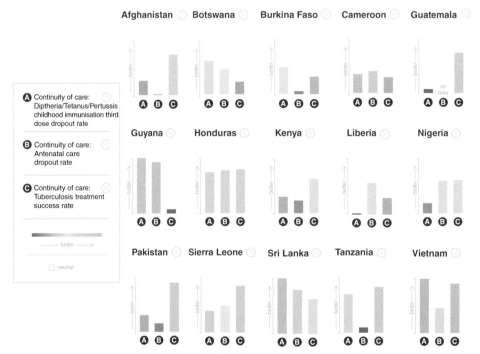

Figure 4.3   Vital signs indicators comparing PHC in different countries.
Source: Bitton et al. (2017).

SPOTLIGHT 4.2

PHC initiatives to reduce maternal mortality in Somaliland

Somaliland has one of the highest maternal mortality rates in the world. Common causes of death include eclampsia, haemorrhage, infection, uterine rupture and complications from female genital mutilation. Many of these deaths occur in women who are nomadic and live in rural or semi-rural areas (Central Statistics Department, Somaliland, 2020). Financial obstacles and distance to health-care centres are barriers to accessing care reported by Somaliland women. The first level of access to health care is the primary health unit, staffed by a trained volunteer community health worker. They are supported by personnel from the nearest maternal and child health centre (MCH), who can refer patients to regional hospitals. Several measures to improve maternal mortality at the MCH level include:

1   funding for midwives provided by non-governmental organisations (NGOs)
2   availability of essential drugs for managing obstetric complications
3   free or subsidised services, including ambulances, surgical interventions and certain medications.

Despite these initiatives, maternal mortality rates remain high due to poor health literacy, negligence by healthcare providers and poor leadership. Other NGO initiatives include training traditional birth attendants, providing them with mobile phones and small incentives for every referral they make, enabling a qualified health worker to attend the delivery, and increasing community engagement through radio, video and outreach drama to promote healthy behaviour.

  (With acknowledgement to Dr Yusuf Ahmed Ali Ardo, Dean of Medicine and Health Sciences, University of Burao, Somaliland.)

QUESTION
Which of the three pillars of PHC described in the Declaration of Astana require strengthening in order to reduce maternal mortality in LMIC countries such as Somaliland? Suggest other interventions that may improve the maternal mortality rates in LMICs.

Effective models of care within PHC

In this section, a range of effective models of care within PHC and community health is examined and discussed. The latest research evidence on innovative models of care from Australia and internationally is also explored.

What are effective models of care?

Effective models of care successfully deliver health services to achieve desired outcomes. There are many examples showing that the translation of an effective model into different settings or into different healthcare systems produces different outcomes. Models of care include multidisciplinary care, integrated care and patient-centred medical homes.

Multidisciplinary care

Multidisciplinary care – comprehensive patient care by health professionals from more than one discipline, provided one-on-one or through case-conferencing.

Interprofessional care – health workers from more than one profession working with individuals and communities to provide health care.

Effective **multidisciplinary care** occurs when health workers from different disciplines collaborate to plan and provide patient-centred care (Mitchell, Tieman & Shelby-James, 2008). Multidisciplinary care is critical in Australia where GPs play a leading role in arranging care in the community and linking with other health sectors (Royal Australian College of General Practitioners, n.d.). The term **interprofessional care** focuses on each individual team member's professional role rather than their disciplinary background. Thistlethwaite and colleagues (2019) emphasise the role of interprofessional education to improve collaborative practice and address workforce issues in order to optimise UHC. Following the Declaration of Astana, a greater emphasis on teaching collaborative care and leadership of interdisciplinary health teams is being promoted in family medicine (GP) training programs (Ponka et al., 2020).

In Australia, Medicare reimburses GPs to prepare management plans and team-led care arrangements designed to foster multidisciplinary care for patients with chronic disease. Completion of such a plan opens access to Medicare-funded rebates for a limited number of sessions with allied health professionals. However, uptake has been patchy, with men and people living in rural and remote areas less likely to be offered multidisciplinary team care arrangements (Harris, Jayasinghe et al., 2011).

There are two key components of multidisciplinary care planning: multidisciplinarity (a range of clinical perspectives and specialist knowledge) and a team-based approach (communication and support), which is underpinned by interaction between care providers, alignment of roles and work practices, and improved organisational arrangements (Mitchell et al., 2008). **Case management**, or enhanced multidisciplinary teamwork, is one effective intervention to improve outcomes, particularly among people with multimorbidity in PC settings (Smith et al., 2012). In a mixed-methods study in South Australia, Bentley and colleagues (2018) described facilitators of interprofessional teamwork comprising co-location of services, communication strategies and a shared PHC culture and commitment. Funding cuts, policy changes and restructuring were found to hinder teamwork.

Case management – a collaborative care process of assessment, organisation, coordination and monitoring to address a patient's comprehensive health needs.

SPOTLIGHT 4.3

Multidisciplinary care to reduce childhood malnutrition in Bolivia

Although progress has been made recently, more than 30 per cent of children under age five in lower socio-economic groups in Bolivia have been found to show stunting, and more than 40 per cent have anaemia. Obesity is also starting to occur more frequently, particularly in higher socio-economic groups (Miranda, Bento & Aguilar, 2020). The Bolivian Ministry of Health provides micronutrients (Vitamin A, zinc, multivitamins, fortified foods) through its health programs, and local municipalities provide a free breakfast for school-aged children, supported by NGOs and PHC personnel. Child-health checks are performed by PHC personnel in health centres as well as on home visits. Another important initiative has been the Salud Familiar Comunitaria e Intercultural (SAFCI) program, whereby mobile multidisciplinary teams including community nurses, dentists, traditional medicine healers and doctors specialised in SAFCI work together with communities to develop educational activities. Strengths of this program include community participation in health promotion and prevention; however, political and budgetary constraints have hindered equitable roll-out.

(With acknowledgement to Dr Javier Rodríguez Morales, public health physician, Instituto Boliviano en Calidad en Salud, Tarija, Bolivia.)

QUESTION

Describe an example of multidisciplinary care in Australian PHC addressing nutritional issues in the community.

Integrated care

Integrated care refers to an approach to overcome fragmentation in health care (Goodwin, 2016), including coordination between different parts of the health system and ensuring continuity across care pathways and care providers. A literature review by Veras and colleagues (2014) found that the use of care plans and case management approaches enabled patients to maintain continuity of community-based care, integrating primary and secondary care, day centres, in-home care and social services. They found that integrated care resulted in cost savings from reduced hospital care, reduced prevalence of functional loss and improved satisfaction and quality of life. The transition following hospital discharge is acknowledged to be a high-risk period, with frequent communication gaps between primary and secondary care services. Freeman, Scott and colleagues (2021), in a stepped-wedged, cluster-randomised controlled trial, found that including a pharmacist in general practices reduced the rate of unplanned re-admissions to hospital. In Australia, Medicare provides rebates for home medication reviews, whereby pharmacists identify medication issues, educate the patient and coordinate care with GPs.

Roles of nurses and other primary health worker-led models of care

Nurses with additional skills, training or scope of practice can enhance delivery of PC to patients with chronic diseases such as diabetes, coronary artery disease or heart failure. The nurse-led primary care model is well established, particularly in the United Kingdom, where nurse-led care has been associated with higher patient satisfaction, investigative tests and medications, and lower rates of hospital admission and mortality (Martinez-Gonzalez et al., 2014). These outcomes were more consistent with nurse practitioners than with registered or licensed nurses. Halcomb and colleagues (2020) describe the key role PHC nurses can play in a global pandemic such as COVID-19, and the supports they require including work safety, self-care, job satisfaction and job security.

The integration of a pharmacist into general practice-based multidisciplinary care teams has been well researched. A meta-analysis of randomised controlled trials showed that pharmacist-led care improved quality use of medicine and clinical outcomes such as blood pressure, glycaemic control and cholesterol (Tan et al., 2014).

Community health workers from different professions can play an important role in health promotion and education in PC and community health settings (Krantz et al., 2013). The community health worker-led model has also been identified as an effective solution to health workforce shortages, particularly in developing countries, where they increase access to and quality of PHC (Liu et al., 2011). Implementation of non-GP-led models requires understanding of the local context, systems management, integration with other primary health facilities, sustainable funding and appropriate workforce skills (Liu et al., 2011).

Patient-centred medical homes

Following the development of patient-centred medical home (PCMH) models of care in the United States, there is growing support in Australia for implementation of this model (Metusela et al., 2020). Transformation from usual PC models to a PCMH requires engaged leadership, quality improvement driven by measurable data, linkage of patients to a specific PC practitioner team, continuing team-based care, organised evidence-based care, patient-centred interactions, enhanced access, care coordination and population management (Wagner et al., 2012). Reported benefits included better patient experience of care, improved work life of healthcare providers, reduced costs and better population health outcomes (Metusela et al, 2020). An Australian government-funded trial of a similar model of care (healthcare homes) aimed to recruit 170 general practices and ACCHS (Department of Health, 2021c). The trial ended in mid-2021 and an evaluation will inform future PHC policy.

Challenges and future directions in PHC

The final section of this chapter provides insights into some of the challenges encountered in strengthening PHC in Australia and globally, and identifies future directions.

Overview of global changes in demographic and disease profile

The 2019 Global Burden of Disease (GBD) Study describes a trend towards increasing life expectancy worldwide (Abbafati et al., 2020). There has been a reduction in infant and maternal mortality, and in the burden from target conditions such as tuberculosis, malaria and HIV/AIDS. The health systems of LMICs are adapting to address increased prevalence of chronic non-communicable diseases and disability. Diabetes and ischaemic heart disease have overtaken diarrhoea and malaria as the leading causes of death in some LMICs (see Figure 4.4). The COVID-19 pandemic superimposed on an epidemic of non-communicable disease has been labelled a 'syndemic' (*The Lancet*, 2020), highlighting the need for national strategies to move beyond a narrow focus on health care to tackling social inequities by addressing education, economic growth, gender and migration issues.

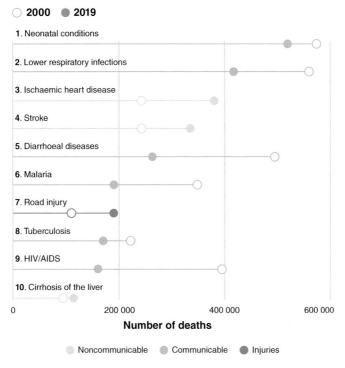

Figure 4.4   Leading causes of death in low-income countries.
Source: WHO (2020).

SPOTLIGHT 4.4

Integrating palliative care into PHC services in Sri Lanka

An emerging health problem in Sri Lanka is the need for palliative care services because of an ageing population and increasing rates of cardiovascular disease and cancer. The Ministry of Health and the Asia Pacific Hospice Network have conducted training for healthcare professionals in palliative care, and the Postgraduate Institute of Medicine now offers a postgraduate diploma in palliative medicine. Local and regional palliative care centres have been formed, and community nurses are delivering palliative care services at patients' homes. Free educational videos have been distributed to raise awareness about palliative care at the community level; however, commitment to a national program with input from PHC professionals is required to enable UHC, including palliative care.

(With acknowledgement to Dr Maithri Rupasinghe, Consultant Family Physician, Ministry of Health, Sri Lanka.)

QUESTION
The WHO (2018b) estimates that 40 million terminally ill adults and children in the world require palliative care, and 86 per cent do not receive it. In what ways are PHC, PC services and community health well placed to provide palliative care at the community level? What are barriers to implementing palliative care in LMICs?

Challenges ahead

Many of the challenges facing PHC systems are common to high-income countries as well as many LMICs.

Increasing health expenditure

Health spending in Australia is around 10 per cent of the gross domestic product (GDP), or $185 billion in 2017–18, with health expenditure continuing to escalate well above the population growth or ageing projection (AIHW, 2020c). The rapid expansion of new technology in health care that produces better precision in diagnosis and therapy, coupled with discovery of new drugs and vaccines, along with community expectations that such treatments be available, are key contributors to the increase in health expenditure.

Multimorbidity

Multimorbidity is the presence of two or more diseases in a person. The prevalence of patients with at least two chronic conditions in Australian GP consultations was 51.6 per cent (Harrison et al., 2017). Best-practice guidelines tend to be single-disease-focused and do not take into account the effects of multimorbidity on the complexity of care (Harris, Dennis & Pillay, 2013). As life expectancy increases, so does the prevalence of multimorbidity and polypharmacy rise, and this has a direct effect on health expenditure. Multimorbidity is also more common and has the greatest effect on quality of life in lower socio-economic settings (Lawson et al., 2013).

Health inequity among disadvantaged communities

Despite Australia having one of the best PHC systems in the world, many communities experience challenges in accessing health care and poorer health outcomes. These communities include Aboriginal and Torres Strait Islander peoples, culturally and linguistically diverse communities, and people living in rural and remote areas (AIHW, 2020b) (see chapters 19, 20 and 21). The four considerations to improving both equity of access to health services and also health outcomes are availability, affordability, acceptability and engagement with the disadvantaged community (Freeman et al., 2011). The COVID-19 pandemic exposed health inequities within many countries. Minority groups were disproportionately affected, and had increased difficulty accessing testing, immunisation and social and economic support during lockdowns (Xafis, 2020). A geospatial mapping study during the COVID-19 infodemic (Stephens, 2020) highlighted regions where conspiracy theories abounded. This misinformation can lead to poorer health outcomes due to a reluctance to accept public health messaging about primary prevention in these areas.

PHC workforce skills and availability

The number of nurses, midwives and medical practitioners practising in Australia is growing (AIHW, 2020d); however, ensuring the optimal distribution of an appropriately skilled workforce across all regions to meet the needs of the population remains a challenge. The lack of access to non-GP specialists and other allied health practitioners in regional and remote areas requires GPs to deliver clinical services beyond the scope of PC in order to meet the needs of the population. Strategies to improve the distribution of the health workforce to address areas of need in Australia include establishing undergraduate and postgraduate training programs for health workers in rural areas, financial incentives, and requirements for overseas-trained doctors to practice in areas of workforce shortage for 10 years. A looming problem in Australia is the increasing specialisation of the medical workforce. Although general practice remains the second most popular career choice for Australian medical graduates (Medical Deans Australia and New Zealand, 2020), fewer graduates choose general practice as a career when compared to hospital specialties (Playford et al, 2020). Similar reductions in generalist physicians are reported in the majority of OECD countries (OECD, 2020).

Beyond Astana

The Declaration of Astana highlighted the importance of PHC in achieving health for all through UHC. Kraef and Kallestrup (2019) encourage health decision-makers to draw upon the 'treasure of historical lessons' learned following Alma-Ata to inform policy and provide evidence for improving PHC. Threats to health identified included conflict, disease outbreaks and insecurity, inadequate monitoring, and inappropriate workforce and funding models. Political commitment is paramount in addressing the needs of the community and addressing equity of health outcomes. In Australia, the government launched a Long Term National Health Plan to build the world's best health system (Department of Health, 2019), which included support for PHC. Informing the implementation of this health reform agenda, the Primary Health Reform Steering Group recommended a range of strategies including funding reform, improved teamwork and greater use of technology (Primary Health Reform Steering Group, 2021), reflecting some of the principles promoted in the Declaration of Astana.

Funding for Australian general practice is based predominantly on a fee-for-service model that encourages high-volume care rather than high-quality, integrated and continuing care. The Practice Incentive Program payment provides a small additional payment for performance; however, approximately 90 per cent of government funding for Australian general practice is derived from fee-for-service payments through Medicare.

Many have called on the Australian government to consider a range of alternative funding models, including voluntary registration of patients, quality incentive programs, activity-based funding, capitation and blended funding models (RACGP, 2019; Australian Medical Association, 2020). The OECD (2020) encouraged a focus on improving health outcomes through use of high-value, patient-centred, team-based multidisciplinary care.

The importance of multidisciplinary teams for successful coordination of PHC is clear. However, there are many barriers to effective teamwork. Baum and colleagues (2020) have identified some of these, including the predominance of medical perspectives and prioritisation of cost-containment that results in the contracting-out of services, which causes fragmentation of care. Community voices that describe lived experience and social perspectives related to health are often unheard. The OECD (2020) recommends restructuring the PC team model of care such that the team leader is not always the physician. The role of the lead is to coordinate and delegate care using digital technology to maximise informational continuity. Another emerging role is that of the health services navigator, who can assist patients to navigate complex health systems.

Rapid evolution in technology has improved the efficiency of management, communication and coordination of care. Areas that have major potential include new biosensor devices, enhanced data management and analytics, and improved data integration and feedback (Chouvarda et al., 2015). Some technologies currently available in Australia include:

- A secure, online, personally controlled electronic health record (My Health Record). Despite various obstacles during the early phase of implementation, the usefulness of e-health records is starting to be realised. These are currently uploaded and viewed by GPs more often than in the ED setting (Mullins et al., 2021); however, accurate and up-to-date e-records can include patient health summaries and useful information about medications dispensed, hospital discharge letters, some hospital pathology and imaging reports, and immunisation records.
- Telehealth has been supported during the COVID-19 pandemic by Medicare reimbursement for video and telephone consultation between patients, specialists, GPs and nurse practitioners. Patients with chronic disease reported that during the COVID-19 pandemic they found telehealth helpful in accessing GPs, pharmacists and pathology services, though less so in providing access to specialist and other allied health practitioners (Javanparast, Roeger & Reed, 2021).
- HealthPathways is a web-based portal enabling GPs to access evidence-based clinical management guidelines and advice regarding local referral services. HealthPathways is becoming a valuable aid for GPs and other practitioners in health service delivery (NSW Health, 2021). Primary and secondary care clinicians work collaboratively to identify best-practice guidelines (such as Choosing Wisely recommendations), and to map local referral networks related to clinical issues (Choosing Wisely Australia, 2020). Some HealthPathways have been extended to provide links to reliable health information for community members.
- Smartphone applications and electronic sensing and tracking tools for self-monitoring of health and physical activity, such as continuous glucose monitoring (Blackberry et al., 2014), are affordable and accessible, although the cost is not yet covered by Medicare. Caution has been advised regarding reliability of the data and potential for data harvesting for commercial benefit.
- A national Real Time Prescription Monitoring system has been implemented in parts of Australia, enabling prescribers to identify patients at risk of harm through dependence, or who may be diverting controlled medications (Department of Health, 2021d).

REFLECTION QUESTION

How did the COVID-19 pandemic demonstrate the importance of PHC? In what ways was PHC involved, or perhaps overlooked, in the response to the pandemic in health systems in different parts of the world?

According to Bishai and Schleiff (2020), '[t]he Astana Declaration identifies PHC as the most effective, efficient, and equitable approach to enhancing health, and foundational to achieving universal health coverage' (p. vii). The thee pillars of Astana are empowering individuals and communities, evidence-based policy to address health determinants, and strengthening PHC and public health. Where these are supported, there is growing evidence for improved health outcomes in populations across the globe. Evidence from the United States demonstrates that implementing PHC principles can improve patient and staff satisfaction, reduce costs including those related to ED and hospital admissions, and improve care-quality for chronic conditions (OECD, 2020). In a six-country comparison, Huston and colleagues (2020) found that countries such as Australia, which initially did well in their response to the COVID-19 pandemic, had UHC as well as up-to-date pandemic plans and good government and public support. However, success in strengthening PHC does not come easily. It will require strong political commitment and leadership, development of good governance and policies, adequate funding allocations and successful community engagement and involvement (Peiris et al., 2021).

SUMMARY

Learning objective 1: Define primary health care, primary care and community health.
PHC is a key strategy enabling people to access affordable and equitable health care in a community setting. The PHC concept was introduced at Alma-Ata in 1978 and revitalised at Astana in 2018, with a focus on UHC. PC is one component of PHC and is the gateway for entry to the health system. Community health refers to services provided at the community level. Despite improvements in health and longer life expectancy, there are health disparities between developed and developing countries, and even between groups within countries.

Learning objective 2: Describe the contexts of primary health care and community health in Australian and global healthcare systems.
PHC is the initial point of contact with the healthcare system for individuals and communities. There have been several PHC reforms in Australia, primarily driven by increased health expenditure, demographic changes and fragmentation of care in the Australian health system. PC is part of PHC and includes GPs, nurses, dentists, pharmacists, other allied health professionals and community and Aboriginal health workers. GPs act as gatekeepers for those seeking specialist care.

Learning objective 3: Discuss effective models of care within primary health care and community health.
PHC is a key component of health care. There is growing evidence for the effectiveness of several models of care (including multidisciplinary care team, integrated care, PCMH models and nurse-led and allied health-led care). However, establishing and embedding effective models of care into routine care remain a challenge. To be effective, care needs to be tailored to individual patient needs and to take into account available local resources, including the workforce.

Learning objective 4: Identify challenges and future directions in primary health care.
The population is ageing and prevalence of multimorbidity is increasing. With higher costs of health care and community expectations of access to the latest technologies and treatments, there is increasing health expenditure and widening health inequity. An adaptive health workforce, supported by a strong PHC system, funding reform and affordable technology, is needed. Integrated care provided by multidisciplinary healthcare teams, evidence-based care pathways and patient empowerment are key to meeting future PHC challenges.

TUTORIAL EXERCISES

1   Compare the characteristics of PHC in Australia with those in other developed and developing countries.
2   Identify an effective PHC model of care from the literature and discuss how this model can be implemented in your local community.
3   Describe the latest initiatives in PHC from the both the Australian government and from your state/territory government in response to changing demographic and non-demographic factors.

FURTHER READING

Australian Institute of Health and Welfare (AIHW). (2020a). *Primary health care*. Release Date: 23 Jul 2020
     Section: Health system. Retrieved https://www.aihw.gov.au/reports/australias-health/primary-
     health-care

Bishai, D and Schleiff, M. (2020). *Achieving Health for All: Primary health care in action*. Johns Hopkins University Press.

OECD. (2020). *Realising the potential of primary health care, OECD health policy studies*. OECD Publishing. Retrieved https://doi.org/10.1787/a92adee4-en.

World Health Organization (WHO). (1978). *Primary health care. Report of the International Conference on Primary Health Care, Alma-Ata, USSR*. WHO.

——(2018). *Declaration of Astana*. WHO. Retrieved https://www.who.int/publications/i/item/WHO-HIS-SDS-2018.61

REFERENCES

Abbafati, C., Abdollahi, M., Abedi, P., Abreu, L.G., Alanezi, F.M., Alizade, H. . . . Lim, S.S. (2020). Five insights from the Global Burden of Disease Study 2019. *The Lancet (British Edition)*, *396*(10258), 1135–59.

Australian Institute of Health and Welfare (AIHW). (2020a). *Primary health care*. Release Date: 23 Jul 2020 Section: Health system. Retrieved https://www.aihw.gov.au/reports/australias-health/primary-health-care

——(2020b). *Australia's health 2020: In brief*. (Australia's Health Series No. 17, Cat. No. AUS 232). AIHW.

——(2020c). *Health expenditure*. Snapshot Release Date: 23 Jul 2020 Section: Health system. Retrieved https://www.aihw.gov.au/reports/australias-health/health-expenditure

——(2020d). *Health workforce snapshot*. Release date 23 Jul 2020. Retrieved https://www.aihw.gov.au/reports/australias-health/health-workforce

Australian Medical Association. (2020). *Delivering better care for patients: The AMA 10-Year Framework for Primary Care Reform*. Retrieved https://www.ama.com.au/articles/delivering-better-care-patients-ama-10-year-framework-primary-care-reform

Baum, F., Ziersch, A., Freeman, T., Javanparast, J. Henderson, T., & Mackean, T. (2020). Strife of interests: Constraints on integrated and co-ordinated comprehensive PHC in Australia. *Social Science & Medicine*, *248*, 112824.

Bentley, M., Freeman, T., Baum, F.& Javanparast, S. (2018). Interprofessional teamwork in comprehensive primary healthcare services: Findings from a mixed methods study. *Journal of Interprofessional Care*, *32*(3), 274–83.

Biggs, A. (2003). *Medicare – Background brief*. Retrieved http://web.archive.org/web/20120207065307/http://www.aph.gov.au/library/intguide/SP/medicare.htm

Bishai, D., & Schleiff, M. (2020). *Achieving health for all: Primary health care in action*. Johns Hopkins University Press. doi:10.1353/book.77991.

Bitton, A., Ratcliffe, H.L., Veillard, J.H., Kress, D.H., Barkley, S., Kimball, M., . . . Hirschhorn, L.R. (2017). Primary health care as a foundation for strengthening health systems in low- and middle-income countries. *Journal of General and Internal Medicine*, 32, 566–71.

Blackberry, I. D., Furler, J. S., Ginnivan, L. E., Manski-Nankervis, J. A., Jenkins, A., Cohen, N., . . . O'Neal, D. N. (2014). An exploratory trial of basal and prandial insulin initiation and titration for type 2 diabetes in primary care with adjunct retrospective continuous glucose monitoring: INITIATION study. *Diabetes Research and Clinical Practice*, *106*(2), 247–55.

Boxall, A., & Gillespie, J. (2013). *Making Medicare: The politics of universal health care in Australia*. UNSW Press.

Central Statistics Department, Ministry of Planning and National Development, Somaliland Government. (2020). *The Somaliland Health and Demographic Survey 2020*.

Choosing Wisely Australia. (2020). *Principles INTO practice 2020 report*. Retrieved https://www.choosingwisely .org.au/assets/Choosing-Wisely-Australia-2020-Annual-Report-Principles-into-Practice.pdf

Chouvarda, I. G., Goulis, D. G., Lambrinoudaki, I., & Maglaveras, N. (2015). Connected health and integrated care: Toward new models for chronic disease management. *Maturitas*, *28*(15), S0378–5122.

Department of Health. (2017). Australia's health landscape infographic. Retrieved https://www.health.gov .au/resources/publications/australias-health-landscape-infographic.

——(2019). *Long term national health plan to build the world's best health system*. Retrieved https://www .health.gov.au/sites/default/files/australia-s-long-term-national-health-plan_0.pdf

——(2021a). *MBS Online Medicare Benefits Schedule*. Retrieved http://www9.health.gov.au/mbs/fullDisplay .cfm?type=item&q=36

——(2021b). *Primary Health Care Research Initiative*. Retrieved https://www.health.gov.au/initiatives-and- programs/primary-health-care-research-initiative

——(2021c). *Health Care Homes*. Retrieved https://www1.health.gov.au/internet/main/publishing.nsf/ Content/health-care-homes

——(2021d). *National Real Time Prescription Monitoring (RTPM)*. Retrieved https://www.health.gov.au/ initiatives-and-programs/national-real-time-prescription-monitoring-rtpm

Duckett S., & McGannon C. (2013). Tough choices: How to rein in Australia's rising health bill. *The Conversation*. Retrieved https://theconversation.com/tough-choices-how-to-rein-in-australias-rising- health-bill-13658

Freeman, T., Baum, F., Javanparast, S., Ziersch, A., Mackean, T., & Windle, A. (2021). Challenges facing primary health care in federated government systems: Implementation of Primary Health Networks in Australian states and territories. *Health Policy*, *125*, 495–503.

Freeman, T., Baum, F., Lawless, A., Jolley, G., Labonte, R., Bentley, M., & Boffa, J. (2011). Reaching those with the greatest need: How Australian primary health care service managers, practitioners and funders understand and respond to health inequity. *Australian Journal of Primary Health*, *17*(4), 355–61.

Freeman, CR., Scott, IA., Hemming, K., Connelly, LB., Kirkpatrick, CM., Coombes, I., . . . Foot, H. (2021). Reducing medical admissions and presentations into hospital through optimising medicines (REMAIN HOME): A stepped wedge, cluster randomised controlled trial. *Medical Journal of Australia*, *214*(5), 212–17.

Goodwin N. (2016). Understanding integrated care. *International Journal of Integrated Care*, *16*(4), 6.

Halcomb, E., Williams, A., Ashley, C., McInnes, S., Stephen, C., Calma, K., & James, S. (2020). The support needs of Australian primary health care nurses during the COVID-19 pandemic. *Journal of Nursing Management*, *28*(7), 1553–60.

Hall, J. J., & Taylor, R. (2003). Health for all beyond 2000: The demise of the Alma-Ata Declaration and primary health care in developing countries. *Medical Journal of Australia*, *178*(1), 17–20.

Harris, M. F., Dennis, S., & Pillay, M. (2013). Multimorbidity: Negotiating priorities and making progress. *Australian Family Physician*, *42*(12), 850–4.

Harris, M. F., Islam, F. M., Jalaludin, B., Chen, J., Bauman, A. E., & Comino, E. J. (2013). Preventive care in general practice among healthy older New South Wales residents. *BMC Family Practice*, *14*, 83.

Harris, M., Jayasinghe, U., Taggart, J., Christl, B., Proudfoot, J., Crookes, P., Beilby, J., & Powell Davies, G. (2011). Multidisciplinary team care arrangements in the management of patients with chronic disease in Australian general practice. *Medical Journal of Australia*, *194*(5), 236–9.

Harrison, C., Henderson, J., Miller, G., & Britt, H. (2017). The prevalence of diagnosed chronic conditions and multimorbidity in Australia: A method for estimating population prevalence from general practice patient encounter data. *PLOS One*, *12*(3): e0172935.

Hendry, D. (2019). Why do patients go to emergency rather than to their GP? *NewsGP*, July 12. Retrieved https://www1.racgp.org.au/newsgp/professional/why-do-patients-go-to-emergency-rather-than-to-the

Huston, P., Campbell, J., Russell, G., Goodyear-Smith, F., Phillips, RL., van Weel, C., & Hogg W. (2020). COVID-19 and primary care in six countries. *BJGP Open*, 4(4).

Javanparast, S., Roeger, L., & Reed, R. L. (2021). Experiences of patients with chronic diseases of access to multidisciplinary care during COVID-19 in South Australia. *Australian Health Review*, *45*(5), 525–32.

Kraef C, Kallestrup P. (2019). After the Astana declaration: Is comprehensive primary health care set for success this time? *BMJ Global Health*, *12*(4), e001871.

Krantz, M. J., Coronel, S. M., Whitley, E. M., Dale, R., Yost, J., & Estacio, R. O. (2013). Effectiveness of a community health worker cardiovascular risk reduction program in public health and health care settings. *American Journal of Public Health*, *103*(1), e19–27.

Lawson, K.D., Mercer, S.W., Wyke, S. et al. (2013). Double trouble: The impact of multimorbidity and deprivation on preference-weighted health related quality of life a cross sectional analysis of the Scottish Health Survey. *International Journal of Equity in Health, 12*, 67.

Liu, A., Sullivan, S., Khan, M., Sachs, S., & Singh, P. (2011). Community health workers in global health: Scale and scalability. *Mt Sinai Journal of Medicine*, *78*(3), 419–35.

Lunnay, BK., McIntyre, E., Oliver-Baxter, J. (2014). *Fact Sheet: Primary Health Care Matters*. Primary Health Care Research and Information Service (PHCRIS). Retrieved https://dspace.flinders.edu.au/xmlui/bitstream/handle/2328/36334/factsheet_primary%20health%20care.pdf?sequence=1&isAllowed=y

Martinez-Gonzalez, N. A., Djalali, S., Tandjung, R., Huber-Geismann, F., Markun, S., Wensing, M.& & Rosemann, T. (2014). Substitution of physicians by nurses in primary care: A systematic review and meta-analysis. *BMC Health Services Research*, *14*, 214.

Medical Deans Australia and New Zealand. (2020). *National Data Report 2020*. Retrieved https://medicaldeans.org.au/data/medical-schools-outcomes-database-reports/

Metusela, C., Usherwood, T., Lawson, K. et al. (2020). Patient centred medical home (PCMH) transitions in western Sydney, Australia: A qualitative study. *BMC Health Services Research*, *20*, 285.

Miranda, M., Bento, A., Aguilar, A.M. (2020). Malnutrition in all its forms and socioeconomic status in Bolivia. *Public Health Nutrition*, *23*(S1), s21–8. doi: 10.1017/S1368980019003896.

Mitchell, G.K., Tieman, J.J., & Shelby-James, T.M. (2008). Multidisciplinary care planning and teamwork in primary care. *Medical Journal of Australia*, *188*(8), S61–4.

Mullins, A.K., Morris, H., Bailey, C., Ben-Meir, M., Rankin, D., Mousa, M., & Skouteris, H. (2021). Physicians' and pharmacists' use of My Health Record in the emergency department: results from a mixed-methods study. *Health Information Science Systems, 9*, 19.

National Aboriginal Community Controlled Health Organisation (NACCHO). (2021). *Core services and outcomes framework: The model of Aboriginal and Torres Strait Islander community-controlled comprehensive primary health care*. NACCHO.

NSW Health. (2021). *HealthPathways*. Retrieved https://www.health.nsw.gov.au/integratedcare/Pages/health-pathways.aspx

OECD. (2020). *Realising the potential of primary health care*. OECD Publishing. Retrieved https://doi.org/10.1787/a92adee4-en.

Peiris, D., Sharma, M., Praveen, D., Bitton, A., Bresick, G., Coffman, M., . . . Mash, R. (2021). Strengthening primary health care in the COVID-19 era: A review of best practices to inform health system responses in low- and middle-income countries. *WHO South-East Asia Journal of Public Health*, *10*(3).

Playford, D., May, JA., Ngo, H., & Puddey, IB. (2020). Decline in new medical graduates registered as general practitioners. *Medical Journal of Australia*, *212*(9), 421–2.

Ponka. D., Arya, N., Malboeuf, V., Leung, C., Wilson, C.R., Israel, K., ... Rouleau, K. (2020). The contribution of family medicine and family medicine leaders to primary health care development in Americas – from Alma-Ata to Astana and beyond. *Cien Saude Colet*, *25*(4), 1215–20.

Primary Health Reform Steering Group. (2021). *Draft recommendations from the Primary Health Reform Steering Group*. Retrieved https://www.racgp.org.au/FSDEDEV/media/documents/RACGP/Reports%20and%20submissions/Consultations/Primary-Health-Reform-Steering-Group-draft-recommendations.pdf

Rasanathan, K., & Evans, T.G. (2020). Primary health care, the Declaration of Astana and COVID-19. *Bull World Health Organisation*, *98*(11), 801–8.

Rifkin, S. B. (2018). Alma Ata after 40 years: Primary health care and health for all-from consensus to complexity. *BMJ Global Health*, *20*(3)(suppl 3), e001188.

Royal Australian College of General Practitioners (RACGP). (n.d.). *What is General Practice?* Retrieved http://www.racgp.org.au/becomingagp/what-is-a-gp/what-is-general-practice

——(2019). *Vision for general practice and a sustainable healthcare system*.

Sathanapally, H., Khunti, K., , Kadam, U., & Seidu, S. (2018). Shared decision making in multimorbidity. *Australian Journal of General Practice*, *47*(6), 397–8.

Schneider, EC., Sarnak, DO., Squires, D., Shah, A., & Doty, MM. (2017). *Mirror, mirror 2017: International comparison reflects flaws and opportunities for better U.S. health care*. Retrieved https://interactives.commonwealthfund.org/2017/july/mirror-mirror/

Smith, S. M., Soubhi, H., Fortin, M., Hudon, C., & O'Dowd, T. (2012). Interventions for improving outcomes in patients with multimorbidity in primary care and community settings. *Cochrane Database Systematic Review*, *4*, CD006560. doi:10.1002/14651858.

Standing Council on Health. (2013). *National primary health care strategic framework*. Commonwealth of Australia.

Stephens, M. (2020). A geospatial infodemic: Mapping Twitter conspiracy theories of COVID-19. *Dialogues in Human Geography*, *10*(2), 276–81.

Talbot, L., & Verrinder, G. (2017). *Promoting health: The primary health care approach* (6th ed.). Elsevier Australia.

Tan, E. C., Stewart, K., Elliott, R. A., & George, J. (2014). Pharmacist services provided in general practice clinics: A systematic review and meta-analysis. *Research in Social and Administrative Pharmacy*, *10*(4), 608–22.

The Lancet. (2020). Global health: Time for radical change? *Lancet*, *396*, 1129.

Thistlethwaite, J. E., Dunston R., & Yassine, T. (2019). The times are changing: Workforce planning, new health-care models and the need for interprofessional education in Australia. *Journal of Interprofessional Care*, *33*(4), 361–8.

United Nations. (2015). Department of Economic and Social Affairs. *Sustainable Development Goals. Ensure healthy lives and promote well-being for all at all ages*. Retrieved https://sdgs.un.org/goals/goal3

Veras, R. P., Caldas, C. P., Motta, L. B., Lima, K. C., Siqueira, R. C., Rodrigues, R. T., ... Guerra, A. C. (2014). Integration and continuity of care in health care network models for frail older adults. *Revis de Saude Publica*, *48*(2), 357–65.

Wagner E. H., Coleman K., Reid R. J., Phillips, K., & Sugarman, J. R. (2012). Guiding transformation: How medical practices can become patient-centered medical homes. *The Commonwealth Fund*. Retrieved https://www.commonwealthfund.org/publications/fund-reports/2012/feb/guidingtransformation-how-medical-practices-can-become-patient.

World Health Organization (WHO). (1978). *Primary health care. Report of the International Conference on Primary Health Care, Alma-Ata, USSR*. WHO.

——(1986). *Ottawa Charter for Health Promotion 2015*. Retrieved http://www.who.int/healthpromotion/conferences/previous/ottawa/en/index4.html

——(2018a). *Declaration of Astana*. WHO. Retrieved https://www.who.int/docs/default-source/primary-health/declaration/gcphc-declaration.pdf

——(2018b). *Integrating palliative care and symptom relief into primary health care: A WHO guide for planners, implementers and managers*. WHO.

——(2020). *The top 10 causes of death*. Retrieved https://www.who.int/news-room/fact-sheets/detail/the-top-10-causes-of-death

World Health Organization and the United Nations Children's Fund (UNICEF). (2018). *A vision for primary health care in the 21st century: Towards universal health coverage and the Sustainable Development Goals*. WHO and UNICEF).

Xafis, V. (2020). 'What is inconvenient for you is life-saving for Me': How health inequities are playing out during the COVID-19 pandemic. *Asian Bioethics Review*, *12*(2), 223–34.

5

Public health ethics

Jane Williams and Stacy M. Carter

LEARNING OBJECTIVES

After studying this chapter, you should be able to:

1   explain what public health ethics is and how it differs from clinical ethics and research ethics
2   understand how utilitarian thinking commonly underpins public health policy, and explain the pros and cons of consequentialist approaches to public health
3   understand different conceptions of liberty and paternalism, and explain the relevance of libertarian thinking for public health
4   understand the complexity of the concept of justice and its relationship to concepts of equity in public health
5   analyse public health ethics frameworks to identify the key values driving them and understand how they can be used to support public health practice.

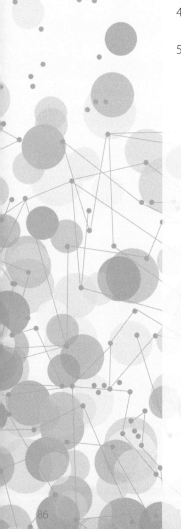

Ethics and vaccination

Measles is a highly infectious viral illness spread by coughing and sneezing. People infected with the measles virus experience fever, coughing, runny nose and a rash. Most do not experience complications, and the virus runs its course, though they may feel very unwell. For some, particularly young children, complications can arise. These include pneumonia (1 in 20 cases) and encephalitis (inflammation of the brain, 1 in 1000). Of every 1000 people who contract measles, one or two will die as a result of complications (Centers for Disease Control and Prevention, 2017a).

Measles may be prevented by a combination vaccine (MMR). It is a highly effective vaccine, with two doses preventing infection in around 97 per cent of vaccinated people (Centers for Disease Control and Prevention, 2016). Despite this, recent years have seen measles outbreaks in many countries known to have robust public health systems and vaccination programs, leading to hospitalisations and deaths (Turner, 2019; Zurcher, 2015; Hall et al., 2017). Countries with low levels of public health infrastructure or disruptions to regular vaccine uptake have seen serious outbreaks (Patel et al., 2020; Petousis Harris, 2019).

If a sufficiently high proportion of the population is vaccinated, the entire population may benefit from 'herd immunity'. It means that even unvaccinated people can be protected from measles if enough people in the community are immune. The level of immunity required for this differs depending on the characteristics of each infectious disease. In the case of measles, the optimal level of vaccination in a population is 95 per cent; a level not often reached.

While the measles vaccine is very safe in general, some individuals have a severe reaction to it. Around one per million vaccinated children develop encephalitis and, of those cases, around 40 per cent result in permanent brain damage and 10 per cent in death. Another 1–3 per million children experience a severe anaphylactic (allergic) reaction to the vaccine (Global Vaccine Safety, 2014). Other reactions have been reported, such as long-term seizures and deafness, but it is not clear whether these are directly attributable to the vaccine.

Population-level vaccination programs are rightly lauded as one of the greatest achievements of public health. They greatly reduce the burden of disease and death in populations and for individuals, at relatively low cost. But they do also cause very rare but potentially catastrophic damage to a tiny number of children. And, as the level of vaccination in a population increases and the incidence of measles decreases, a minority of parents begin to question whether they should vaccinate their children.

Consider: should vaccination against measles be compulsory? Should parents be penalised for not getting their children vaccinated? Should they be offered inducements to vaccinate? Should unvaccinated children be excluded from those aspects of public life in which they may be more likely to spread measles, such as daycare or school? What is gained and what is lost in these scenarios? What might we owe those children (and their parents) who are harmed by the vaccination itself?

Introduction

Public health practice involves protecting the public from ill health and promoting conditions that help people to live healthy lives (Turnock, 2016; Fleming, 2019; see also Chapter 1).

When utilitarianism is used in public health, the 'good' that is maximised is generally some sort of positive health outcome. Utility is worked out by calculating the difference between the sum of the good things produced (aggregated benefits) by an action or policy and the sum of the bad things (population harms) (Bellefleur & Keeling, 2016).

Proponents of utilitarianism often describe it as being impartial or objective (Bellefleur & Keeling, 2016) because each individual in a population is, generally speaking, given the same weight or importance in the calculation. The population is thus conceived as being a group of individuals, and the total utility produced results from the aggregation of the good and bad outcomes for all those individuals. The aim is to maximise good outcomes, on balance, rather than for specific groups or individuals.

Utilitarianism in public health

Utilitarian thinking commonly underlies public health policy. In its simplest terms, utilitarianism is concerned with maximising population good; since health is a good, public health seeks to protect and promote health for the population (Bellefleur & Keeling, 2016).

We see evidence of utilitarian thinking in public health through a strong focus on outcomes, and where it prioritises small gains for a large 'easy-to-reach' population, rather than more resource-intensive interventions in smaller, 'hard-to-reach' populations. There is widespread use of measures such as quality adjusted life years (QALYs) and disability adjusted life years (DALYs) gained (or lost), and cost–benefit analyses (Hyder, Puvanachandra & Morrow, 2012). These tools seek to find a universal reductive measure of outcome that can be applied to diverse human experience, then aggregate outcomes over the entire (diverse) population. These measures are commonly used to inform policy (Hyder et al., 2012).

Utilitarianism has some strengths and weaknesses as a justification for whether public health actions are morally right (Bellefleur & Keeling, 2016). It may indicate the most appropriate course of action *when a single outcome is agreed by all as the most important.* An example is when the risk of death from a disease is one in 1000 and the risk of death from vaccinating against that disease is one in 1 million. Comparing like outcomes makes for a fairly simple calculation. The question of outcomes is not always so simple, however. Imagine a road expansion project that aims to ease traffic congestion with the goal of fewer road accidents. For this road expansion to happen, some popular parks and old trees need to be removed. What outcome matters more? Fewer traffic accidents or good access to green open spaces for people in crowded communities? Importantly, who gets to decide what outcomes matter? Comparing different things to average them into an aggregated good is difficult and involves taking into account different values.

In theory, utilitarianism aims to treat all individuals as equal in calculating outcomes. The idea of fairness built into utilitarianism – that outcomes for each individual should be equally weighted – is intuitively appealing. It is also a value judgement, however, and we may want to question whether it is always appropriate. Different individuals and different populations have different needs and may thus benefit from, or be harmed by, policies in different ways. Aiming for improved outcomes for the majority may mean shaping interventions to target the mainstream, thereby making it less likely that disadvantaged communities receive predicted benefits, due to logistical, economic or cultural reasons.

SPOTLIGHT 5.1

Utilitarianism and vaccination

In the vignette at the beginning of this chapter, we introduced the idea of weighing benefits and harms of public health interventions by using the example of vaccination. In act utilitarian terms, vaccination is justifiable because the health benefits that accrue to a population with high vaccination levels are significant and outweigh the damage caused by vaccination to a small number of individuals. Basically, the number of lives saved by vaccinating the population is greater than the number of lives lost. In many countries, there are no-fault compensation schemes for people damaged by vaccines. Such programs may be expensive but they are increasingly viewed as being 'an important component of successful vaccination programs' (Looker & Kelly, 2011, p. 375).

QUESTIONS

1   Why, if utilitarianism can justify the sacrifice of a few for the greater good, are compensation programs sometimes seen as morally necessary?

2   What does this suggest is missing from act utilitarian reasoning?

Liberty and paternalism: The role of the state in public health

Public health is fundamentally a political endeavour (see also Chapter 10). For the most part, it involves the state making decisions about the behaviour of its citizens. As we saw in the previous section, utilitarianism emphasises aggregated outcomes across a population, not the means for achieving them or the effect on individuals. There are other ways of thinking about public health ethics that are not primarily focused on outcomes. By contrast to utilitarianism, **libertarianism** is centrally concerned with individual freedoms. In this section we look at the role of basic liberties and the extent to which the state can enforce public health measures.

> **Libertarianism** – a political philosophy based on the premise that negative liberty is the most important consideration in how we live our lives.

Liberty

There are two main ways of conceptualising liberty, or freedom. Most commonly, when the idea of liberty or rights is invoked, it is in the sense of negative liberty. **Negative liberty** is freedom from the interference of others (particularly the state) in how people live their lives (Carter, 2018). On this view, people are most free to act in accordance with their values when the state is minimally involved in their lives. A simple example is the use of bicycle helmets. Many jurisdictions require cyclists to wear a helmet while they are cycling. Some object to this, saying that it ought to be the cyclist's own choice whether they want to wear a helmet. They are objecting to an infringement of their negative liberties and want *freedom from* outside interference.

> **Negative liberty** – freedom from interference by other people or the state.

Positive liberty, on the other hand, requires that people have the capacity to live in accordance with their values and goals (Carter, 2018). This is likely to require some input

> **Positive liberty** – freedom and capacity to act in accordance with one's preferences and values.

from the state to provide the conditions necessary for people to be able to flourish. For example, for people to be able to eat a varied and plentiful diet, simply choosing to do so may be insufficient. The negative liberty view that would say 'eat what you want, no one is stopping you' does not help people who cannot afford, or do not have access to, the varied and plentiful diet they want or need. In that case, the state may need to assist people to achieve their preferences. In contrast to the *freedom from* idea that is negative liberty, positive liberty seeks *freedom to* act in accordance with beliefs and values. We will pick up this idea again in the next section. Usually, when people invoke liberty arguments in the context of public health, they mean negative liberty and are protesting the involvement of the state in people's affairs; this fails to understand that *freedom to* sometimes requires external structures and supports.

Many public health interventions seek to enforce health-promoting behaviours through restrictions. Examples include not being allowed to drive a car without wearing a seatbelt or to ride a motorcycle without a helmet. Smoking may be restricted to certain locations, and the purchase of alcohol is restricted by age. While utilitarians may argue that these restrictions are a reasonable price to pay for a good outcome, people focused on individual negative liberties may disagree.

Libertarianism and objections to public health

Libertarianism is a political philosophy based on the premise that ensuring negative liberty is the most important consideration in how we live our lives (van der Vossen, 2018). Libertarians most often lead the cry against government interference in people's health-related behaviours. In the context of public health, a libertarian is likely to object to any government interventions that compel or even strongly encourage people to undertake activities to improve health. This is usually framed using the 'harm principle' (Powers, Faden & Saghai, 2012). The harm principle is derived from the work of John Stuart Mill, who made a case for when it was permissible for the state and society to intervene in individuals' lives (Mill, 1974). Broadly, the harm principle says that the state (and individual people) should leave adult individuals to live their lives in accordance with their own preferences and values, as long as individuals' actions do not harm others. If an individual's actions are causing harm to others, then that person's liberty may be restricted to prevent that harm. Note that the harm principle allows for *persuasion* of people to live their lives in accordance with social norms, even where their actions do not harm others.

While the harm principle provides the basis for libertarian thinking and underpins some arguments for how public health interventions should be carried out, it is important to note that some readings of Mill argue for the allowance of relatively broad government interference. Powers and colleagues (2012) claim that Mill argued that different types of liberties required different treatment. They posit that some basic liberties, such as freedom of conscience and expression, should be exempt from interference or should enjoy the presumption of non-interference. Other liberties, however, do not have the same protections. Government should be able to regulate in certain areas where people have a common interest. This suggests that a careful reading of the harm principle might not support the threat to public health policy that libertarians claim.

Paternalism and 'the nanny state'

One common criticism of public health – especially by libertarians – is that it is paternalistic (Dworkin, 2018). The word **paternalism** comes from the idea that, historically, men made decisions for family members and others considered to be less capable than themselves. Individuals or collectives (such as states) sometimes act paternalistically towards others. What does it mean to say that an action is paternalistic? In the most commonly used definition (Dworkin, 2018) there are three main conditions that define a paternalistic act:

Paternalism – an action is paternalistic if it restricts the freedom of another person without their consent for their own good.

1 It somehow restricts or limits the freedom, autonomy or liberty of a person.
2 This is done without that person's consent.
3 It is done only for that person's good.

Criticisms of paternalistic policies are often couched in the language of the 'nanny state'. This term is shorthand for the (libertarian) idea that the state ought not interfere with people's private lives. These criticisms are presented as though paternalism is always morally indefensible. However, some paternalistic policies may be justifiable.

One way in which political philosophers have distinguished between more and less-justifiable paternalism is to demarcate 'hard' and 'soft' paternalism. In 'soft' paternalism, it is not clear whether the person whose action is being restricted fully understands the negative consequences of the choices they are making. In 'hard' paternalism, the restriction is in place even when the person can demonstrate full understanding and responsibility. The assumption behind the distinction is that soft paternalism is more justifiable than hard paternalism (Dworkin, 2018).

There is another way of thinking about the justifiability of paternalistic actions, which has to do with the values about and views of the responsibilities of the state that implicitly underpin the critique. Accepting that paternalistic policies or actions are bad means accepting that limiting someone's freedom for their own good without their consent is always bad. This assumes that liberty is more important than outcomes or other considerations, and comes back to a central issue in public health ethics of what a 'good' is and who might define it. When we talk about what kinds of liberties are important enough to be always paramount, we tend to move into discussion of rights. A discussion of human rights is beyond the scope of this chapter, but it is useful to consider the kinds of liberties or rights that are often said to be absolute (see also Chapter 11). Childress (2015) suggests the following: bodily integrity, privacy, freedom of movement, freedom of association, and freedom of religion and conscience. Note, however, that some of these may be legitimately curtailed during a public health emergency in which measures such as quarantine are deemed necessary for public safety. Other liberties, such as the freedom to travel in a car without a seatbelt, are much easier to justify interfering with. This suggests that the justifiability of paternalistic actions may need to be considered on a case-by-case basis.

REFLECTION QUESTION

Responses to the COVID-19 pandemic infringed on at least one of the 'absolute' liberties suggested above. Lockdowns, quarantine and border closures meant that many people went through sometimes long periods of not being able to move freely. Under what conditions might it be justified to impose on this liberty? Can you think of ways that some of the other absolute liberties that Childress (2015) lists were curbed in response to the pandemic?

SPOTLIGHT 5.2

New York City 'soda ban'

In 2012, then-mayor of New York City, Michael Bloomberg, announced new legislation that would restrict the size of soft drinks and other sugary drinks for sale at food service establishments to 16 oz (about 500 mL). The rationale for the ban was to reduce people's sugar intake to help curb rising rates of obesity. The proposed ban was widely opposed and ridiculed, and ultimately struck down in court. Among others, liberty-based arguments were put forward against limiting serving sizes. In the hearing that turned down the ban, the judge said that he feared the health department would have an 'almost limitless authority' if it were allowed to restrict the purchase of sugary drinks (Weiner, 2013). Critics of the proposal said overturning the ban was a 'win for freedom' and argued that government should not be allowed to get involved in the minutiae of daily life.

The United States has by far the highest per-capita daily sugar intake of any country, with corresponding rates of obesity (Ferdman, 2015). Obesity can lead to health consequences that make people more likely to suffer heart disease and stroke, diabetes and some cancers. In high-income countries, obesity is also associated with disadvantage (Adams, 2020).

The 'soda ban' debate raises questions about what goods are important and who decides what matters. Is the freedom to drink very large single-serves of sweetened soft drinks an important one? If not, how did it garner such support? Note here that the opposition to the ban was financed by the soda industry (Huehnergarth, 2012), which is much more likely to be concerned with financial loss than liberties. This introduces the question of who controls public debate and why: an 'individual liberty' argument is much more likely to gather public support than one with a profit motive.

QUESTIONS

1   Is it the role of the state to restrict what people eat and drink, if the aim is to improve people's health?
2   If not, what might some more acceptable approaches be to reduce the prevalence of obesity? Are there any?

Justice

In the previous section we distinguished between positive and negative liberties and looked at critiques of public health that assume the primacy of negative liberties. In this section we look at positive liberties and their connection to justice and **equity** in public health.

Equity – a principle underlying a commitment to reduce or eliminate socially patterned disparities in health.

Health outcomes are not evenly distributed in society (Marmot, 2007). Some of the variation seen across individuals and populations is likely unavoidable; where physiological differences mean that a disease behaves differently or is more prevalent, for example. Most variation is avoidable. Patterns of socially driven disadvantage and poor health repeat across and within countries. This is true for countries all over the world and at all levels of income (Marmot, 2007; see also chapters 1, 7 and 11).

Life expectancy is often used as a proxy for population health. In Australia in 2020, life expectancy for a boy born in 2016–18 was around 80 years, comparable with other top

10 OECD countries (AIHW, 2020). For an Aboriginal and/or Torres Strait Islander boy born in Australia in the same year, life expectancy was around 10 years less (AIHW, 2020; see also Chapter 19), about the same as a boy born the same year in Bangladesh (World Health Organization (WHO), 2021). In England, boys born in the wealthiest postcodes in London have a life expectancy more than 9 years longer than boys born in Blackpool, a city characterised by low-socio-economic status (SES), and inequalities are increasing (Office for National Statistics, 2020). Beyond the measure of life expectancy, patterned differences in health outcomes are seen in non-communicable diseases such as diabetes, heart disease and many cancers (Goldberg, 2017).

In response to systematic distribution of disadvantage, many approaches to public health call on policies that promote justice or equity, or reduce inequality (Smith, 2015). It is often not clear how these concepts are being defined, and they are sometimes used interchangeably. At the core, however, they indicate a belief that the state has a moral responsibility to provide the circumstances for all people to be able to be healthy. That is, as mentioned in the section above, the state should be responsible for supporting the conditions that provide for people to have the *freedom to* act in accordance with their choices, and should ensure that all people – whatever their position in society – have these opportunities. Public health that focuses on justice and related ideas is thus connected with valuing positive liberties.

Social determinants of health

Some public health ethicists argue that justice should be the core concern of public health (Sen, 2002; Powers & Faden, 2006; Daniels, 2008). Justice, they claim, is a matter of addressing social issues that sit outside of what is traditionally considered to be the sphere of health, because social determinants influence population health outcomes. According to the WHO (n.d.), the social determinants of health are:

> the conditions in which people are born, grow, live, work and age. These circumstances are shaped by the distribution of money, power and resources at global, national and local levels. The social determinants of health are mostly responsible for health inequities – the unfair and avoidable differences in health status seen within and between countries.

There is empirical evidence that a wide variety of social conditions affect health outcomes (Liamputtong, 2019; see also Chapter 7). Broadly, these include income, education, housing quality, class, employment type and self-determination (having control over how you live) (Sreenivasan, 2018). Empirical evidence describes the way the world is, but it is the job of ethics to take a normative position on what, if any, actions should be taken to change the status quo.

Equality and equity

Equity is a concept that is used in different ways, and is often central to arguments about justice in public health ethics (Smith, 2015). Equity as it pertains to justice might involve identifying deficits in some people's circumstances and altering social conditions so that those deficits may be erased. This may mean helping individuals or groups, or it may mean changing structural conditions altogether so that the same populations are not consistently disadvantaged. Remember that intervening for equality and intervening for equity are not the same thing. If people have different needs but are treated equally, they are likely to have very different outcomes. If those same people receive different types of support according to their particular needs, they are more likely to enjoy similar outcomes. In other words, they could enjoy equal outcomes or opportunities not by being treated equally, but by being treated equitably.

Opportunities and outcomes

Generally speaking, there is a difference between theories of justice that focus on opportunities (Sen, 2002) and those that focus on outcomes (Powers & Faden, 2006). Theories of justice that focus on the promotion of meaningful opportunity tend to argue that poor health limits one's opportunities to achieve wellbeing, and that the freedom to achieve wellbeing is of primary moral importance. Taking this view, the minimal conditions for good health must be accessible, such that people can be self-determining, or have the genuine opportunity to live or act in accordance with their own values. In these accounts, health is not generally an end in itself; rather, being able to access the means to be in good health is a necessary condition for social justice (see Chapter 7). The best-known of these theories is the capability approach, particularly the version developed by Amartya Sen (2002). In this approach, what matters is that people have the *capability* – the real opportunity or freedom – to live lives that they have reason to value. These capabilities, and the resources required to develop them, determine wellbeing; their availability indicates a more just society.

Powers and Faden (2006) focus on different ends in their theory of social justice: for them, it is the *achievement* of wellbeing that is morally important, rather than (or as well as) the opportunity to achieve it. They outline six interconnected dimensions of wellbeing, of which health is one. As with the capabilities approach, the role of justice in this theory is not to improve public health as an end goal, but rather that 'the foundational moral justification for the social institution of public health is social justice' (p. 80). An analysis of a public health intervention using this theory of justice requires thinking about its effects on all six dimensions of wellbeing: health, personal security, reasoning, respect, attachment and self-determination. Powers & Faden (2006) consider that a just society will ensure at least a threshold level of sufficiency of each dimension in all members of that society.

SPOTLIGHT 5.3

Cashless cards for welfare recipients

Since 2016, trials of 'cashless cards' for most welfare recipients have been undertaken in some Australian states and territories. Under this scheme, people receiving a welfare payment (with the exception of aged and veteran's pensions) receive 80 per cent of their money on a debit card. The remaining 20 per cent is deposited to the recipient's bank account. The card may not be used to purchase goods from vendors selling alcohol or gambling products, or to withdraw cash. It may be used online, but only at approved sites. Participation is compulsory but others in the community, such as those who receive some income from other sources, such as employment, or who are on excepted pensions, may also volunteer to take part in the trial.

The stated aim of the trial is to assess whether reduced access to cash could 'reduce the overall harm caused by welfare fuelled alcohol, gambling and drug misuse' in communities in which 'high levels of welfare dependence co-exist with high levels of social harm' (Department of Social Services, 2018). A large majority of participants in the trial are Aboriginal and/or Torres Strait Islander people.

An evaluation of the 12-month trial found mixed support and results from the cashless card initiative (Orima Research, 2017). Crime statistics remained unchanged, but participants reported lower rates of alcohol and illegal drug use and gambling. Qualitatively, community leaders and stakeholders reported increased perceived community safety. However, more participants reported that their own and their children's lives were negatively affected by the card than reported a positive effect. The Australian government extended the trial to more locations and for a longer period, including into late 2020.

Cashless cards arguably give welfare recipients the opportunity to live healthier lives by restricting their capacity to spend their income on products that could lead to ill health. It is not yet clear whether these opportunities translate to improved health outcomes. Beyond opportunity and outcomes, there are further ethical considerations associated with compulsory income management. These include whether it is reasonable to curtail freedoms by restricting what people choose to do with their income, and whether it is reasonable to implement such programs that disproportionately affect Aboriginal and/or Torres Strait Islander people.

QUESTIONS

1   Are cashless cards a justifiable method for trying to improve health by reducing alcohol, drug and gambling-related harms? If so, should such measures be compulsory?

2   What are the assumptions underpinning income management for welfare recipients? How might those assumptions undermine the wellbeing of the communities in question?

Putting it all together: Can public health ethics frameworks help?

In this chapter we have introduced three key approaches and sets of concepts in public health ethics. These come from moral philosophy and ethics, but once you know about them you can see them operating implicitly across many public health plans and programs (and also in common criticisms of public health). The first approach is utilitarian, in which the right thing to do is that which produces the best outcome (the highest aggregated good). The second approach focuses on liberty, especially libertarianism, whereby negative liberty – freedom from interference – is taken to be the most important principle for organising society. If this approach is accepted, then most public health action becomes illegitimate. Finally, we considered different ways of thinking about justice.

Each of these sets of concerns or approaches to moral reasoning prioritises different values and they can, at times, be incompatible. What to do with these sometimes competing or incompatible approaches? Some key figures in public health ethics have published frameworks to help practitioners think about the justifications for, and implications, of proposed policies or interventions. While there is no definitive framework, nor any single definitive model for how to 'do' public health ethics, the frameworks we outline here may help you to apply your thinking to real-life situations.

But first, two important notes

Concepts and terminology

It is important to note that people can use the same concepts in quite different ways. It is good practice to be very clear in your thinking and your language when you use terms such as benefit, liberty or justice to justify your thinking about a public health intervention. For example, ask yourself 'what do I mean when I say this is a benefit?'

Autonomy

You may notice that we have not included a discussion of autonomy in this chapter. For those of you who are familiar with ethical concepts, this may appear to be an oversight. Autonomy is conceptualised in a variety of different ways, and its place in public health ethics is highly complex. Traditionally, autonomy is thought of as an individual's capacity to govern themselves – to make their life go in the way they want it to. It tends not, in common usage, to take account of context, and cannot easily accommodate discussion about populations. Some conceptualisations of autonomy may be useful for public health ethics. Where autonomy is used in the frameworks in this section, it is taken to mean something like (negative) liberty, covered earlier in this chapter. However, many theorists of autonomy would resist equating autonomy with negative liberty: autonomy is a much more complex concept.

Frameworks

Ethics frameworks take ethics concepts and turn them into principles for use. Public health ethics frameworks are different to those used in and for other healthcare settings. Bioethics frameworks such as the Four Principles developed by Beauchamp and Childress (2013) are not suitable for use in public health because their unit of concern is the individual, and public health is a collective endeavour. The public health ethics frameworks we introduce here are commonly used; they differ but have some key concepts in common.

Goals and outcomes in public health interventions

Nancy Kass (2001) wrote one of the first public health ethics frameworks in 2001, summarised here.

The following questions are to be posed in order:

1 'What are the public health goals of the proposed program?
2 How effective is the program in achieving its stated goals?
3 What are the known or potential burdens of the program?
4 Can burdens be minimised? Are there alternative approaches?
5 Is the program implemented fairly?
6 How can the benefits and burdens of a program be fairly balanced?' (Kass, 2001)

This framework upholds basic utilitarian values, with the addition of others. The first concern is the anticipated outcome, and there is a strong focus on benefits and burdens. It is not entirely consequentialist, however. Question 5 is concerned with process, specifically distributive justice (that is, who gets the benefits and burdens). In this framework, who gets what and why is important.

For another example of a framework that balances a focus on utilitarian outcomes with process and negative liberty, see James Childress and colleagues' 2002 publication. Like Kass, Childress and colleagues' key concerns lie with producing population benefits, and balancing benefits and harms such that positive utility is produced. They also focus on protecting liberty, encouraging transparent processes and promoting such values as honesty and truthfulness.

Least infringement/the harm principle

The Nuffield Council on Bioethics published an 'Intervention Ladder' as part of a longer consideration of ethical issues in public health (Nuffield Council on Bioethics, 2007). The ladder is predicated on the idea that the key concern about public health intervention is state infringement on personal liberties. Each rung on the ladder represents the level of effect, from least (at the bottom) to greatest, that a proposed policy is likely to have on individuals' lives. The higher the intervention sits on the ladder, the greater the justification required to carry it out. Another early and frequently cited framework, by Ross Upshur (2002), similarly focuses on individual liberties with a foundation in the harm principle. Upshur also introduces the idea of reciprocity to public health ethics; that the state (or public health entity in question) is obligated to help people if they face burdens while complying with public health requests. As with most frameworks, process is also considered ethically important.

Frameworks can be a useful start when you are considering a public health problem. Public health ethics is often highly contextual, however, and frameworks may not respond well to nuance. Many frameworks also do not provide guidance about what to do when principles are incompatible. We have seen that prioritising justice as equity may not lend itself to maximising utility, for example. Frameworks can prompt you to ask good questions about public health problems, and applying ethical principles can help you form a normative response to those questions in a way that is sound and considered.

SUMMARY

Learning objective 1: Explain what public health ethics is and how it differs from clinical ethics and research ethics.

Public health ethics is the basis for the analysis of moral problems in a public health setting. It involves using evidence (scientific, epidemiological, sociological) and normative argument to make claims about the ethical justifiability of public health activity. Public health ethics is primarily focused on groups, communities and populations; it differs from clinical and research ethics in its focus and thus employs different principles.

Learning objective 2: Understand how utilitarian thinking commonly underpins public health policy, and explain the pros and cons of consequentialist approaches to public health.

Utilitarianism in public health aims to produce aggregate health benefits for the population. It is concerned with outcomes, but not necessarily how they are achieved. It focuses on aggregated effects in whole populations, so smaller, vulnerable and 'hard-to-reach' segments of the population may be overlooked. It can also be difficult to weigh different types of benefits and harms against each other.

Learning objective 3: Understand different conceptions of liberty and paternalism, and explain the relevance of libertarian thinking for public health.

Liberty can be positive or negative. Positive liberty can be thought of as having the freedom *to* do something and negative liberty is freedom *from* interference. Arguments about negative liberty are used to criticise public health campaigns for 'nanny statism' or paternalism. A paternalistic action is one that restricts someone's freedom without their consent and is done for their 'own good'. Paternalism may be more or less easy to justify, depending on the nature of the freedom that is being restricted.

Learning objective 4: Understand the complexity of the concept of justice and its relationship to concepts of equity in public health.

Health outcomes are not evenly distributed across society. In response, there is a move to look beyond healthcare access to other social factors that affect health outcomes, such as housing, education and self-determination, or the 'social determinants of health'. Such approaches to public health increasingly refer to ideas like justice, fairness, equity and inequality. These concepts are not used uniformly, and it is important to qualify meanings within context. There is debate about whether opportunities or outcomes are what matter when it comes to human flourishing.

Learning objective 5: Analyse public health ethics frameworks to identify the key values driving them and understand how they can be used to support public health practice.

Public health ethics frameworks tend to apply several different principles to public health problems. The most commonly used frameworks are based on either utilitarian or liberty promoting principles, but they also include principles of fairness, particularly distributive and procedural fairness. Frameworks can provide the public health practitioner with good starting points and questions to ask, but public health ethics tends to be highly contextual and must account also for evidence.

TUTORIAL EXERCISES

1   Imagine that your parents have told you of their plan to buy you a property in Sydney. You currently rent a room in a student flat and receive income from a part-time job and your parents while you study. One night at a party, a friend tells you that you should urge your parents not to buy the property but instead to give that money to proven charities that work in low-income countries. He says the money from your investment property alone could build 25 community health clinics or 950 toilets, and this

would have a much greater effect on human wellbeing than your parents buying you a property. What should you do? Why? What sorts of problems does this scenario raise for utilitarianism?

2 Find an article in the media that uses a libertarian or 'nanny state' argument against a public health program or intervention. Does the intervention meet the paternalism criteria you learned about in this chapter? What freedom(s) are being infringed upon? Are they important?

3 Compulsory drug testing for welfare beneficiaries is a topic that regularly comes up for debate in the federal parliament in Australia. The aim of this policy is twofold: to get drug users into treatment (and subsequently into paid work); and to assure the public that public funding does not go towards funding illegal drug use. What are some of the ethical issues with this proposal? What principles might you use, and what questions might you ask to make up your mind about its justifiability?

FURTHER READING

Barrett, D., Ortmann, L., Dawson, A., Saenz, C., Reis, A., & Bolan, G. E. (2016). *Public health ethics: Cases spanning the globe*. Springer Open.

Chapman, A. R. (2015). The social determinants of health: Why we should care. *American Journal of Bioethics*, *15*(3), 46–7.

Dawson, A. (Ed.) (2011). *Public health ethics: Key concepts and issues in policy and practice*. Cambridge University Press.

Holland, S. (2007). *Public health ethics*. Polity.

MacDonald, M. (2015). *Introduction to Public Health Ethics 3: Frameworks for Public Health Ethics*. Retrieved http://www.ncchpp.ca/docs/2015_Ethics_Intro3_Final_En.pdf

REFERENCES

Adams, J. (2020) Addressing socioeconomic inequalities in obesity: Democratising access to resources for achieving and maintaining a healthy weight. *PLoS Medicine*, *17*(7): e1003243.

Australian Institute of Health and Welfare (AIHW). (2020). *Reports and data: Life expectancy and death*. Retrieved https://www.aihw.gov.au/reports/life-expectancy-death/deaths-in-australia/contents/life-expectancy

Bayer, R., & Fairchild, A. L. (2004). The genesis of public health ethics. *Bioethics, 18*(6), 473–92.

Beauchamp, T., & Childress, J. (2013). *Principles of biomedical ethics* (7th ed.). Oxford University Press.

Bellefleur, O., & Keeling, M. (2016). *Utilitarianism in public health*. Retrieved http://www.ncchpp.ca/127/Publications.ccnpps?id_article=1527

Carter, I. (2018). Positive and negative liberty. In E. N. Zalta (Ed.), *The Stanford Encyclopedia of Philosophy* (Winter 2019). Retrieved https://plato.stanford.edu/archives/win2019/entries/liberty-positive-negative/

Centers for Disease Control and Prevention. (2016). Measles (rubeola): Measles vaccination. Retrieved https://www.cdc.gov/measles/vaccination.html

——(2017a, March). Measles (rubeola): Complications of measles. Retrieved https://www.cdc.gov/measles/about/complications.html

——(2017b). *Public health 101: Introduction to public health*. Retrieved https://www.cdc.gov/publichealth101/public-health.html

Childress, J. F. (2015). Public health and civil liberties. In J. D. Arras, E. Fenton, & R. Kukla (Eds.), *The Routledge companion to bioethics*. Routledge.

Childress, J. F., Faden, R. R., Gaare, R. D., Gostin, L. O., Kahn, J., Bonnie, R. J., . . . Nieburg, P. (2002). Public health ethics: Mapping the terrain. *Journal of Law Medicine & Ethics*, *30*(2), 170–8.

Daniels, N. (2008). *Just health: Meeting health heeds fairly*. Cambridge University Press.

Department of Social Services. (2018). *Welfare quarantining: Cashless debit card*. Retrieved https://www.dss .gov.au/families-and-children/programmes-services/welfare-conditionality/cashless-debit-card-overview

Dworkin, G. (2018) Paternalism. In E. N. Zalta (Ed.) *The Stanford encyclopedia of philosophy* (Fall 2020). Retrieved https://plato.stanford.edu/archives/fall2020/entries/paternalism/

Ferdman, R. A. (2015). Where people around the world eat the most sugar and fat. *Washington Post*. Retrieved https://www.washingtonpost.com/news/wonk/wp/2015/02/05/where-people-around-the-world-eat-the-most-sugar-and-fat/?utm_term=.e0f57341cef4

Fleming, M. L. (2019). Defining health and public health. In M. L. Fleming (Ed.), *Introduction to public health* (4th ed.) (pp. 3–15). Elsevier.

Global Vaccine Safety. (2014). *Observed rate of vaccine reactions: Measles, mumps and rubella vaccines*. World Health Organization.

Goldberg, D. S. (2017). *Public health ethics and the social determinants of health*. Springer Briefs in Public Health.

Hall, V., Banerjee, E., Kenyon, C., Strain, A., Griffith, J., Como-Sabetti, K., . . . Ehresmann, K. (2017). Measles outbreak – Minnesota April–May 2017. *CDC Morbidity and Mortality Weekly Report, 66*(27), 713–17.

Huehnergarth, N. (2012, September 2). The masterminds behind the phony anti-soda tax coalitions. *Huffington Post*. Retrieved https://www.huffingtonpost.com/nancy-huehnergarth/soda-ban-new-york_b_1644883.html

Hyder, A., Puvanachandra, P., & Morrow, R. (2012). Measuring the health of populations: Explaining composite indicators. *Journal of Public Health Research, 1*(e35).

Kass, N. E. (2001). An ethics framework for public health. *American Journal of Public Health*, *91*(11), 1776–82.

Liamputtong, P. (Ed.) (2019). *Social determinants of health*. Oxford University Press.

Looker, C., & Kelly, H. (2011). No-fault compensation following adverse events attributed to vaccination: a review of international programmes. *Bulletin of the World Health Organization, 89*, 371–8.

Marmot, M. (2007). Achieving health equity: From root causes to fair outcomes. *Lancet, 370*(9530), 1153–63.

Mill, J. S. (1974). *On liberty*. Penguin.

Nuffield Council on Bioethics. (2007). *Public health: Ethical issues*. Cambridge Publishers Ltd.

Office for National Statistics. (2020). Health state life expectancies by national deprivation deciles, England: 2016–2018. Retrieved https://www.ons.gov.uk/peoplepopulationandcommunity/healthandsocialcare/healthinequalities/bulletins/healthstatelifeexpectanciesbyindexofmultipledeprivationimd/latest

Orima Research. (2017). *Cashless debit card trial evaluation: Final evaluation report*. Retrieved https://apo.org .au/node/104916

Patel M. K., Goodson, J. L., Alexander, J. P. Jr., et al. (2020) Progress toward regional measles elimination – worldwide, 2000–2019. *MMWR Morbidity and Mortality Weekly Report*, *69*, 1700–5. Retrieved http://dx .doi.org/10.15585/mmwr.mm6945a6

Petousis Harris, H. (2019) Samoa's devastating measles epidemic – why and how bad? Retrieved https:// sciblogs.co.nz/diplomaticimmunity/2019/11/28/samoas-devastating-measles-epidemic-why-and-how-bad/

Powers, M. & Faden, R. (2006). *Social justice: The moral foundations of public health and health policy*. Oxford University Press.

Powers, M., Faden, R. & Saghai, Y. (2012). Liberty, Mill and the framework of public health ethics. *Public Health Ethics, 5*(1), 6–15.

Razai, M., Osama, T., McKechnie, D., & Majeed, A. (2021). Covid vaccine hesitancy among ethnic minority groups. *British Medical Journal, 372*(513).

Sen, A. (2002). Why health equity? *Health Economics, 11*(8), 659–66.

Smith, M. J. (2015). Health equity in public health: Clarifying our commitment. *Public Health Ethics, 8*(2), 173–14.

Sreenivasan, G. (2018). Justice, inequality, and health. In E. N. Zalta (Ed.), *The Stanford Encyclopedia of Philosophy* (Fall 2018). Retrieved https://plato.stanford.edu/archives/fall2018/entries/justice-inequality-health/

Sze, S., Pan, D., Nevill, C.R., Gray, L.J., Martin, C.A., Nazareth, J., . . . Pareek, M. (2020). Ethnicity and clinical outcomes in COVID-19: A systematic review and meta-analysis. *EClinicalMedicine*, (29–30), 100630.

Turner, N. (2019). A measles epidemic in New Zealand: Why did this occur and how can we prevent it occurring again? *New Zealand Medical Journal, 132*(1504), 8–11.

Turnock, B. J. (2016). *Public health: What it is and how it works* (6th ed.). Burlington, MA: Jones & Bartlett Learning.

Upshur, R. (2002). Principles for the justification of public health intervention. *Canadian Journal of Public Health, 93*(2), 101–3.

van der Vossen, B. (2018). Libertarianism. In E. N. Zalta (Ed.), *The Stanford encyclopedia of philosophy* (Spring 2019 ed.). Retrieved https://plato.stanford.edu/archives/spring2019/entries/libertarianism/

Weiner, R. (2013). The New York City soda ban explained. *The Washington Post*. Retrieved https://www.washingtonpost.com/news/the-fix/wp/2013/03/11/the-new-york-city-soda-ban-explained/?utm_term=.be787c610176

White, R. (2000). Unravelling the Tuskegee Study of untreated syphilis. *Archives of Internal Medicine, 160*(5), 585–98.

World Health Organization (WHO). (n.d.). Social determinants of health. Retrieved http://www.who.int/social_determinants/sdh_definition/en/

——(2021). Global health estimates: Life expectancy and healthy life expectancy. Retrieved https://www.who.int/data/gho/data/themes/mortality-and-global-health-estimates/ghe-life-expectancy-and-healthy-life-expectancy

Zurcher, A. (2015). Measles outbreak at Disney raises vaccination questions. Retrieved http://www.bbc.com/news/blogs-echochambers-30942928

6

Advocacy and the workforce

Gemma Crawford, Jonathan Hallett, Tina Price,
Toni Hannelly and Christina Pollard

LEARNING OBJECTIVES

After studying this chapter, you should be able to:

1 describe the structure and resourcing of public health activities in Australia
2 critically identify the features of the public health workforce
3 articulate the rationale for advocacy as a key requirement for public health action
4 describe theories and evidence that underpin effective public health advocacy
   and activism.

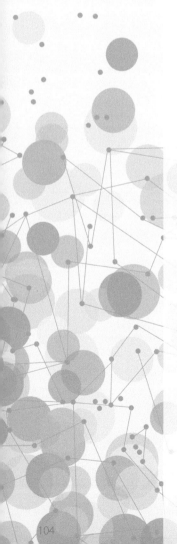

VIGNETTE

The case for stronger public health systems in Australia

Winslow (1920) defined public health as 'the science and the art of preventing disease, prolonging life and promoting physical health and efficiency through organized community efforts' (p. 30). Almost 100 years later, the World Federation of Public Health Associations, supported by the World Health Organization (WHO), launched the Global Charter for the Public's Health (the Charter), which highlighted the role of protection, prevention and promotion, ('services') governance, advocacy, capacity and information ('functions') in public health. The Charter called for resilient public health systems, in recognition of the fragmented nature of public health governance, funding and leadership. The COVID-19 pandemic has amplified growing inequalities and the need for strong public health systems and structures, with sufficient investment to build the capacity of the public health workforce.

While Australia's prevention and health promotion efforts have long been admired, our investment in public health is lower than the Organisation for Economic Co-operation and Development (OECD) average. Treating illness, rather than protecting and promoting health, remains the focus of public health. Many countries were insufficiently prepared to respond to the pandemic, and this has exacerbated economic, social and health disparities. The fact that health systems are overwhelmed highlights the need for well-planned and resourced public health efforts that can be scaled up as required.

Australia is the only OECD country that does not have a specific national authority to provide scientific coordination, research and leadership for disease control and prevention; these tasks are managed jointly by departments across jurisdictions. While countries deliver these functions in different ways, a common and necessary feature is that science and technical professionals are not directly involved in the political process but are accountable to the public and governments. The Public Health Agency of Canada, the Centers for Disease Control and Prevention in the United States, the Robert Koch Institute in Germany, and the National Institute for Health and Welfare in Finland apply such models. Their focus is on major national public health problems, and their work in policy implementation and resource allocation is based on scientific evidence. The International Association of National Public Health Institutes suggests that the key functions of public health systems include investigating and controlling outbreaks; undertaking disease surveillance, detection and monitoring; laboratory science; research; analysis of health information to develop policy; health promotion and education; and workforce capacity building.

Successive Australian governments have resisted calls to establish and set aside funding for such an institution. Attempts to establish a national office for preventive health, for example, have not withstood the forces of changing political priorities. Key stakeholders, including the Public Health Association of Australia, the Australian Health Promotion Association, the Australian Medical Association (AMA) and the Australian Healthcare and Hospitals Association (AHHA), have called for a centralised institution for public health governance, driven by reflections on Australia's pandemic response (AHHA, 2020; AMA, 2017).

A national agency should be established in Australia to support implementation of public health action across functions and services, as articulated in the Charter. Such an agency would serve to keep public health action squarely on the agendas of decision-makers, which is critical if public health infrastructure is to withstand future, inevitable and widescale threats to public health.

Introduction

To tackle complexity in public health, a capable, appropriately qualified workforce of sufficient scope and size is required. The public health workforce is multidisciplinary and applies public health principles and methods across a range of areas, including program management, policy development, research and surveillance (Dhavan & Reddy, 2017). Public health practitioners may work in the public or private sector, within government, non-profit organisations or international agencies.

Working in public health requires multi-sectoral collaboration, a willingness to tackle challenging issues and a desire to improve the health of populations (Dhavan & Reddy, 2017). Consequently, public health practitioners must cultivate their knowledge and competencies in politics and advocacy (Kreuter, 2005; Moore et al., 2013). It has been argued that countries whose 'government cannot perform core public health functions cannot truly meet the health needs of its citizens' (Bloland et al., 2012); therefore, strengthening systems, structures and capacity towards public health objectives is critical. Collective effort is needed to call governments and institutions to act with urgency and to prioritise public health action so that growing social and health disparities may be addressed.

Building capacity for public health

As emphasised in the opening vignette, the COVID-19 pandemic highlights the need for enhanced public health capacity through systems, structures and institutions. Capacity building is a mechanism by which the public health workforce can effectively achieve its intentions for existing and emerging health issues (Beaglehole & Dal Poz, 2003). Six consistent domains for building public health were identified by Aluttis and colleagues (2014), building:

  i)   capacities for adequate information and monitoring systems
 ii)   a knowledgeable and skilled public health workforce
iii)   capacity for research and development
 iv)   sufficient resources and infrastructures
  v)   collaboration between various actors
 vi)   adequate policy, planning and management systems
vii)   country-specific context (p. 40).

Several of these domains are explored in detail here.

Institutions and organisations for public health

Institutions – structures or mechanisms that organise relations across society.

Institutions are the formal and informal rules, norms and codes of conduct that organise economic, social and political relations (North, 1991). Examples of institutions that influence public health include property rights and labour laws, redistributive public expenditure and rights-based anti-discrimination legislation, and the WHO Framework Convention on Tobacco Control.

If institutions are the 'rules of the game', how we 'structure ourselves to play' is through organisations (DFID, 2003). At the global level, the WHO, the United Nations (UN), the World Trade Organization and the World Bank influence public health. Universities, professional associations and non-government public health organisations can also play a role. These organisations are made up of players brought together for a common purpose and responsible for governance and the enactment of rules and norms.

The Charter (World Federation of Public Health Associations, 2016) highlights the importance of institutions and organisations in providing governance on key public health functions such as legislation, policy, strategy and financing. There have been assertions that public health governance has been weakened as the leadership and resources of global organisations such as the WHO have diminished, coordination capacity of the UN has been challenged, relationships between nations and multilateral organisations have fractured and a lack of coherent strategy and resourcing have occurred at the local level (Kruk, 2012; Lisk & Šehović, 2020; Gostin, Moon & Meier, 2020).

The 2030 Sustainable Development Agenda (UN, n.d.) argues that 'weak institutions and limited access to justice remain a great threat to sustainable development.' Sustainable Development Goal 16 is for 'Peace, justice and strong institutions'.

The WHO points to opportunities to strengthen the health system and institutions, with a greater focus on delivery of core public health services: health promotion, disease prevention and health protection. This requires the establishment of several structural platforms, including public health institutes with strong institutional capacity to support multi-sectoral action (WHO EMRO, n.d.).

Resourcing public health

Financing public health may be politically challenging as its benefits can take time to manifest and may be difficult to quantify, given that the outcome is prevention and capacity building with long-term access and equity. More immediate, visible and politically salient outcomes, such as reductions in hospital waiting lists, attract attention and draw funds away from public health. Despite estimates of the economic benefits of prevention being four times that of direct clinical services, OECD countries allocate less than 5 per cent of their health expenditure to disease prevention and health promotion (Collins et al., 2020).

Beyond the overall expenditure towards preventive health, consideration of economic, social and political factors can reveal influences on financing decisions. Examining differences in expenditure allocations across geographic areas and health issues, as well as sources of funding and where responsibility for financing lies, can indicate priorities and pressures.

In Australia, all levels of government as well as the private sector are involved in resourcing and providing healthcare services, along with significant out-of-pocket contributions by consumers. The health system includes tertiary medical services and hospitals, primary health care and public health. This spans a wide range of services from promotion and prevention through to treatment and continuing care (AIHW, 2020a; AIHW, 2018).

Overall health spending in Australia has more than doubled over the past two decades, at a rate higher than population growth, resulting in increased health expenditure per person (AIHW, 2020a; AIHW 2020b). If we look at this in terms of the federal budget, spending on health has hovered around 16 per cent of total government expenditure in recent years, including expenditure on public hospitals, capital expenses and dental care (AIHW, 2018). Only 1.3 per cent of all health spending is on prevention: just $89 per person each year (Jackson & Shiell, 2017). The argument is that increasing expenditure on prevention would improve health system cost-effectiveness, since preventable, chronic disease-related tertiary health system costs would reduce. The problem is that the outcome requires longer-term, bipartisan support, which often is not the approach of governments looking for short-term political wins.

A workforce for the public's health

The structure and scope of public health services vary between countries and offer a diversity of roles that can be categorised as either part of the 'core' workforce or the broader workforce. This core consists of those who perform public health activities as a major part of their role and who possess and develop consistent core competencies. There is also a broader range of individuals who contribute to public health action as part of their work but who may not identify as part of the public health workforce (WHO, 2020).

A public health profession and discipline

To understand public health, it is useful to define the workforce, and examine how staff are trained, what roles they take on and how they think about their professional identity. This is challenging due to public health's interdisciplinary, heterogenous nature. Public health has relatively porous professional boundaries, with a range of occupations undertaking public health functions. For example, think about physicians, health administrators, town planners and statisticians. They may all work in public health, but their professional values and ideology may be connected to their initial training, so they may not see themselves as part of a public health profession or discipline. The increasing professionalisation of public health serves to develop a distinct identity and to move public health beyond a limited field of practice or scope of action (Czabanowska et al., 2014). Understanding the definitions specific to a discipline, profession and identity is helpful as a starting point.

Profession – a collection of like-minded individuals united in developing the science and art of practice and its members.

Professional identity is how an individual defines themselves as a member of a **profession** (Ibarra, 1999). A profession has been defined as a collection of individuals who are like-minded and who unite in the development of the science and art of practice and its members (Hendrick, 2004). For a workforce to be considered a profession, a specific knowledge base is required, including advanced formal education and training, significant self-regulation and autonomy (Evashwick et al., 2013). Additional criteria have been suggested as part of the identity of health professionals, including providing a service that is valued and trusted by society, conducting research and technical competence (Freegard & Isted, 2012).

In contrast, a discipline can be considered an 'ordered field of study' (Davies, 2013, p. 5), dedicated to producing original and robust knowledge used by professions (Dubois, 2016). But a discipline is more than just knowledge. A disciplinary identity is the vehicle for its production, dissemination and, to some extent, its control. Bailey (1977) imagined disciplines as diverse 'academic tribes', suggesting that 'each tribe has a name and territory, settles its own affairs, goes to war with others, has a distinct language or at least a distinct dialect, and a variety of symbolic ways of demonstrating its apartness from others'. For a field such as public health to be considered a discipline, it needs to have a set of unifying features. Davies (2013) suggests that these include a value base, knowledge domain, history and traditions, preferred research methods and systems for development of competencies and capacity-building.

A **discipline** may be recognised through organisations such as academies, societies (e.g. the Royal Society for Public Health), conferences (e.g. the World Congress on Public Health) and journals (e.g. *Critical Public Health*), and research and higher degree programs (Dubois, 2016).

Discipline – a field of study dedicated to producing original and robust knowledge.

REFLECTION QUESTION

1 Public health advocates have called for increases to the public health component of health budgets for many years. What are the implications of not doing this? Why should government increase the proportion of the health budget spent on public health?

2 What would be the implications of a reduced public health workforce? Should public health workforce planning consider the breadth of skills required, or only those of 'core' professions? Why or why not?

Competencies for public health

Those working in public health require specific knowledge and skills. Public health interventions and priorities are diverse, and often complex. For example, tasks may range from developing a policy to provide new immigrants with access to health services upon arrival in a country, to designing a campaign to increase awareness of the benefits of vaccination, to researching the effects of climate change on community food security. It is helpful if there is consistency in the way these tasks are approached, by having a guide or 'road map' to collective public health efforts. To consistently perform public health actions at an appropriate level, practitioners require a set of **competencies**.

Competencies may be described as the 'building blocks' common within a discipline or profession. They are often articulated through a framework, which provides the structure and minimal standards expected to perform a role or for graduates to be able to demonstrate upon completion of their degree. Competency frameworks are useful in guiding workforce development for organisations and government departments, and offer a valuable tool for human resources functions such as recruitment and professional development.

Competencies – attributes and capabilities such as knowledge, skills, values and attitudes that enable an individual to perform a set of tasks to an appropriate standard required in a particular context.

The WHO-ASPHER (Association of Schools of Public Health in the European Region) Competency Framework has been developed to strengthen Europe's core public health workforce. These competencies are arranged to work across levels and systems, and point to developing expertise across content and context (e.g. law, policies and ethics), relations and interactions (e.g. leadership and systems thinking), and performance and achievement (e.g. governance and resource management) (Association of Schools and Programs of Public Health (ASPPH), n.d.; WHO, 2020).

The US Council on Education for Public Health (2016) developed core competencies as part of accreditation requirements for tertiary public health programs of study. These include foundation knowledge regarding the profession and science of public health (e.g. public health history, philosophy and values) and factors relating to human health (e.g. the social, political and economic determinants of health) as well as foundational competencies, which are:

- evidence-based approaches to public health
- public health and healthcare systems

- planning and management to promote health
- policy in public health
- leadership
- communication
- interprofessional practice
- systems thinking.

The Australian Council of Academic Public Health Institutions Australasia (CAPHIA) developed a set of foundation competencies for public health graduates (CAPHIA, 2016). These are arranged into the following areas of practice:

- health monitoring and surveillance
- disease prevention and control
- health protection
- health promotion
- health policy, planning and management
- evidence-based professional population health practice (p. 8).

Educating, training and regulating the public health workforce

There is a lack of global consistency in formal qualifications, training and the degree to which practice is regulated. This is concerning, given the wide-ranging nature of the roles and the skills and experience required in public health. The Master of Public Health is a commonly recognised postgraduate qualification that covers the core competencies described earlier. In the United States and Europe, competency-based training that links education and practice is widespread, but this is less consistent in other parts of the world, including in Australia. In the United States, course accreditation for masters and doctoral programs is common, and accreditation is often paired with a process of practitioner registration or regulation. This is not the case in Australia.

There are several approaches to regulation. The first is statutory regulation, whereby the government is responsible for enforcing legislation and penalising non-compliance. Forms of regulation may include registration, licensing, accreditation or certification. In Australia, many health professions are regulated by government; for example, Aboriginal and Torres Strait Islander health practitioners, medical, nursing and midwifery, optometry and paramedical practitioners. Some health professions are **self-regulated**, such as dietetics and social work. Public health is generally self-regulated, although health promotion practitioners and public health nutritionists are among the few exceptions that are also self-regulated (see e.g. NSA 2021). Spotlight 6.1 profiles accreditation and a workforce development initiative in the health promotion profession in Australia.

Self-regulation – involves a professional association (rather than government) determining the rules and requirements that regulate the conduct of its individual members.

SPOTLIGHT 6.1

Building graduate capacity through health promotion scholarships

Health promotion is a core service of public health, and in the years since the Ottawa Charter, efforts have been made to formalise the workforce and profession. These efforts include developing ethical values for practice, a knowledge base and internationally agreed competencies (International Union for Health Promotion and Education [IUHPE], 2016). Tertiary degrees have been instituted alongside their global accreditation through the IUHPE. At the country level, national accreditation organisations oversee individual practitioner registration (e.g. Australian Health Promotion Association [AHPA], n.d.). A global network of health promotion foundations has been established (INHPF, 2021), offering national and international conferences, and development of guiding charters and declarations through the WHO and the health promotion community, including the most recent, the Shanghai declaration on promoting health in the 2030 Agenda for Sustainable Development.

As with other areas of public health, on-the-job training provides a complementary strategy to the conceptual knowledge gained in tertiary-level courses. Such training can also support transition to, and retention within, the workforce and can contribute to boosting capacity. However, such programs in the Australian context are relatively limited.

For almost 30 years, the Health Promotion Foundation of Western Australia (Healthway) has funded the AHPA to offer competitive scholarships to health promotion graduates and Aboriginal and Torres Strait Islander people. The scholarships provide individuals with the opportunity to experience a supported training experience while working on a project in a health promotion agency. During their training, recipients build required competencies to maintain their registration as an IUHPE Health Promotion Practitioner.

Since 1991, more than 120 scholarships have been awarded. Agency placements have resulted in sustained initiatives, such as the Public Health Advocacy Institute's (PHAIWA) Children's Environment and Health Local Government Policy Awards (PHAIWA, n.d.). In an evaluation of the program, around two-thirds of recipients were still working in the health sector; this suggests that the scholarships have enabled the commencement of long-term careers in health promotion (Crawford et al., 2019). The program represents a long-term partnership model that contributes to public health capacity and strengthens systems towards health promotion and prevention. The program also contributes to the development of the health promotion profession and discipline. Given the relatively modest investment and positive outcomes, the initiative has the potential for replication and scale-up, including to other jurisdictions, to complement existing public health training programs.

QUESTION

What contribution can a program such as the Healthway AHPA scholarships make to public health?

Other key public health professions include:

- Epidemiologists: Epidemiologists are employed by departments of health, universities and research institutions. They usually have qualifications in public health or specialist masters degrees, such as in applied epidemiology. The Australian National University runs the accredited Australian Field Epidemiology Training Program (Master of Philosophy in Applied Epidemiology). The Centers for Disease Control and Prevention (CDC) in the United States began the first training program in applied epidemiology in 1951. The CDC's Epidemic Intelligence Service is a two-year training program to develop the workforce of applied or field epidemiologists.

- Aboriginal and Torres Strait Islander Health Workers and Practitioners: The Aboriginal and Torres Strait Islander health workforce is critical to public health outcomes, particularly in reducing health inequalities for Aboriginal and Torres Strait Islander people. Individuals are employed in a range of settings, including Aboriginal Community Controlled Health Organisations (ACCHO), government general practice and non-government organisations. There are two roles specifically designed for Aboriginal and Torres Strait Islander people: Aboriginal and Torres Strait Islander Health Workers and Aboriginal and Torres Strait Islander Health Practitioners.

- Environmental Health Officers: In Australia, environmental health professionals who undertake compliance and enforcement roles that can lead to prosecution need to have undertaken courses accredited by Environmental Health Australia (EHA). In addition to determining an adequate level of academic support from universities, the accreditation process also ensures that academic and professional skills align with the enHealth Environmental Health Officer Skills and Knowledge Matrix (Environmental Health Australia, 2014). Graduates of accredited courses are recognised as having the skills, knowledge and attributes required to practise as Environmental Health Officers throughout Australia and in countries with reciprocal recognition arrangements.
- Public Health Physicians: Public health efforts are supported by Public Health Physicians who are fellows of the Australasian Faculty of Public Health Medicine (AFPHM). AFPHM provides training and continuing education for public health medicine fellows and trainees in Australia and Aotearoa New Zealand. Public health medicine fellows are medical doctors with postgraduate clinical experience, a Master of Public Health and three years of advanced training in public health medicine and continuing professional development. Training is completed in settings such as ACCHOs, sexual health clinics and departments for communicable disease control.

In most countries, on-the-job training supports formal qualifications in public health. The New South Wales (NSW) Public Health Training Program provides trainee Public Health Officers a three-year workplace experience to support public health careers following completion of a Master of Public Health. Trainees undertake a range of population health placements within the NSW health system. The program enhances the capacity of the NSW health system to meet sudden increases in demand for health services (e.g. during a pandemic) (NSW Health, 2016). The CDC administers the two-year, paid public health associate program (PHAP), which supports frontline public health efforts across public health agencies and non-government organisations in the United States and its territories (Schneider et al., 2011).

Public health: A political priority?

Responding to the COVID-19 pandemic, the Australian National Cabinet agreed to a plan to enhance Australia's public health capacity and support a sustainable public health workforce for future public health efforts (Morrison, 2020). Proposed actions included a national program to train a surge workforce, and a review of the organisation and structure of public health units. However, the federal budget allocated very little for the workforce and at the time of writing there is no national public health strategy for Australia.

In Australia, from 1987 to 2010, the Public Health Education and Research Program (PHERP) coordinated efforts to ensure a well-trained, quality public health workforce. PHERP oversaw a scale-up of public health education and research training across Australia and the establishment of a competency framework through the Australian Network of Academic Public Health Institutions (ANAPHI, now CAPHIA). A decade later, this level of investment is still required to enable sufficient workforce capacity to respond to existing and emerging public health threats, including infectious and communicable diseases, non-communicable diseases, climate change and social determinants of health such as racism.

We are in need of visionary public health leaders, advocates, policy-makers, researchers and practitioners. Gould and colleagues (2012) have suggested that 'many health practitioners appreciate the need for advocacy but do not have the requisite skills...' (p. 165). Recent iterations of competency frameworks for public health have included advocacy as part of their goals. For example, Australian competencies include a unit to 'Develop an advocacy strategy regarding a population health issue to influence public policy' and an element of this to 'Articulate the role of public policy in promoting and protecting health and preventing disease' (CAPHIA, 2016). These frameworks guide teaching and training of public health practitioners, and there is a growing number of degree courses and continuing professional development that provide education on advocacy and politics (see e.g. Spotlight 6.2). This is the focus of the next section on public health advocacy.

The need for advocacy for public health

Public health is inherently political (see Chapter 10). Initiatives to improve road safety, promote immunisation, support safe drug use through harm reduction and reduce tobacco use have all faced vehement opposition from various sectors and individuals (Chapman, 2001). Unequal power relationships in society represent a key driver of health inequality. It is possible for government policies and systems to be agents in redistributing power, increasing access to resources and, in doing, so to address health inequity. Farrer and colleagues (2015) state that advocacy is a way to improve health equity through promoting polices that address social determinants of health through universal service provision and a focus on the health of disadvantaged populations through targeted interventions. This is a critical opportunity for public health practitioners who are well-placed to facilitate advocacy efforts, both at the community and structural levels. Dissatisfaction with the perceived lack of strength, focus and representation of many multilateral organisations that influence global public health action has led to calls to challenge the status quo and diffuse power through new mechanisms, such as the sustainable development agenda, the New Development Bank (Lisk & Šehović, 2020) and greater participation from civil society and citizens (Kickbusch & Gleicher, 2012) .

REFLECTION QUESTION

Why do you think health is political? Can you think of a public health topic that that may require action by both governments and communities to address a power imbalance?

What is public health advocacy?

Public health advocacy aims to change upstream determinants of health such as laws and regulations, and organisational or corporate practices and standards (Chapman, 2001). Moore and colleagues (2013) define **advocacy** as 'persuading decision makers of the need

Advocacy – a range of strategies to influence those in power to implement desired changes.

for change through identifying desired public health outcomes and effective and feasible methods of achieving that change' (p. 5). Planning for advocacy can involve a range of tools, tactics and techniques to protect population health through influencing and holding to account the actions and decisions of those in power (such as government or corporations) (Brinsden & Lang, 2015). The Ottawa Charter identified advocacy as one of the three basic health promotion actions (WHO, 1986) and it is a key element of the strategic plans of many public health organisations (Moore et al., 2013).

A defining feature of advocacy is that it occurs in the face of opposition and resistance, and therefore needs to harness or influence power in some way. Laverack (2013) described 'hard power' as the capacity of some to have 'power-over' others, an ability to generate intended or unintended consequences for others through coercive or direct measures, and 'soft power' as working through persuasion and co-option through voluntary means. Changes proposed may be effective but unpopular, hence the need to advocate. Opposition can be expressed in many ways, including neglect of issues perceived as insignificant (Chapman, 2001). Some corporations generate negative effects on health as a direct result of their promotion, production and sale of goods (Kreuter, 2005). Terms such as 'manufacturers of disease' and 'corporate disease promotion' have been used by advocates to describe these activities and industries (Kreuter, 2005). Government reluctance to act, and strong opposition to proposed or existing public health measures, can often reveal the powerful influence of business or industry. As the power of corporations, organisations and industry has increased relative to governments, so too has their influence on public policy (Mays, 2017).

Advocacy can be described as either facilitative or representative; the key difference being whether the aim is to protect or to empower (Carlisle, 2000). In a facilitative approach, the aim is for individuals and communities to develop skills that enable them to advocate for themselves. A representative approach sees public health professionals advocating on behalf of individuals. In many contexts, moving away from representative towards facilitative advocacy is consistent with social health promotion, by equipping communities with skills in political advocacy. Yet, there remains a role for 'top-down' advocacy, such as health advocacy for policy reform, whereby the specific knowledge and influence of advocates can be harnessed to effect social change.

Public health advocacy can also be described and categorised according to who or what is being advocated for, or in relation to the function an advocate is performing. Carlisle (2000) defines four types of advocacy: representation, community development, community activism and social policy reform (see Figure 6.1). *Representation* focuses on representation at the individual level, with the goal being to counter power imbalances and uphold rights. *Social policy reform* advocacy operates further upstream against structural and systemic determinants. *Community activism* calls out and opposes powerful health-damaging entities. *Community development* advocacy arises from individuals having become effective policy advocates attaining greater control over their own health (Carlisle, 2000).

It is important to consider the reasons we do advocacy. Often, in the cases presented here, advocacy is discussed in the context of democratic governments, but this is not always the case. Advocacy is often linked to a rights-based agenda, which assumes that people have rights (whether that is access to health care, employment, housing or a clean environment) and works to ensure these rights are enforced, respected and realised (International Council of Nurses, 2008).

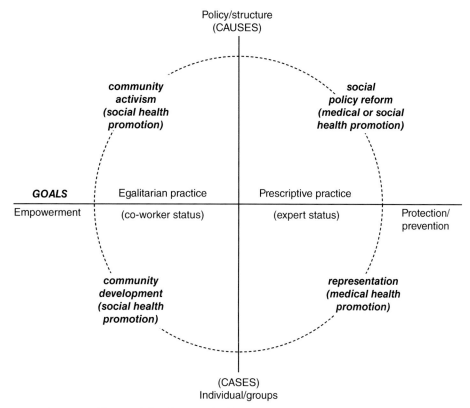

Figure 6.1   A conceptual framework for advocacy in health promotion.
Source: Carlisle, 2000, p. 372.

SPOTLIGHT 6.2

Building capacity for advocacy: A toolkit for public health professionals

Building the capacity of the public health workforce to engage in advocacy is vital – both for adequate resourcing of public health activity and in driving changes in policy to address health inequalities. The Public Health Advocacy Institute (PHAI, formerly PHAIWA), based at Curtin University in Western Australia, aims to influence, build, promote and support advocacy for public health priorities through innovation in education, applied research, engagement and practice. PHAI's suite of capacity building activities includes tools, resources and skills-based professional development for organisations and individuals to improve their ability to achieve effective health promotion and public health advocacy. PHAI's e-mentoring program for public health professionals builds advocacy skills and knowledge through skills-based activities and mentoring by experienced public health advocates (O'Connell, Stoneham & Saunders, 2016). The online resource 'Advocacy in Action' (https://www.phaiwa.org.au), now in its 4th edition, is a toolkit that aims to demystify advocacy through case studies that demonstrate how advocacy strategies can be applied across different issues, tips to work effectively with the media and practical tools to help practitioners to engage in advocacy. Central to the toolkit is a planning framework to guide advocacy strategies (Figure 6.2) that integrates theories of change, including the advocacy coalition theory.

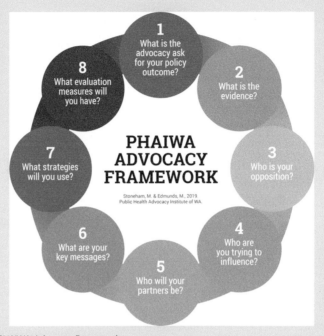

Figure 6.2   The PHAIWA Advocacy Framework.

Source: Stoneham, Vidler & Edmunds (2019). © Public Health Advocacy Institute, Curtin University.

QUESTION

What are some examples of political changes that could have public health benefits in the prevention of chronic disease? Choose a section on the advocacy framework and consider what might be your first steps.

Theories for public health advocacy

Effective advocacy often results from a planned and strategic approach. This approach should consider the cultural and political contexts, empower and engage with communities, examine possible tactics and actions, and build alliances, in addition to presenting evidence (David et al., 2020; Kreuter, 2005). Using a framework to develop an advocacy approach can offer clarity, efficiency and improved results (Moore et al., 2013). When selecting a framework, we are in effect considering a theory of change. This is informed by our worldviews and values, and describes our assumptions about how change can occur and what tactics will drive this change, and in which circumstances (Stachowiak, n.d.). These theoretical roadmaps can guide our advocacy work, and there is consensus that advocacy and its evaluation cannot be done effectively without a theory of change that is grounded in both social science and real-world experience (Klugmann, 2011).

Many theories have been developed to help us understand how influencing policy may work, but no theory can always explain all change. The following three political science theories provide an understanding of how public policy processes are influenced and offer insights to developing effective advocacy strategies.

- Advocacy Coalition Framework (ACF): The ACF attempts to unravel public policy processes, particularly in relation to controversial issues. It contends that individual 'policy actors' come together regarding shared beliefs, forming coalitions that compete with others who hold different beliefs, for the goal of achieving policy change (Cairney, 2019). Shared beliefs are central to actions taken by coalitions. The ACF conceptualises beliefs into three levels: deep core, policy core and secondary aspects that are each respectively more amenable to change. Coalitions articulate and promote their beliefs, cooperate or compete with others, and learn and adapt their beliefs and actions. According to the ACF, policies and programs are essentially reflections of the beliefs of members of the dominant advocacy coalitions. Coalition actions are restricted or facilitated by larger structural elements such as social values, government configurations, political systems as well as system-level 'events' such as socio-economic change and shifts in power. The ACF suggests that policy change can be effected by a combination of significant events (external or internal to the policy's subsystem), learning and negotiations between coalitions (Weible & Sabatier, 2006).

- Multiple Streams Framework (MSF): Unlike the ACF, which has beliefs at its centre, the MSF is more about ideas. The MSF contends that three separate streams must come together at the same time for a significant policy change to occur: (1) problem; (2) policy; and (3) politics (Kingdon, 1984). A problem grabs attention, a solution to that problem (a policy) is available and the political climate is right (policy-makers have motive and opportunity to adopt it). These converging streams create a 'window of opportunity'; favourable conditions that are short-lived. Problems may garner attention because of how they are 'framed', or perhaps due to a crisis or significant event that changes the scale of a problem. Attention is frequently temporary, meaning advocates need to be attuned and ready to act quickly and in anticipation of future problems. The MSF describes 'policy entrepreneurs' as influential actors who use framing and advocacy, and who leverage their power, knowledge and connections to promote ideas and capitalise upon 'windows of opportunity'. Presenting the evidence is not enough; translating evidence into crafted messages to appeal to shared beliefs or values (framing) is more powerful in persuading the target audience to act. Developing solutions cannot wait until the problem gains attention, so feasible solutions must be already prepared. Finally, the broader political environment is a key driver of which strategies to select and when. Cairney (2019) likens this to 'surfers waiting for the big wave'.

- Punctuated Equilibrium Theory (PET): PET helps to explain how agendas are set, why some problems receive attention and others are ignored. It is common for policy to remain stable over time, subject to only minor changes. Yet, occasionally, policy does undergo major change. PET attempts to explain this stability (stasis) and change (punctuations) in public policy processes (Cairney, 2019). PET describes these two states as affected by bounded rationality, selective attention, policy monopolies and venue shopping. It is not possible for policy-makers to constantly examine all issues, and therefore many are ignored and remain relatively static. Selective attention also arises from the

Marginalised groups in low socio-economic status (SES) areas are more likely than residents of medium to high-SES areas to be exposed to environmental contaminants, and to live in overcrowded and sub-standard housing. They are also less likely to have the financial resources to be able to adapt or modify their accommodation circumstances, and more likely to lack access to health care, either due to being unable to afford services or lack of enabling infrastructure such as public transport. These disparities may lead to increased sickness and disease when compared to wealthier communities (NIEHS, 2021). When global disasters such as the COVID-19 pandemic occur, the spread of inequities can be widened and specific vulnerabilities emerge (Zota & Shamasunder, 2021). On a global scale, the COVID-19 pandemic has exacerbated many inequalities; higher-income countries generally managed outbreaks more successfully in terms of access to healthcare facilities, appropriate treatment protocols and vaccines, with corresponding lower case and death rates.

Another example of inequity emerging between groups comes with resource development in developing countries. Economic growth, coupled with urbanisation and rapid technological progress, has led to an increased demand for raw materials, which in turn has led to increased investment in mining operations for various minerals and other commodities. Much of this investment has occurred in lower-income regions such as Latin America, Africa and parts of Asia where environmental regulations and development conditions are often less restrictive. While this investment creates employment and contributes to the local and national economies, there are frequently trade-offs, including widespread environmental damage. Mining operations require huge areas of land to be excavated, which may cause soil erosion and site contamination from leakage of chemicals and poor drainage. They also usually require intensive use of water resources, which may lead to loss of access to water supplies as well as widespread water and air pollution. These adverse effects can lead to the displacement of whole communities and to social conflicts (Antoci, Russu & Ticci, 2019). Several humanitarian groups, such as Amnesty International and Global Citizen, advocate for environmental justice and the protection of human rights in many countries in which resource developments are causing detrimental health and environmental effects and the forced displacement of whole communities. Examples of mining operations that have led to disparity and conflict include coal mining in South Africa, and cobalt and coltan mining in the Democratic Republic of the Congo (Morrice & Colagiuri, 2013).

QUESTION

Research the source of mineral components of personal electronic devices (phones, tablets etc.) such as tantalum (coltan), cobalt and others. Where are these minerals mined and what are the local conditions in terms of employment, environment etc.? What progress has been made? Are the manufacturers advocating for the workers?

SUMMARY

In this chapter you have learnt about the diverse public health workforce, some of the challenges in resourcing our public health responses and why advocacy is an important skill needed to address this and health inequalities more broadly.

Learning objective 1: Describe the structure and resourcing of public health activities in Australia.
A multitude of organisations, institutions and individuals, both within, outside and at all levels of government, work towards improving public health. Public sources of funding are significant in resourcing public health activities, yet are subject to competing priorities and economic, social and political influences that limit greater investment in prevention.

Learning objective 2: Critically identify the features of the public health workforce.
The public health workforce encompasses a range of professions and disciplines. Competency frameworks exist for public health with continuing education and training being key to workforce development. Accreditation and the regulation of public health professionals may contribute to the field of public health becoming recognised as a distinct profession and discipline.

Learning objective 3: Articulate the rationale for advocacy as a key requirement for public health action.
Public health action involves politics and power. Measures attract support or opposition from individuals, groups and organisations, depending on their positions, stakes, values and beliefs. Some have substantially more power than others. Advocacy is an essential skill that public health practitioners can develop to exert influence and contribute to change.

Learning objective 4: Describe theories and evidence that underpin effective public health advocacy and activism.
Effective advocacy is planned, strategic and underpinned by frameworks or theories of change. ACF, MSF and PET are just three examples that can help practitioners understand how public policy processes are influenced and then identify how advocacy and activism strategies can be productively applied.

TUTORIAL EXERCISES

1   Review the CAPHIA Foundation Competencies for Public Health Graduates (https://caphia.com.au/resources) and consider the units you are enrolled in. Can you map the content of your degree against the competencies, and identify any gaps for further training?

2   Australia is developing a National Preventive Health Strategy. Similar strategies have been developed in the past, with relatively little attention paid to the social determinants of health. Discuss in groups: What is the role of government, public health practitioners and civil society in prioritising a public health equity focus in such strategies?

3   There has been increasing recognition of the role of climate change on health and the role of health-related institutions in driving the agenda for change. Despite this, progress is slow. Review the PHAI Advocacy Toolkit (https://www.phaiwa.org.au) and use the advocacy framework to develop your own plan for advocacy action on climate and health.

4   Consider the Black Lives Matter movement. It developed from previous social justice and human rights action related to racism and civil rights, particularly in the United States, but has grown across the globe using both non-violent and confrontational strategies. In Australia it has linked systemic racism with deaths in custody of Aboriginal and Torres Strait Islander people. Discuss: Why is systemic racism a

public health issue? What type of advocacy does it demonstrate? What theory or theories underpin the development of the Black Lives Matter movement?

FURTHER READING

Council of Academic Public Health Institutions in Australia (CAPHIA). (2016). Foundation Competencies for Public Health Graduates in Australia (2nd ed.). Retrieved http://caphia.com.au/testsite/wp-content/uploads/2016/07/CAPHIA_document_DIGITAL_nov_22.pdf

Laverack, G. (2013). *Health activism: Foundations and strategies*. SAGE Publications Ltd.

People's Health Movement. Global Health Watch. (n.d.). Retrieved https://phmovement.org/global-health-watch/

Stoneham, M., Vidler, A., & Edmunds,M. (2019). *Advocacy in action: A toolkit for public health professionals* (4th ed.). Retrieved https://www.phaiwa.org.au/wp-content/uploads/2019/09/2019_Advocacy-in-Action-A-Toolkit-for-Public-Health-Professionals-1.pdf

World Federation of Public Health Associations. (2016). *The Global Charter for the Public's Health*. Retrieved https://www.wfpha.org/document-upload/the-global-charter-for-the-public%E2%80%99s-health.pdf

REFERENCES

Aluttis, C., den Broucke, S. V., Chiotan, C., Costongs, C., Michelsen, K., & Brand, H. (2014). Public health and health promotion capacity at national and regional level: a review of conceptual frameworks. *Journal of Public Health Research*, *3*(1), 199.

Antoci, A., Russu, P., & Ticci, E. (2019). Mining and local economies: Dilemma between environmental protection and job opportunities. *Sustainability*, 11, 6244.

Association of Schools and Programs of Public Health (ASPPH). (n.d.) *MPH Core Competency Model*. Retrieved https://www.aspph.org/teach-research/models/mph-competency-model/

Australian Health Promotion Association (AHPA). (n.d.). *Health promotion practitioner registration*. Retrieved https://www.healthpromotion.org.au/our-profession/practitioner-registration

Australian Healthcare and Hospitals Association (AHHA). (2020). *An Australian centre for disease control*. Retrieved https://ahha.asn.au/sites/default/files/docs/policy-issue/australian_centre_for_disease_control_position_statement_final_1.pdf

Australian Institute of Health and Welfare (AIHW). (2018). *Australia's health 2018. Cat. No. AUS 221.* AIHW.

——(2020a). *Health expenditure Australia 2018–19. Cat. No. HWE 80.* AIHW.

——(2020b). *Australia's health 2020: Data insights. Cat. No. AUS 231.* AIHW.

Australian Medical Association (AMA). (2017). *Australian National Centre for Disease Control (CDC) – 2017*. Retrieved https://www.ama.com.au/position-statement/australian-national-centre-disease-control-cdc-2017

Bailey, F. G. (1977) *Mortality and expediency*. Blackwell.

Baum, F. (2016). *The new public health* (4th ed). Oxford University Press.

Baum, F., Sanders, D., & Narayan, R. (2020). The global people's health movement. What is the people's health movement? *SciELO Public Health*, 44(Spe1).

Beaglehole, R., & Dal Poz, M.R. (2003). Public health workforce: Challenges and policy issues. *Human Resources in Health* 1, 4.

Bloland, P., Simone, P., Burkholder, B., Slutsker, L., & De Cock, K.M. (2012). The role of public health institutions in global health system strengthening efforts: The US CDC's perspective. *PLOS Medicine*, *9*(4), e1001199.

Brinsden H., & Lang T. (2015). *An introduction to public health advocacy: Reflections on theory and practice.* Food Research Collaboration. Retrieved http://foodresearch.org.uk/wp-content/uploads/2015/10/BrinsdenLang_PublicHealthAdvocacy_FRC_briefing_FINAL2_19_10_15.pdf

Cairney, P. (2019). *Understanding public policy: Theories and issues.* (2nd ed.) Red Globe Press.

Carlisle, S. (2000). Health promotion, advocacy and health inequalities: A conceptual framework. *Health Promotion International, 15*(4); 369–76.

Chapman, S. (2001). Advocacy in public health: Roles and challenges. *International Journal of Epidemiology, 30*(6), 1226–32.

Collins, T., Akselrod, S., Bloomfield, A., Gamkrelidze, A., Jakab, Z., & Placella, E. (2020). Rethinking the COVID-19 pandemic: Back to public health. *Annals of Global Health, 86*(1), 133.

Council of Academic Public Health Institutions in Australia (CAPHIA). (2016). Foundation competencies for public health graduates in Australia (2nd ed.). Retrieved http://caphia.com.au/testsite/wp-content/uploads/2016/07/CAPHIA_document_DIGITAL_nov_22.pdf

Council on Education for Public Health. (2016). Accreditation criteria: Schools of public health & public health programs. Retrieved https://storage.googleapis.com/media.ceph.org/wp_assets/2016.Criteria.pdf

Crawford, G., Hallett, J., Barnes, A., Cavill, J. L., Clarkson, J., & Shilton, T. R. (2019). Twenty years of capacity building and partnership: A case study of a health promotion scholarship program. *Health Promotion Journal of Australia, 30*(2), 281–4.

Czabanowska, K., Laaser, U., & Stjernberg, L. (2014). Shaping and authorising a public health profession. *South Eastern European Journal of Public Health*, 2.

David, J.L., Thomas, S.L., Randle, M. & Daube, M. (2020). A public health advocacy approach for preventing and reducing gambling related harm. *Australia and New Zealand Journal of Public Health, 44*, 14–19.

Davies, J. K. (2013). *Health Promotion: A unique discipline?* Retrieved http://www.hauora.co.nz/assets/files/Occasional%20Papers/Health%20Promotion%20is%20a%20Discipline%2027%20Nov(1).pdf

Department for International Development (DFID). (2003). *Promoting Insitutional & Organisational Development.* Retrieved http://www.kalidadea.org/castellano/materiales/evaluacion/DFID%20promoting%20institutional%20develpment%20guide.pdf

Dhavan, P., & Reddy S. K. (2017). Public health professionals. *International Encyclopedia of Public Health* (2nd ed.), 210–16.

Dubois, P. (2016). Science as vocation? *Discipline, Profession and Impressionistic Sociology*, 69, 21–39.

Environmental Health Australia. (2014). *Environmental Health University Course Accreditation Policy.* Retrieved https://www.eh.org.au/workforce/course-accreditation-policy

Evashwick, C. J., Begun, J. W., & Finnegan, J. R., Jr. (2013). Public health as a distinct profession: Has it arrived? *Journal of Public Health Management and Practice, 19*(5), 412–19.

Farrer, L., Marinetti, C., Cavaco, Y.K., & Costongs, C. (2015). Advocacy for health equity: A synthesis review. *Milbank Quarterly*, 93, 392–437.

Freegard, H. C., & Isted, L. (2012). What is a health profession? In H. C. Freegard, & L. Isted (Eds.), *Ethical practice for health professonals.* Cengage Learning Australia.

Gostin, L. O., Moon, S. & Meier, B. M. (2020). Reimagining global health governance in the age of COVID-19. *American Journal of Public Health*, 110, 1615–19.

Gould, T., Louise Fleming, M., & Parker, E. (2012). Advocacy for health: Revisiting the role of health promotion. *Health Promotion Journal of Australia*, 23, 165–70.

Hendrick, J. (2004). *Law and ethics.* Nelson Thomas Ltd.

Ibarra, H. (1999). Provisional selves: Experimenting with image and identity in professional adaptation. *Administrative Science Quarterly, 44*(4), 764–91.

International Council of Nurses. (2008). *Promoting health advocacy guide for health professionals*. World Health Communication Associates Ltd.

International Network of Health Promotion Foundations (INHPF). (2021). *Who we are*. Retrieved https://inhpf .net/2018/01/15/about/

International Union for Health Promotion and Education (IUHPE). (2016). *IUHPE core competencies and professional standards for health promotion*. Retrieved http://www.ukphr.org/wp-content/uploads/ 2017/02/Core_Competencies_Standards_linkE.pdf

Jackson, H., & Shiell, A. (2017). *Preventive health: How much does Australia spend and is it enough?* Foundation for Alcohol Research and Education.

Keleher, H., & MacDougall, C. (2015). *Understanding Health*. (4th ed.). Oxford University Press.

Kickbusch, I., & Gleicher, D. (2012). *Governance for health in the 21st century*. World Health Organization. Retrieved https://apps.who.int/iris/bitstream/handle/10665/326429/9789289002745- eng.pdf

Kingdon, J. (1984, 1995) *Agendas, alternatives and public policies* (1st and 2nd eds.). Harper Collins.

Klugmann, B. (2011). Effective social justice advocacy: A theory-of-change framework for assessing progress. *Reproductive Health Matters, 19*(38), 146–62.

Kreuter, M. W. (2005). Commentary on public health advocacy to change corporate practices. *Health Education & Behavior, 32*(3), 355–62.

Kruk, M. E. (2012). Globalisation and global health governance: Implications for public health. *Global Public Health*, 7: Sup1, S54–62.

Lisk, F. & Šehović, A.B. (2020). Rethinking global health governance in a changing world order for achieving sustainable development: The role and potential of the 'rising powers'. *Fudan Journal of the Humanities and Social Sciences, 13*, 45–65.

Laverack, G. (2013). *Health activism: Foundations and strategies*. SAGE Publications Ltd.

Martin, B. (2007). *Activism, social and political*. In Anderson, G. L., & Herr, K. (Eds.) *Encyclopedia of activism and social justice* (pp. 20–27). SAGE Publications, Inc.

Mays, N. (2017). Interest groups and civil society in public health policy. *International Encyclopedia of Public Health* (2nd ed.) *4*, 296–303.

Moore, M., Yeatman,H., & Pollard, C. (2013). Evaluating success in public health advocacy strategies. *Illawarra Health and Medical Research Institute*. 390.

Morrice, E. & Colagiuri, R. (2013). Coal mining, social justice and health: A universal conflict of power and priorities. *Health & Place, 19*(1), 74–9.

Morrison, S. (2020). Media statement: 26 June. Retrieved https://www.pm.gov.au/media/national-cabinet- statement-0

Musolino, C., Baum, F., Freeman, T., Labonté, R., Bodini, C., & Sanders, D. (2020). Global health activists' lessons on building social movements for Health for All. *International Journal for Equity in Health, 19*, 116.

National Institute of Environmental Health Sciences (NIEHS). (2021). *Environmental health disparities and environmental health justice*. Retrieved https://www.niehs.nih.gov/research/supported/translational/ justice/index.cfm

North, D. (1991) *Institutions, institutional change and economic performance*. Cambridge University Press.

NSW Health (2016). *NSW public health training program*. Retrieved https://www.health.nsw.gov.au/training/ phot/Pages/default.aspx

Nutrition Society of Australia (NSA). (2021). *Applying for registration*. Retrieved https://www.nsa.asn.au/nsa- registration/applying-for-registration

O'Connell, E., Stoneham, M., & Saunders, J. (2016). Planning for the next generation of public health advocates: evaluation of an online advocacy mentoring program. *Health Promotion Journal of Australia, 27*(1), 43–7.

Public Health Advocacy Institute of WA (PHAIWA). (n.d.). *Local government policy awards*. Retrieved https://www.phaiwa.org.au/local-government-report-card-project/

Schneider, D., Evering-Watley, M., Walke, H. & Bloland, P.B. (2011). Training the global public health workforce through applied epidemiology training programs: CDC's experience, 1951–2011. *Public Health Reviews*, *33*, 190–203.

Stachowiak, S. (n.d.). Pathways for change: 10 theories to inform advocacy and policy change efforts. ORS Impact. Retrieved http://www.evaluationinnovation.org/sites/default/files/Pathways%20for%20Change.pdf

Stoneham, M., Vidler, A., & Edmunds, M. (2019). *Advocacy in action: A toolkit for public health professionals* (4th ed.). Retrieved https://www.phaiwa.org.au/wp-content/uploads/2019/09/2019_Advocacy-in-Action-A-Toolkit-for-Public-Health-Professionals-1.pdf

United Nations. (n.d.). Goal 16: Promote just, peaceful and inclusive societies. Retrieved https://www.un.org/sustainabledevelopment/peace-justice/

United States Environmental Protection Authority (USEPA). (2021). *Environmental Justice*. Retrieved https://www.epa.gov/environmentaljustice

Weible, C. M., & Sabatier, P. A. (2006). *A guide to the advocacy coalition framework: Handbook of public policy analysis*. Routledge.

Winslow CEA. (1920). The untilled fields of public health. *Science*, *51*(1306), 23–33.

World Federation of Public Health Associations. (2016). *The global charter for the public's health*. Retrieved https://www.wfpha.org/document-upload/the-global-charter-for-the-public%E2%80%99s-health.pdf

World Health Organization (WHO). (1986). *The Ottawa charter for health promotion*. Retrieved https://www.who.int/publications/i/item/ottawa-charter-for-health-promotion

——(2020). *WHO-ASPHER competency framework for the public health workforce in the European region*. Retrieved https://www.euro.who.int/__data/assets/pdf_file/0003/444576/WHO-ASPHER-Public-Health-Workforce-Europe-eng.pdf

World Health Organization Regional Office for Eastern Mediterranean (WHO EMRO). (n.d.). *Assuring effective health governance, public health legislation, financing and institutional support*. Retrieved http://www.emro.who.int/about-who/public-health-functions/effective-health-governance.html

Wyatt, K. (2021). *Applications open for remote store food security grants*. Retrieved https://www.indigenous.gov.au/news-and-media/announcements/applications-open-remote-store-food-security-grants

Zota, A. R., & Shamasunder, B. (2021). Environmental health equity: Moving toward a solution-oriented research agenda. *Journal of Exposure Science & Environmental Epidemiology*, 31, 399–400.

PART 2

Determinants of health

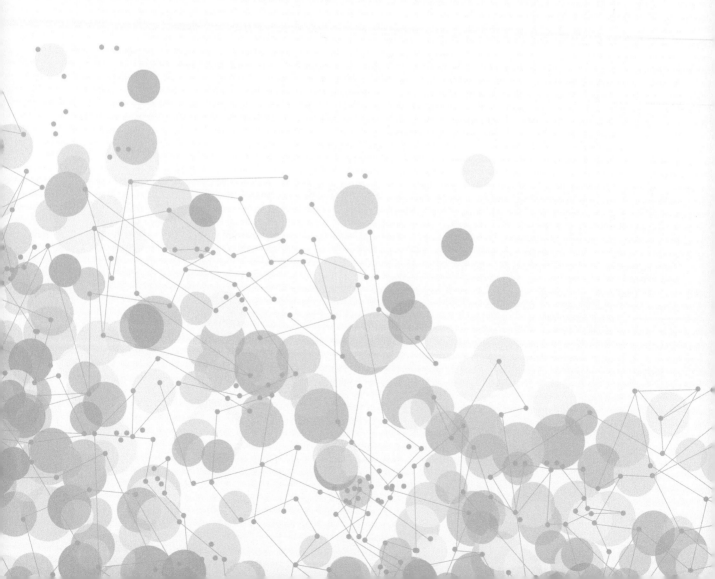

Social determinants of health

7

John Oldroyd

LEARNING OBJECTIVES

After studying this chapter, you will be able to:

1 describe the relative contribution of individual behaviours, the healthcare sector and structural determinants in the generation of health
2 describe health inequities
3 explore explanations for ethnic disparities in health
4 understand the concept of social justice
5 explain the social gradient in health
6 expound a key social determinant of health from *The Solid Facts*.

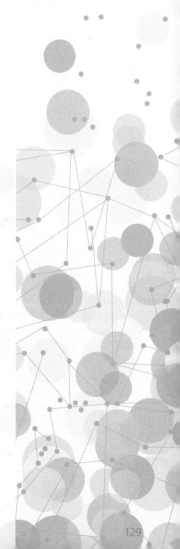

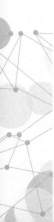

VIGNETTE

The social determinants of health at work – *Struggle Street*

Struggle Street (SBS On Demand, 2015) was a 'fly on the wall' Australian documentary series, broadcast on SBS TV in 2015. The series poignantly illustrated how individuals are only as healthy as the communities in which they live. What emerged from this series is that disadvantage clusters in individuals, families and communities. How do these inequities cause ill health? People who are unemployed are more likely to have poor housing and limited social support, which can lead to experiences of stress, anxiety and depression. They are also more likely have poor diets, to be inactive and smoke. All of which is linked to poorer health. Further, this disadvantage is often intergenerational. This means that children who experience poor parenting are likely to have little knowledge about how to parent well when they grow up. This complex web of factors is called the 'social determinants of health'. They include employment (whether a person works, where they work, the type of work they do, the stress experienced at work), early life experiences (maternal health, breastfeeding, parental attachment) and social exclusion (the lack of social supports). Addressing them involves developing healthy communities. By gaining employment, a person has income to purchase healthy food and to pay for educational and material resources. These material resources improve physical health and increase self-confidence, which improves mental health. Self-confident people are more likely to engage in health-promoting behaviours, to develop strong social networks and to have respectful relationships. Healthy adults are more likely to be better parents and provide a healthy start to life for their children who, in turn, will be better equipped to be good parents. *Struggle Street* was filmed in the western suburbs of Sydney. It provided an eye-opening glimpse of the social determinants of health at work in disadvantaged Australian communities.

Introduction

Evidence accumulates on a daily basis that health is generated by far more than individual behaviours. Individuals are members of communities. Geoffrey Rose (1926–93), a professor of epidemiology in the London School of Hygiene and Tropical Medicine in the United Kingdom, articulated the idea that an *individual's* risk of illness cannot be considered separately from the risk of the illness of the *population* in which the person lives. Rose suggested that interventions should aim to shift the entire distribution of risk by targeting whole populations (called a 'population strategy'). Social epidemiology has taken this a step further, suggesting that we can apply the distribution of traditional risk factors within populations to social factors such as social cohesion and socio-economic status (Berkman & Kawachi, 2000; see also Chapter 13). Thus, a person's social context becomes a determinant of their health. The implication of this is that the greatest benefits to population health will occur by improving the health of the *communities* in which people live. The degree to which people interact with each other, are integrated into society and support each other makes the community a healthy place to live. In turn, the health of communities influences the health of individuals living in the community. Today, the concept that health is influenced by **social determinants** is widely accepted. There is more and more evidence, using increasingly sophisticated measures of socio-economic status, pointing to the importance of the social determinants of health. Societies that support the most disadvantaged and are respectful of their indigenous peoples have better health outcomes. Improving the social context means that contemporary public health has to be cross-disciplinary, encompassing not only medicine, but also sociology, psychology, anthropology, ecology, urban planning, architecture, engineering, social work, political science and economics. This chapter introduces the social determinants of public health. It discusses the relative contribution to health of individual behaviours and the factors external to individuals, such as the healthcare sector and structural racism. Then it introduces the concepts of social justice and health equity, which underpin healthy societies. Finally, it introduces a social determinant of health that has been identified by key workers in the field as having a profound influence on health, namely unemployment. Spotlight case studies are provided throughout to give a practical understanding of the social determinants of health.

Social determinants of health – the social and economic conditions in which people are born, grow, live, work, play and age, and which influence their health, such as poverty, unemployment, civic participation and social relationships (World Health Organization, 2008).

SPOTLIGHT 7.1

Indigenous ways of knowing as a social determinant

Aboriginal and Torres Strait Islander people in Australia experience health disparities as a result of colonisation. How colonisation causes illness in Aboriginal and Torres Strait Islander people is suggested to be through historical trauma, comprising such things as intergenerational political disempowerment, loss of collective identity, genocide, forced separation of children and denigration of culture (Paradies, 2016). Addressing these continuing inequities is complex but involves non-Indigenous Australians forming genuine partnerships with Aboriginal and Torres Strait Islander peoples. The public discourse should approach these inequities with cultural humility, and should value and embed the knowledges and perspectives of Aboriginal and Torres Strait Islander peoples into Australia's social fabric, using a strengths-based approach. In 2017, a roadmap as to how to reduce inequities was provided by Aboriginal and Torres Strait Islander peoples in the form of the Uluru Statement from the Heart.

The Uluru Statement from the Heart was written by Aboriginal and Torres Strait Islander people who attended the 2017 National Constitutional Convention (Uluru Statement from the Heart, 2017). A key element identified in the statement is that they were the first **sovereign** nations of the Australian continent, a sovereignty that has never been relinquished ('ceded'). This sovereignty coexists with the sovereignty of the Australian government (the Crown). Here, Aboriginal and Torres Strait Islander people are speaking about power imbalances in relation to governance in Australia. Consistent with this notion, the document also calls for constitutional reforms that would empower Aboriginal and Torres Strait Islander peoples to manage their own affairs, and for the correction of imbalances in outcomes (e.g. incarceration and suicide).

Sovereign – having power or authority.

The statement also calls for a 'truth-telling' mechanism (a Makarrata Commission) that would permit sovereign Aboriginal and Torres Strait Islander nations to negotiate their own respective treaties and oversee a process of truth-telling. Similar truth-telling commissions have been established in Canada, Aotearoa New Zealand and South Africa.

Truth-telling is an important part of the healing process in which past injustices experienced by Aboriginal and Torres Strait Islander people are brought to light. Describing Aboriginal and Torres Strait Islander history, in an honest way, is an important step towards genuine reconciliation.

The statement also speaks searingly of the disproportionate representation of Aboriginal and Torres Strait Islander young people in the criminal justice system ('. . . our youth languish in detention in obscene numbers . . .'). It highlights that structural changes are needed to correct this (Uluru Statement from the Heart, 2017). These observations underline the urgency with which changes are needed.

The Uluru Statement from the Heart has set out a clear agenda for healing in Australia. It has been endorsed by the *Medical Journal of Australia* (Talley, 2018). In 2021, it was awarded the Sydney Peace Prize, in recognition that it offered a 'powerful and historic offering of peace' (Zhou, 2021).

QUESTION

What is meant by 'The public discourse should approach these inequities with cultural humility?'

Where is health created?

Public perceptions about where health is generated (that is, the determinants of health; see Figure 7.1) usually focus on individual behaviours (e.g. an individual's physical activity or diet, or their alcohol or tobacco consumption) or on healthcare systems (e.g. hospital treatments). However, there is increasing evidence that only about half of our health can be attributed to

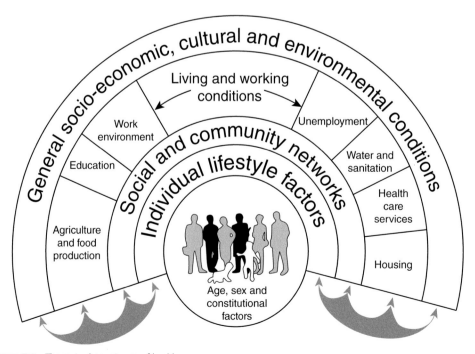

Figure 7.1   The main determinants of health.

Source: Dahlgren & Whitehead, 1991.

either the healthcare sector or to individual behaviours (Blue Cross and Blue Shield of Minnesota Foundation, 2010). This means that almost half of health is not due to causes that we often use to explain differences in health. Half is driven by forces external to the individual including education, work environments, unemployment, the built environment, government policy and other 'structural' factors. It follows that if we seek to address differences in health by improving the healthcare system or changing people's lifestyle choices alone, we only have the potential to influence about 50 per cent of health. To address the remaining fraction we need to go to higher-level factors, which are called 'structural determinants'.

SPOTLIGHT 7.2

How social movements such as #metoo have exposed structural determinants of health

What do we mean by 'structural determinants' of health? To answer this question, let's look at a social movement that has been highly visible in recent years, namely the #metoo movement. It has laid bare certain structural determinants of health.

The #metoo movement has its origins in the United States and on social media, when advocates sought to support victims of sexual assault. In 2006, sexual assault survivor and activist Tarana Burke first posted the hashtag #metoo on MySpace and later, in 2017, advocate Alyssa Milano posted on Twitter: 'If you've been sexually harassed or assaulted write "me too" as a reply to this tweet' (Garcia, 2017a). Their reasoning was that if all the women who had been victims of sexual assault identified themselves, the world would get a sense of how widespread the problem was. An avalanche of stories of assault followed on social media. The hashtag #metoo became a way for users to identify with the movement, to share their experiences of sexual violence and to stand in solidarity with other survivors.

The #metoo movement exposed structural power imbalances between men and women in society culminating in men getting away with sexually predatory behaviours against women. These imbalances are hidden; they are known as *structural determinants of health*, masked by overtures to equality such as well-publicised appointments of women to high-level positions of employment. However, underneath this, women continue to experience unequal pay, poor representation in the corporate and other sectors, and bear a disproportionate burden of responsibility for child care and family. Sexual abuse is a symptom of these imbalances. That men have not been held to account for the sexual abuse of women for so long has now been uncovered. The #metoo movement prepared the ground for allegations in 2021 about sexual harassment and sexual assault in the Australian Parliament House. The Australian government and others have made promises to examine the practices that have enabled it to be acceptable for sexual abuse to occur in workplaces. This coincides with the appointment in 2018 of a Sex Discrimination Commissioner, who is leading initiatives at the Australian Human Rights Commission, including the National Inquiry into Sexual Harassment in Australian Workplaces (Australian Human Rights Commission, n.d.). Power imbalances such as those that occur between men and women are structural determinants of health. They persist even after legislation to outlaw discriminatory practices and policies. People who are powerless have poorer health outcomes than those in power.

QUESTION

What does the #metoo movement mean to you? How do you think it can bring about meaningful, sustained change to structural sexism?

Health inequities

In 2008, the World Health Organization (WHO) published a seminal report titled *Closing the Gap in a Generation: Health Equity through Action on the Social Determinants of Health*, which described an investigation into the social determinants of health. The report identified that:

> ... the high burden of illness responsible for appalling premature loss of life arises in large part because of the conditions in which people are born, grow, live, work, and age. In their turn, poor and unequal living conditions are the consequence of poor social policies and programmes, unfair economic arrangements, and bad politics... (WHO, 2008).

The report cites examples of health differences that result from such poor policies. These examples cross all age groups and ethnicities, and affect rich and poor countries alike. They include outcomes such as the following:

a The life expectancy for Aboriginal and Torres Strait Islander men is 10.6 years less than for non-Indigenous men. Indigenous women can expect to live on average 9.5 years less than their non-Indigenous counterparts (Australian Institute of Health and Welfare [AIHW], 2017).

b Maternal mortality is three to four times higher among poor people, compared to the rich in Indonesia (WHO, 2008).

c There is a 2.5-fold difference in adult mortality between least and most deprived areas in the United Kingdom (WHO, 2008).

d A baby born to a Bolivian mother with no education has a 10 per cent chance of dying, while one born to a woman with at least secondary education has a 0.4 per cent chance of dying (WHO, 2008).

Health inequity – an avoidable disparity between health resources and outcomes across populations.

These differences in health outcomes are tragic because so many of them are avoidable. Differences in health outcomes that are avoidable are called **health inequities**. There is no biological reason for these differences. Health inequities are not just caused by the poor distribution of health care; they reflect deeper structural factors that shape the organisation of societies, such as poor government policies and unfair economic arrangements that enable imbalances to flourish. They can result in differences in health between countries, between cities in a country, and even between suburbs within a city. These structural factors are examples of the social determinants of health. They operate overtly within countries, supported by governments, as well as between countries as a result of globalisation. They are largely responsible for the health inequities experienced by large numbers of people throughout the world (WHO, 2008).

REFLECTION QUESTION

List two health inequities in the country in which you live. Why are they inequities?

SPOTLIGHT 7.3

Health inequities – the twin cities

Minneapolis and St Paul – referred to as the 'twin cities' – make up the largest metropolitan area in the state of Minnesota in the United States. The region is widely recognised as a national leader in health-related quality of life, with high household income, home ownership, educational attainment and access to health care. Unfortunately, the region does not do as well on issues of poverty, school performance and life expectancy. The proximity of good health and bad health, *within a few kilometres of each other,* is striking. Residents of the highest-income areas in the twin cities have an average life expectancy of 82 years, while residents of the neighbouring lowest-income areas have an average life expectancy of 74 years, a full 8-year difference (Blue Cross and Blue Shield of Minnesota Foundation, 2010). On average, every US $10 000 increase in an area's median income appears to buy its residents an extra year of life. In relation to educational attainment, mortality rates among 25–64-year-olds in areas where less than 12 per cent of the population has a college degree are about twice as high as areas with greater than 40 per cent degree-educated residents. These disparities are arguably avoidable and are examples of health inequities (Blue Cross and Blue Shield of Minnesota Foundation, 2010).

QUESTION

Disparities in the twin cities suggest that health is determined by living conditions in high-income and low-income areas. How could a poor neighbourhood be revitalised to break the cycle of poverty?

Ethnic disparities in health

Ethnicity, as used in epidemiology, refers to the 'group' to which people belong by virtue of certain shared characteristics. These include language, religion, culture, country of birth and ancestry. Ethnicity is best ascertained through self-identity, although this means it may change over time and in different settings. Ethnic groups are highly heterogeneous – ethnicity is personal – and this heterogeneity makes it difficult to account for the causes of ethnic variations in health. Despite these observations, there is considerable evidence of disparities in health by ethnicity in conditions as diverse as maternal care, coronary heart disease, diabetes and cancer. In the case of maternal care, for example, data from the United Kingdom suggests that, between 2014 and 2016, maternal deaths in pregnancy were 8 per 100 000 white women, 15 per 100 000 Asian women and 40 per 100 000 Black women (MBRRACE-UK, 2018). There are also ethnic differences in COVID-19 outcomes. For example, in the United Kingdom, infection and mortality rates have also been found to be much higher among Black, Asian and minority ethnic (BAME) communities than non-BAME groups (Fenton et al., 2021). In the United Kingdom, poor access to healthcare services among ethnic minorities have been documented and may account for some of these dispar-ities. However, there is growing evidence that the higher burden of these diseases cannot be attributed to differences in access to health care, or other factors such as genetic attributes, alone. The National Health Service is taking this seriously: in 2020 it announced that a Race and Health Observatory would be established to address the health inequalities facing people from ethnic minority backgrounds (Kmietowicz, 2020). Now, more than ever, it is important to find out why these disparities exist. Could it be that policies and processes in health care and other 'structures' account for the disparities in health seen in ethnic minorities? One such structure that has gained purchase within the Black Lives Matter movement is that of structural racism. This is best described within the paradigm of critical race theory.

Ethnicity, structural racism and critical race theory

Critical race theory is an analytic framework 'based on the premise that race is not a natural, biologically rounded feature of physically distinct subgroups of human beings but a socially constructed (culturally invented) category that is used to oppress and exploit people of colour' (Britannica, n.d.). The theory asserts that racial disparities reproduced by the legacies of historical racism can persist even after legislation against discriminatory racial policies and practices. The central premise of critical race theory is that racism is structural, rather than just prejudice harboured by individuals. In fact, *structural racism* is racial inequality embedded in structures in ways that individuals are very often unaware of.

The Black Lives Matter movement, which resulted in the biggest civil rights protests in American history, was sparked by the murder of a Black man in Minneapolis by white police officers on 25 May 2020. The movement is important because it has highlighted structural racism in law enforcement. A public institution, the police force, which is overwhelmingly a force for good, was enabled by structural racism to murder a Black man in plain sight.

The concepts of structural racism and critical race theory are not simply the domain of liberal journalism. In February 2021, the *New England Journal of Medicine*, a highly prestigious journal within the medical establishment, published a review titled 'How structural racism works – racist policies as a root cause of U.S. racial health inequities' (Bailey et al., 2021). The authors said that there is 'growing recognition that racism has a structural basis and is embedded in long-standing social policy. This framing is captured by the term "structural racism"' (Bailey et al., 2021). The article gave examples of structural racism, mainly in the United States, but also with wider applicability, namely 1) 'red-lining', which is segregation in residential housing on the basis of race, in which 'red lines' were drawn on maps to highlight communities with a high density of Black people, for the purposes of issuing home loans; 2) police violence; and 3) inequalities in health care. In relation to health care, historically people of colour have tended to be cast as more susceptible to disease than white people, and this characterisation persists to this day. For example, a study involving white medical students and junior doctors found that participants believed Black patients' pain to be less severe than that of white patients, which in turn influenced pain management decisions for Black patients (Hoffman et al., 2016).

The idea that societies are structurally racist is disputed by many groups (Donegan, 2021). Many politicians in the United States and the United Kingdom are vocal in their opposition and have banned the teaching of critical race theory in schools. In the United Kingdom, the Sewell Report from the Commission on Race and Ethnic Disparities concludes that structural racism 'did not contribute to poor health outcomes among ethnic minority groups during the COVID-19 pandemic' (Commission on Race and Ethnic Disparities, 2021). The report states that deprivation, family structures and geography, not ethnicity, are key risk factors for health inequalities (Commission on Race and Ethnic Disparities, 2021). This conclusion has been criticised by other health groups (e.g. the UK Royal College of Psychiatrists), who say that blaming disparities in mental health on families, rather than structures and policies, will be detrimental (Gopal & Rao, 2021). As public health practitioners we need to read the scientific literature and make up our own minds.

REFLECTION QUESTION

How is it possible for there to be disagreement in the scientific community about the presence or absence of a structural factor such as structural racism? Surely the 'facts are the facts' and are not open to interpretation?

Social justice

Health inequities, however they may arise, are a matter of social justice. Social justice refers to fairness and respect for the dignity of all people, concepts that are underpinned by human rights. It includes moral judgement (see also chapters 1 and 11). Traditionally, science has been very good at describing differences in risk factors and health outcomes from a perspective of moral neutrality, given the origins of science in describing 'objective' reality. It is more difficult, but important, to place a moral value on these differences. Morality refers to what is right or wrong. Spotlight 7.4 illustrates this point.

Social justice – the equitable distribution of benefits and burdens among populations.

SPOTLIGHT 7.4

The Forgotten Children report – a case of science versus morality

In February 2014, Professor Gillian Triggs, who was then president of the Australian Human Rights Commission, published a report on an inquiry into children in detention in Australia, titled *The Forgotten Children* (Australian Human Rights Commission, 2014). At the time of its release, 257 children were being held in detention, including 119 held on behalf of Australia by the island nation of Nauru. The report identified that children living in detention are at high risk of developing emotional and developmental disorders. Between January 2013 and March 2014, there were several cases among children in detention of self-harm, sexual assault by adults and starvation. Australia is one of the only countries in the world that detains the children of asylum seekers. Children may be held indefinitely if their parents are under investigation by the Australian Security Intelligence Organisation. *The Forgotten Children* report criticised the two major political parties and called for a royal commission into the continuing use of mandatory detention. The Australian government responded by calling for Professor Triggs's resignation, stating that the publication of the report was a 'blatantly partisan, politicised exercise' (Australian Human Rights Commission, 2014). Professor Triggs responded that the report's findings were based on 'credible and objective evidence' (Australian Human Rights Commission, 2014) and did not single out any one side of politics. Further, she said, the concern was not about who was responsible for mandatory detention – the policy has bipartisan support – but about the policy itself.

Professor Triggs threatened to sue the government, a threat that was subsequently withdrawn, as was the government's request for her resignation. This case illustrates the contentious nature of scientific research, particularly when it involves moral judgement. The report described the health disparities of children held in detention, and Professor Triggs also concluded that this was morally wrong:

> It is imperative that Australian governments never again use the lives of children to achieve political or strategic advantage. The aims of stopping people smugglers and deaths at sea do not justify the cruel and illegal means adopted. Australia is better than this (Australian Human Rights Commission, 2014).

QUESTIONS

Read the Foreword to the report, *The Forgotten Children*. What disparities are described? Which age groups of children are affected? Do you agree that the disparities are inequitable? If not, why not?

The social gradient in health

Social gradient in health – differences in measures of health due to social status and different access to, and security of, resources such as education, employment and housing.

Socio-economic status – a person's economic and social position in relation to others. It is traditionally measured by income, education and occupation. Measures of relative socio-economic disadvantage can be used to identify regions or communities that require greater funding and resources (Australian Bureau of Statistics, 2011).

The **social gradient in health** refers to inequalities in population health that are related to differences in **socio-economic status**. The social gradient results from different access to, and security of, resources such as education, employment and housing, as well as different structural factors. Its outcomes include that people who have less access to these resources (relative disadvantage) have worse health than those who have ready access to them. While unemployment itself is not a biological factor that causes ill health, unemployment results in low income, which is connected to such factors such as worse housing, less access to health services, lower health literacy, less-healthy diets and higher smoking rates. These factors are more strongly associated with illness. The social gradient is found in all population groups in all countries, irrespective of the instrument used to measure disadvantage.

The social gradient in health affects people in rich and poor countries alike. In developed countries, mortality rates vary in a continuous way along with the degree of deprivation. For example, Figure 7.2 illustrates the age-standardised avoidable mortality rates by 'decile' (that is, 10ths) of socio-economic deprivation in men and women in England in 2018 (decile 1 = most deprived; decile 10 = least deprived) (Office for National Statistics, 2018; Romeri et al., 2006). It is evident that those in decile 1 of deprivation (most deprived) have substantially higher avoidable mortality rates than those in decile 10 (least deprived). It is also evident that people in the *second-highest decile* of deprivation (decile 2) also have higher mortality than those in decile 10. In other words, there is a linear relationship between deprivation and avoidable mortality. Greater social disadvantage results in worse health. This is the social gradient. The steepness of the gradient differs between countries and may change over time (WHO, 2008).

The situation among people in poorer countries who have been disadvantaged by 'historical exploitation and persistent inequity in global institutions of power and policy-making' is more complex (WHO, 2008, p. 31). Most people in developed countries who are deprived are still wealthy by global standards. They have good sanitation, clean water, accessible education and relatively good food supplies. They will still be better off than the deprived in poor

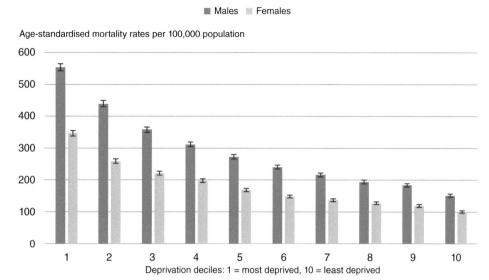

Figure 7.2 Age-standardised avoidable mortality rates by sex and decile, England, 2018.
Source: Office for National Statistics, 2018.

countries – the greater the social disadvantage, the worse the health. Countries in socio-economic transition (such as Bangladesh) are doubly affected: they have high rates of death among those of low socio-economic status and high rates of chronic disease in people of high socio-economic status. The causes of chronic diseases such as heart disease, cancer and diabetes are the same wherever these diseases occur, suggesting there is a need for a coherent framework for global health action (WHO, 2008).

SPOTLIGHT 7.5

Global vaccine equity – a case study of unequal access to COVID-19 vaccines between countries

By 1 November 2021, more than 3.9 billion people worldwide had received a dose of a COVID-19 vaccine, or 50.8 per cent of the global population (Holder, 2021). The global distribution of vaccines, however, illustrates how poorer countries continue to be disadvantaged relative to high-income countries (HIC). For example, the vast majority of vaccine doses has been administered in HIC (e.g. Australia, United States, United Kingdom have two-dose vaccination rates of 58–68 per cent, and booster vaccines (third doses) began to be administered by mid-2021) (Holder, 2021). In contrast, less than 2 per cent of people in many low-income countries – including in several countries in Africa – have been vaccinated (Feinmann, 2021). The reasons for this inequity in distribution include low-income countries not manufacturing vaccines locally and a lack of a cold-supply chain (most vaccines need to be stored in very cold conditions). Leaders of low and middle-income countries are requesting an overhaul of vaccine production 'to break the cycle of dependency on a highly concentrated global vaccine market' (Feinmann, 2021, p. 1). However, there are more immediate solutions, including that the oversupply of vaccines in HIC could fix the distribution problem relatively quickly. For example, in early 2022, several HICs including the United States, the United Kingdom, the European Union and Canada had 1.2 billion doses in excess, which could have been redistributed to poor countries (Feinmann, 2021). Global vaccine production continues in excess of requirements (1.5 billion doses per month). The resulting stockpiles are enough to achieve WHO vaccination targets. Clearly, this is not a supply problem; it is a distribution problem. We have the tools to bring the pandemic under control, if we share them fairly. 'Vaccine equity' will accelerate the end of the pandemic by increasing global population immunity, reducing the burden on the health care systems, enabling economies to resume trading and putting downward pressure on the emergence of new variants of the virus.

QUESTION
Do you think it is best to supply vaccines to poor countries at affordable prices, or to support them to build manufacturing infrastructure so they can produce their own vaccines?

A key social determinant of public health from *The Solid Facts*

The Solid Facts – a publication by the Centre for Urban Health at the WHO's Regional Office for Europe, edited by Richard Wilkinson, Professor Emeritus of Social Epidemiology at the University of Nottingham and Professor Sir Michael Marmot, Chair of the Commission on Social Determinants of Health, University College London.

A collaboration between the WHO Centre for Urban Health and the International Centre for Health and Society at University College London in 2003 resulted in the publication of a seminal document about the social determinants of health, entitled *The Solid Facts* (Wilkinson & Marmot, 2003). It included contributions from numerous scientists in the United Kingdom and provided a focal point for discussion about the social determinants of health and advancement of thinking on the topic. Importantly, it remains relevant today.

The Solid Facts identified 10 social determinants of health, namely the social gradient, stress, early life, social exclusion, work, unemployment, social support, addiction, food and transport (Wilkinson & Marmot, 2003).

Earlier in this chapter we reviewed the social gradient. In this section, we examine unemployment as a social determinant, as outlined in *The Solid Facts*. Students are encouraged to read *The Solid Facts* in its entirety for coverage of the other social determinants.

Unemployment

Neo-liberal economic policies, which encourage free markets, free trade, strong property rights for individuals and minimal government interference, have resulted in intensified global economic competition. This has, in turn, resulted in labour-market deregulation and increased use of flexible forms of employment. Other neo-liberal policies, such as the privatisation of industry and streamlining and outsourcing to cheaper suppliers, have also reduced opportunities for secure employment. Technology is increasingly used to perform many of the jobs that people used to do, thereby further reducing job security. In addition, although physical job demands are diminishing for many workers, there is growing complexity in work environments. Unskilled workers are particularly vulnerable to redundancy. This has been the case during the COVID-19 pandemic, when a high proportion of workers in service industries such as the hotel and food sectors, have lost work (Marmot et al., 2021).

These trends are occurring at the same time as businesses are demanding better health from employees, to maximise their output without necessarily investing in the health of their employees. These changes have modified patterns of employment, such that jobs are increasingly unstable and insecure. Research suggests that job insecurity is strongly associated with ill health. For example, a meta-analysis showed that workers in jobs with low security were about 20 per cent more likely to get coronary heart disease relative to those in secure jobs, even after adjustment for socio-economic circumstances (Virtanen et al., 2013).

Unemployment is an extreme form of job insecurity. It results in absolute poverty, with reduced financial means to purchase material goods such as food, clothing and other resources. This has direct, adverse effects on physical and mental health. Absolute poverty also results in debt and financial difficulties such as inability to pay for transport, telephone and utility bills. Eventually, absolute poverty results in social isolation and reduced means to seek employment. Unemployed people may relocate to cheaper areas to live but these tend to be poorer areas, resulting in a further 'locational' disadvantage.

Unemployment and job insecurity are chronic stresses. The longer they are sustained, the greater the ill effect. How might stress cause poor health? In healthy individuals, stressful situations result in the release of the hormone cortisol from the hypothalamus, as well as catecholamine secretion. These hormones cause an increase in heart rate, blood pressure and circulating glucose, assisting with the 'fight or flight' response; that is, they prepare us to deal with stressful situations. However, when stress is prolonged (that is, chronic stress), it is damaging to our health because psychological resources are diverted to dealing with the perceived constant emergency and away from processes that are needed for maintenance of health. The immune system is affected, and the person becomes more susceptible to a range of inflammatory conditions such as depression, cardiovascular disease, diabetes and obesity.

Unemployment is associated with increased morbidity and a 20–30 per cent excess mortality (Morris et al., 1994). Unemployment also has effects on mental health. Long-term unemployment (unemployed for one year or more) affects families and children. Children in these households are more likely to leave school early, have teenage pregnancies and be reliant on income support. Thus, there is a cumulative disadvantage in families of the long-term unemployed.

SPOTLIGHT 7.6

A case study of long-term unemployment – living on the breadline

Mike was a labourer on a building site. Four years ago, he fell from scaffolding while on a 'work for the dole' scheme. He was badly injured and, as a result, has chronic low back pain, is unable to walk far and has trouble with normal activities of daily life. This is a high level of disability for a 32-year-old. Mike lives in a caravan park with his long-term partner. After his housing costs are paid, Mike has $250 per week to live on.

Mike feels he is trapped in a cycle of unemployment. There are recurring appointments with agencies to find work, but he is not fit to work because of his disabilities and so feels this is futile. He has no choice as payment of his welfare benefits are conditional on providing evidence of seeking employment. Mike is unskilled, having spent most of his working life as a labourer on building sites, so even if he could work he does not have the skills or experience for many of the available jobs. The employment agencies also know the jobs they are presenting to Mike are not suitable for him but they, too, 'go through the motions'. Every fortnight Mike has these obligatory activities: IT training programs, volunteering, evidence of internet searches, mandatory training and so on, but all for jobs that disregard his disabilities.

Financially, everything is a balancing act for Mike, who is doing without now so that he can afford essential items later. He buys 'in bulk', as this means he will have food on the table, but bulk food tends to be of poorer quality. Hence, Mike is putting on weight, which he knows is not good for someone with back problems. Mike has so little to live off that he goes without many things. Purchasing alcohol is out of the question. He does not go to the movies or participate in normal social activities. He just hunkers down. The money he has must be used to pay for essential medical bills, transport to appointments, electricity and gas. He does not own a car and feels he will never be able to afford one in his current circumstances.

Mike is amazed at how dependent he is on the generosity of others. He stores furniture, his fridge and other household items in the garage of his partner's parents. He does not like being dependent on others but has no choice.

Among his circle of family and friends, no one directly criticises him but there is an unspoken stigmatisation of the unemployed. The welfare officers are ever-present, threatening to cut off benefits if he does not comply with the conditions of those benefits. Personally, Mike feels swept aside, in the 'too-hard basket', abandoned. He cannot make plans for a future. Starting a family is out of the question in his current circumstances. His partner is very patient and supportive, but their relationship is becoming increasingly strained. Mike is beginning to suffer bouts of depression and anxiety, adding further to his burden.

QUESTION
What are some of the health effects of long-term unemployment?

SUMMARY

This chapter has discussed salient issues relevant to the social determinants of health. These determinants are important factors that can influence the health and wellbeing of individuals, communities and societies. The determinants are summarised here.

Learning objective 1: Describe the relative contribution of individual behaviours, the healthcare sector and structural determinants in the generation of health.

Only a small proportion of health is attributable to either the healthcare system or to individual behavioural choices. A far greater proportion of health is due to factors external to individuals, such as employment, education and the environment in which a person lives. Structural determinants are the complex social, economic political systems that influence a person's health. Examples are the knowledges and perspectives of Aboriginal and Torres Strait Islander people and the power imbalances between men and women exposed by the #metoo movement

Learning objective 2: Describe health inequities.

Differences in health status that are avoidable are called health inequities.

Learning objective 3: Explore explanations for ethnic disparities in health.

There is evidence of disparities in health by ethnicity in many health areas. It is postulated that these disparities may be due to structural racism. This is best described within the paradigm of critical race theory, which is an analytic framework asserting that racial disparities reproduced by the legacies of historical racism can persist even after legislation to ban discriminatory racial policies and practices. Critical race theory suggests that racism is structural, rather than just individual prejudice. The medical establishment is increasingly recognising the role that structural racism has played in health care. The idea that societies are structurally racist is disputed by many groups.

Learning objective 4: Understand the concept of social justice.

Health equity is a matter of social justice: an approach that values human rights and that recognises the dignity of every human being.

Learning objective 4: Explain the social gradient in health.

The social gradient in health refers to the fact that inequalities in population health status are related to differences in social status and different access to, and security of, resources. It results in those who are disadvantaged having worse health than those who are advantaged.

Learning objective 5: Expound a key social determinant of health from *The Solid Facts*.

A seminal report on the social determinants of health, *The Solid Facts*, identified social gradient, stress, early life, social exclusion, work, unemployment, social support, addiction, food and transport as having substantial influences on population health. Unemployment has effects on physical and mental health and results in excess mortality.

TUTORIAL EXERCISES

1   Rank the importance of the social determinants in terms of their potential to influence health. Justify your ranking.

2   What government policies related to social determinants could be implemented to most dramatically improve population health?

3 Discuss the 'double disadvantage' referred to in countries undergoing socio-economic transition, in which disadvantaged people *and* the most well-off experience ill health.

FURTHER READING

Berkman, L. F., Kawachi, I., & Glymour, M. M. (2014). *Social epidemiology* (2nd ed.). Oxford University Press.
Blue Cross and Blue Shield of Minnesota Foundation. (2010). *The unequal distribution of health in the twin cities*. Retrieved https://www.wilder.org/sites/default/files/imports/BlueCross_HealthInequities_10-10.pdf
Marmot M. (2016) Boyer lectures on inequality and health. Retrieved http://www.abc.net.au/radionational/programs/boyerlectures/series/2016-boyer-lectures/7802472
Robert Wood Johnson Foundation. (2010). *Commission to build a healthier America*. Retrieved http://www.commissiononhealth.org
World Health Organization (WHO). (2008). *Closing the gap in a generation: Health equity through action on the social determinants of health. Final report of the Commission on the Social Determinants of Health.* WHO. Retrieved http://apps.who.int/iris/bitstream/10665/43943/1/9789241563703_eng.pdf

REFERENCES

Australian Bureau of Statistics. (2011). SEIFA 2011. Retrieved http://www.abs.gov.au/ausstats/abs@.nsf/mf/2033.0.55.001
Australian Human Rights Commission. (n.d.) Sex Discrimination Commissioner Kate Jenkins. Retrieved https://humanrights.gov.au/about/commissioners/sex-discrimination-commissioner-kate-jenkins
——(2014). The forgotten children: National inquiry into children in immigration detention. Retrieved https://www.humanrights.gov.au/our-work/asylum-seekers-and-refugees/publications/forgotten-children-national-inquiry-children
Australian Institute of Health and Welfare. (2017). Deaths in Australia. Retrieved https://www.aihw.gov.au/reports/life-expectancy-death/deaths-in-australia/contents/life-expectancy
Bailey, Z.D., Feldman, J.M., & Bassett, M.T. (2021). How structural racism works – racist policies as a root cause of US racial health inequities. *New England Journal of Medicine, 384*(8), 768–72.
Berkman, I.F., & Kawachi, I. E. (2000). *Social epidemiology.* Oxford University Press.
Blue Cross and Blue Shield of Minnesota Foundation. (2010). The unequal distribution of health in the twin cities. Retrieved https://www.wilder.org/sites/default/files/imports/BlueCross_HealthInequities_10-10.pdf
Commission on Race and Ethnic Disparities. (2021). The report. Retrieved https://assets.publishing.service.gov.uk/government/uploads/system/uploads/attachment_data/file/974507/20210331_-_CRED_Report_-_FINAL_-_Web_Accessible.pdf
Dahlgren, G., & Whitehead, M. (1991). *Policies and strategies to promote social equity in health.* Institute for Futures Studies.
Donegan, M. (2021). What the moral panic about 'critical race theory' is about. *The Guardian*, 17 June. Retrieved https://www.theguardian.com/commentisfree/2021/jun/17/critical-race-theory-republicans-moira-donegan
Britannica, The Editors of Encyclopaedia. (n.d.). Critical race theory. Retrieved https://www.britannica.com/topic/critical-race-theory

Feinmann, J. (2021). Covid-19: global vaccine production is a mess and shortages are down to more than just hoarding. *British Medical Journal*, 375, 2375.

Fenton, K., Pawson, E., & de Souza-Thomas, L. (2021). Beyond the data: Understanding the impact of COVID-19 on BAME groups. *Public Health England*. Retrieved https://assets.publishing.service.gov.uk/government/uploads/system/uploads/attachment_data/file/892376/COVID_stakeholder_engagement_synthesis_beyond_the_data.pdf

Garcia, S.E. (2017). The woman who created #metoo long before hashtags. *The New York Times*, 20 October. Retrieved https://www.nytimes.com/2017/10/20/us/me-too-movement-tarana-burke.html

Gopal, D.P., & Rao, M. (2021). Playing hide and seek with structural racism. *British Medical Journal*, *373*, n988

Hoffman, K.M., Trawalter, S., Axt, J.R., & Oliver, M.N. (2016). Racial bias in pain assessment and treatment recommendations, and false beliefs about biological differences between blacks and whites. *Proceedings of the National Academy of Science USA*, *113*, 4296–301.

Holder, J. (2021). Tracking coronavirus vaccinations around the world. Retrieved https://www.nytimes.com/interactive/2021/world/covid-vaccinations-tracker.html

Kmietowicz, Z. (2020). NHS launches race and health observatory after BMJ's call to end inequalities. *British Medical Journal*, 369.

Marmot, M., Allen, J., Boyce, T., Goldblatt, P., & Morrison, J. (2021). *Building back fairer in Greater Manchester: Health equity and dignified lives*. Institute of Health Equity. Retrieved https://www.instituteofhealthequity.org/resources-reports/build-back-fairer-in-greater-manchester-health-equity-and-dignified-lives/build-back-fairer-in-greater-manchester-executive-summary.pdf

MBRRACE-UK. (2018). Saving lives, improving mothers' care. Lessons learned to inform maternity care from the UK and Ireland Confidential Enquiries into Maternal Deaths and Morbidity 2014–16. Retrieved https://www.npeu.ox.ac.uk/assets/downloads/mbrrace-uk/reports/MBRRACE-UK%20Maternal%20Report%202018%20-%20Web%20Version.pdf

Morris, J.K., Cook, D.G., & Shaper, A.G. (1994). Loss of employment and mortality. *British Medical Journal*, *6937*, 1135–9.

Office for National Statistics. (2018). Socioeconomic inequalities in avoidable mortality in England: 2018. Retrieved https://www.ons.gov.uk/peoplepopulationandcommunity/birthsdeathsandmarriages/deaths/bulletins/socioeconomicinequalitiesinavoidablemortalityinengland/2018

Paradies, Y. (2016). Colonisation, racism and indigenous health. *Journal of Population Research*, *33*, 83–96.

Romeri, E., Baker, A., & Griffiths, C. (2006). Mortality by deprivation and cause of death in England and Wales, 1999–2003. Retrieved http://www.ons.gov.uk/ons/rel/hsq/health-statistics-quarterly/no-32-winter-2006/mortality-by-deprivation-and-cause-of-death-in-england-and-wales-1999-2003.pdf

SBS on Demand. (2015). *Struggle Street* (TV program). Retrieved http://www.sbs.com.au/shop/product/category/DVDs/11253/Struggle-Street-Digital-Download

Talley, N.J. (2018). The *Medical Journal of Australia* endorses the Uluru Statement. *Medical Journal of Australia*, *209*(1), 15.

Uluru Statement from the Heart. (2017). Retrieved https://www.referendumcouncil.org.au/sites/default/files/2017-05/Uluru_Statement_From_The_Heart_0.PDF

Virtanen, M., Nyberg, S. T., Batty, G. D., Jokela, M., Heikkilä, K., Fransson, E. I., Alfredsson, L., Bjorner, J. B., . . . Consortium, I.-W. (2013). Perceived job insecurity as a risk factor for incident coronary heart disease: Systematic review and meta-analysis. *British Medical Journal*, *347*, 14746.

Wilkinson, R., & Marmot, M. (2003). *Social determinants of health: The solid facts* (2nd ed.). Retrieved WHO http://www.euro.who.int/__data/assets/pdf_file/0005/98438/e81384.pdf

World Health Organization (WHO). (2008). Closing the gap in a generation: Health equity through action on the social determinants of health. Final report of the Commission on the Social Determinants of Health. WHO. Retrieved http://apps.who.int/iris/bitstream/10665/43943/1/9789241563703_eng.pdf

Zhou, N. (2021). Uluru Statement from the Heart awarded 2021 Sydney Peace Prize. *The Guardian*, 26 May. Retrieved https://www.theguardian.com/australia-news/2021/may/26/uluru-statement-from-the-heart-awarded-2021-sydney-peace-prize

Behavioural, nutritional and environmental determinants and public health

8

Jonathan Hallett, Gemma Crawford, Christina Pollard and Toni Hannelly

LEARNING OBJECTIVES

After studying this chapter, you should be able to:

1 describe key concepts informing behavioural change in health and the strengths and limitations of behavioural approaches in public health
2 identify the major nutritional determinants of health and discuss how they affect populations in low, middle and high-income countries
3 identify the major environmental determinants of health and discuss how they affect populations in low, middle and high-income countries.

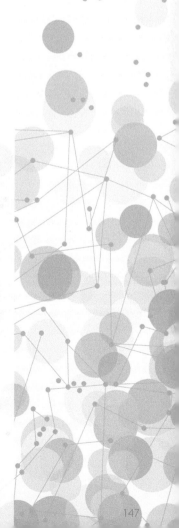

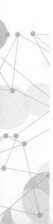

VIGNETTE

Behaviour and contexts matter: The case of non-communicable diseases

Twenty-year-old university student Emily lives in a metropolitan suburb of Perth, Western Australia, with a high density of new housing, young families and fast-food and alcohol outlets. Emily studies full-time and drives to university as public transport takes two hours. Petrol and other living expenses require her to work two part-time jobs. She rarely has enough time to cook the types of meals she would like, and finds it hard to shop to ensure there is fresh food in the fridge. When she finishes work and university at night, Emily is usually very hungry. Getting fast food for dinner from a drive-through outlet is cheap and convenient, and she saw on TV that they are getting healthier. At work, Emily spends most of her day sitting, often eating her lunch at her desk. There is often cake to celebrate birthdays and easy access to junk food and soft drinks in vending machines. Emily has gained weight since she started living out of home, and her friends are constantly talking about new diets. She gets frustrated when her mum tells her to use willpower to eat better, as she does try to buy low-fat and 'diet' foods when she can get to the supermarket. Emily belongs to a netball team but can no longer make it due to her busy schedule. She has thought about joining a gym but it costs so much and she's not sure if she could get there, anyway. There are no lights on her street, and Emily is concerned about her safety at night.

Over the past three decades there has been an unprecedented increase in the prevalence of non-communicable diseases such as cancer, cardiovascular disease and type 2 diabetes in many countries, including Australia. As the above scenario indicates, increasing urbanisation and cheap and widely available, energy-dense foods, combined with progressively more sedentary lifestyles and changing modes of transportation, create significant challenges for public health.

The causes and determinants of poor health are complex. Social norms, culture and environments influence individual behaviours, which in turn shape the health of a population. For example, food purchasing is an individual behaviour, but it is driven by certain contexts including pricing, marketing, industry influence, time scarcity and urban design. Responses that focus on an individual's responsibility to change their behaviour are palatable to governments and industry, but often neglect key determinants. Effective public health approaches interrogate not only behavioural risk and motivation, but also the broader environmental context in which those behaviours occur.

Introduction

Many factors influence the health status of individuals or communities and create health inequalities. They are known as 'determinants of health' (World Health Organization [WHO], 2004). These determinants can affect a person's health status positively or negatively, and include biological (e.g. age), behavioural (e.g. alcohol consumption), environmental (air quality) and social (employment status) factors.

The following conceptual framework highlights the many determinants that influence our health (Figure 8.1). Societal and environmental determinants can influence socio-economic characteristics, for example, which affect health behaviours and subsequently biomedical factors such as body weight, which in turn can affect overall health (Australian Institute of Health and Welfare [AIHW], 2014). The framework suggests that these determinants can help to inform our understanding of why different groups of people have different health outcomes. Many of these determinants of health can be influenced through interventions and healthcare measures to improve health and wellbeing (AIHW, 2014).

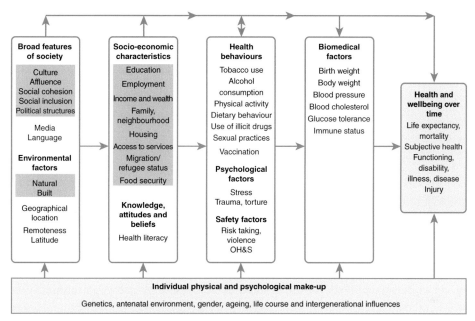

Figure 8.1   A conceptual framework for determinants of health.

Note: Blue shading highlights selected social determinants of health.

Source: AIHW (2014).

Behavioural determinants include a range of behaviours that may directly cause disease, such as tobacco smoking and alcohol consumption, while other determinants, such as socio-economic status, act further up in the causal chain (and may be thought of as 'causes of the causes'). It has been suggested that individuals have a certain level of control over some of the determinants (such as sedentary behaviour), while others are beyond an individual's control (such as environmental determinants like poor sanitation and climate change) (AIHW, 2014).

In reality, most determinants are the result of a combination of factors. Take, for example, **nutritional determinants of health**. Poor diet is often considered the result of individual choices and preferences. However, an individual's food choices are heavily influenced by social and cultural norms, which are shaped by food marketing and promotion, availability, affordability and access (Lawrence et al., 2019; Raza et al., 2020).

Determinants of an individual's health are fundamentally interrelated, and are often described as a 'web of causes' (AIHW, 2014); they are perhaps better termed as 'patterns of determinants' (Kindig & Stoddart, 2003) that cannot be addressed in isolation. Effective public health interventions therefore need to identify and understand individual behaviours, and also look further to wider determinants.

Interventions can be 'upstream' or 'downstream'. Upstream interventions address big-picture determinants at the levels of society and policy, whereas downstream interventions target individual determinants such as biological risk factors, lifestyle and education (Watt,

Behavioural determinant – a personal attribute or behaviour that influences an individual's risk of experiencing poor health.

Nutritional determinants of health – diet-related factors that affect human health, such as nutrition, food availability and access.

2007; Lorenc et al., 2012). Figure 8.2 provides examples of interventions along this spectrum. Upstream interventions address the structural determinants of health equity and have greater potential for reducing social inequalities (Watt, 2007; Lorenc et al., 2012).

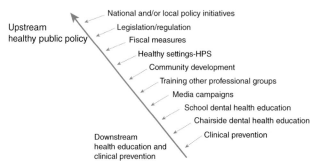

Figure 8.2   Upstream and downstream intervention approaches.
Source: Watt (2007).

As explored in Chapter 7, health is heavily influenced by our social structures that create inequalities and influence our available choices (Smith et al., 2018). A socio-ecological view of health (Whitehead & Dahlgren, 1991) focuses on both individual and population-level health determinants, which can only be effectively addressed by looking to domains external to the health sector, such as housing, agriculture and education (Fisher et al., 2017).

This 'ecosystem' situates the individual and their personal characteristics within their living and working conditions, the social and economic resources and opportunities available, and the built and natural environment (Figure 8.3) (Barton, 2005). Not all of these determinants have an equal effect on health outcomes. Some determinants may be affected by personal choices, while others require policy or structural interventions, which can take significantly more time to achieve and high levels of political will (Shi & Zhong, 2014).

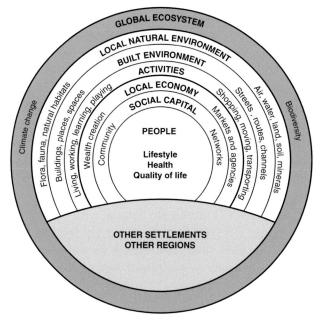

Figure 8.3   A conceptual model of the settlement as an ecosystem.
Source: Barton (2005).

Identifying the factors that influence health is important in preventing disease and promoting health. It is also necessary to differentiate the factors about which little can be done (e.g. age and genetic inheritance) from those that may be modified (e.g. built environments, social norms and individual behaviours). This chapter explores behavioural, nutritional and environmental determinants, and describes the different levels of influence of these on health outcomes, to illustrate key considerations when developing effective public health responses.

Behavioural determinants of health

Behavioural determinants of health encompass individual behavioural patterns that may increase or decrease the risk of positive or negative health outcomes, as well as personal attributes (e.g. values and beliefs) and personality characteristics (including emotional states) that underlie or inform these behaviours (Glanz, Rimer & Viswanath, 2015). These include risk or protective *behaviours* such as alcohol and other drug use (licit and illicit), dietary behaviours, breastfeeding or sexual practices; as well as *individual responses to health problems*, such as help-seeking, adherence to medical treatment and healthcare service use (NSW Department of Health, 2010). Traits, actions or exposures that *increase* the likelihood that an individual will develop a disease or injury are known as 'risk factors'. 'Protective factors' are those that *reduce* this likelihood (Murray et al. 2020).

Behavioural change

Motivation to engage in certain behaviours is not static, so behavioural change should be viewed as a complex process, not an event (Glanz, Rimer & Viswanath, 2015). The 'risk' of developing disease or incurring injury may motivate some individuals to change their behaviour. For example, some people may respond to road-safety messages about the risk of serious injury or death when not wearing a seatbelt while driving. However, many people continue to practise a range of behaviours even when they know that they can be harmful. Individuals vary in their perceptions, understanding and assessment of risk, depending on their personal experience and social context (Prestage et al., 2013).

Determining the factors that underpin an individual's decision to undertake a behaviour, or not, is important (Lobo et al., 2020). For example, over the past decade Australia has experienced an increase in HIV infection among immigrants and travellers (Crawford et al., 2016). Australian men who have reported acquiring HIV overseas, primarily in South East Asia, differ in their experiences and perceptions of risk. For some, infection has occurred because the cultural context provided extensive opportunities for sexual interactions that were previously unavailable. For others, greater risk occurred if a practice of inconsistent condom use in Australia was continued in a country with higher HIV prevalence (Brown et al., 2014).

Theories of behavioural change can improve our understanding of such complexities by explaining behaviours and suggesting ways to create or enhance change (Glanz et al., 2015). No single theory or model can explain human behaviour. Knowledge about the risks and consequences of a behaviour does not ensure that an individual will change that behaviour. The individual also needs to be willing to adopt a new behaviour and have the skills to carry it out. An environment that is health-enhancing and supportive makes this change more likely. Even when all of these elements are present, the individual may still choose not to change their behaviour (Egger, Spark & Donovan, 2013). Understanding the process of behavioural change and the context in which it operates is critical if public health is to better respond to complex health issues.

REFLECTION QUESTION

You find yourself sharing a lift with a public health policy advisor in the Department of Health. What would your 'elevator pitch' be to the policy advisor on the relationship between socio-ecological perspectives and health behaviour?

Health behaviour: A 'lifestyle choice'?

The use of the term 'lifestyle choice' to describe behaviours has often led to 'victim-blaming', and may distract us from addressing the root causes of poor health (Baum & Fisher, 2014). Victim-blaming occurs when individuals are solely held responsible for their poor health, instead of assigning responsibility to the significant environmental, social and systemic factors that affect health outcomes (Laverack, 2017). Health-promoting and compromising behaviours (Watt & Sheihan, 2012) are formed over time, and are deeply embedded within the individual's cultural and environmental contexts (National Institute for Health and Care Excellence, 2014) and history. They are not 'solely the result of current conditions and individual lifestyle choices' (Sundmacher et al., 2010, p. 2).

SPOTLIGHT 8.1

Online alcohol interventions for university students

Around half of Australian university students report binge drinking and that they experience greater alcohol-related problems than their non-student peers. These include individual harms such as academic impairment, personal injury and unintended sexual activity, harms to others (e.g. interpersonal violence) and harms to their institution (e.g. property damage, student attrition) (Tanudjaja et al., 2021). Men are more likely to experience 'public domain' consequences (e.g. aggression and property destruction) and women are more likely to experience personal harms, which frequently go unreported (Hallett et al., 2014).

University environments contribute to high levels of alcohol consumption. High concentrations of young people, many of whom have only recently been able to purchase alcohol legally, a shift of influence from parents to peers, the accessibility of cheap alcohol on campus, social events focused on drinking, and study-related stress all contribute (Hallett et al., 2014).

University students are typically reluctant to seek help for their drinking. Online services provide opportunities to address barriers to help-seeking (Pretorius, Chambers & Coyle, 2019). THRIVE, developed at Curtin University, is an online alcohol intervention that assesses individual alcohol consumption and provides personalised feedback. It comprises a hazardous-drinking score, feedback about individual risk, comparison to peers, alcohol facts and tips, and referral for medical and counselling support (Hallett et al., 2009). At Curtin University, THRIVE has reduced alcohol consumption among heavy drinkers and prompted students with a range of drinking patterns to seek help (Kypri et al., 2009). It has been rolled out in other institutions nationally and globally.

QUESTION

On their own, programs like THRIVE that focus on individual motivation may not eliminate harmful drinking behaviours among university students. Why might this be the case?

Nutritional determinants of health

Food is a basic human need, and access to adequate food – regular supply of safe, nutritious and affordable food – is a fundamental human right. People who regularly eat a nutritious diet are more likely to be healthy and have a reduced risk of diet-related chronic disease. Defining a nutritious diet is challenging because nutritional needs change over the life course (Black et al., 2013; Coulston et al., 2017) and also depend on factors including physical activity levels, health status and sex.

Dietary recommendations for populations

The strength of evidence for dietary advice for health and wellbeing is strong and increasing (Allman-Farinell et al., 2014). This has led the WHO to call for countries to develop food-based, culturally specific dietary guidelines and food selection guides based on the latest scientific evidence and the available food supply (WHO, 2004). Dietary guidelines provide credible and reliable dietary advice at population, local and individual levels, and provide the basis for nutrition education, programs and policies. They aim to prevent and manage diet-related chronic diseases including obesity, cardiovascular disease, diabetes and some cancers.

Generally, dietary patterns to promote health include eating plenty of vegetables including legumes and nuts, fruit and whole-grain cereal foods, moderate amounts of lean meats and/or meat alternatives, and reduced-fat dairy foods while at the same time limiting foods and drinks that are energy-dense and nutrient-poor (e.g. alcohol, sugar-sweetened beverages and foods containing added salt and/or sugar and saturated fat) (D'Innocenzo, Biagi & Lanari, 2019; Nanri et al., 2017; Miller et al., 2017; World Cancer Research Fund International, 2018).

Within a country, dietary behaviours tend to be relatively homogenous due to cultural norms and the available food supply. However, as countries become wealthier, a transition can occur, resulting in a double burden of malnutrition: the stunting of growth and deficiencies in essential nutrients alongside micronutrient deficiencies in obesity and increasing diet-related chronic diseases (Black et al., 2013).

Food environments

Food environments shape dietary intake and burden of disease. Modifying the external environment in which people live supports individual dietary change (Raza et al., 2020).

Food environment – the physical and social settings in which the cost and availability of food and its cultural associations influence what people eat.

An ecological approach can address the social, cultural and economic factors contributing to the formation and maintenance of dietary habits (Lang & Rayner, 2007). For example, the NOURISHING framework (Hawkes, Jewell & Allen, 2013) outlines policy options and actions to improve nutrition by focusing on:

- food environments:
  - **N**utrition labels
  - **O**ffering healthy foods
  - **U**sing economic tools
  - **R**estricting food advertising
  - **I**mproving the quality of the food supply and
  - **S**etting incentives and rules for a healthy retail environment
- food systems:
  - **H**arnessing supply chain actions to ensure health coherence and
- behavioural change:
  - **I**nform people
  - **N**utrition advice
  - **G**iving public education and skills.

Nutritional priorities

To achieve a food system that is safe, nutritious, accessible, secure and sustainable, key nutritional priorities include:

1 improving diet quality while reducing total energy intake to maintain a healthy body weight
2 good maternal nutrition and the breastfeeding of infants exclusively until around six months and then further for about six months as solids are introduced
3 ensuring a safe and sustainable food supply, and
4 **food security** (FAO et al., 2020)

Continuing action is required to address these priority areas at a population level, and also to assist those most in need. Government leadership and multisectoral action are required to create demand for healthy food environments that reduce the risk of overweight, obesity and related chronic diseases (Swinburn et al., 2015; Mason-D'Croz et al., 2019).

Food security – having physical, social and economic access to a sufficient quantity of safe, affordable, nutritious and culturally appropriate food that meets dietary needs and food preferences for an active and healthy life.

SPOTLIGHT 8.2

'Go for 2&5'

The United Nations designated 2021 as the International Year of Fruits and Vegetables. Increasing fruit and vegetable intake is considered the single most-important dietary change to improve health. The Western Australian 'Go for 2&5' fruit and vegetable campaign was a comprehensive social marketing approach to increasing consumption, currently used as a sponsorship message for sports and arts activities. Theory guided the campaign's development, and concepts were tested with target audiences; it was found that although improving nutrition was important, it was not the highest priority for consumers (Pollard et al., 2008).

The goal was to increase population-average fruit and vegetable consumption by one serve over five years, by targeting 'household food shoppers/meal preparers'. 'Go for 2&5' aimed to increase awareness of the need to eat more fruit and vegetables, improve perceptions of the ease of preparing and eating vegetables, and encourage increased consumption. It provided solutions for quick, easy, convenient, tasty and good-value meal preparation by integrating multiple strategies, through:

- high-reach mass communication (TV, radio, press, website)
- point-of-sale promotions
- publications/cookbooks
- school activities/curriculum resources
- sports and arts sponsorships
- FOODcents budgeting, shopping and cooking skills development program and
- uniting agriculture, health, education, retail, producers, and non-government organisations.

The World Cancer Research Fund International featured the campaign as a successful example for global food policy because of its potential for international replication. 'Go for 2&5' achieved its objectives (Pollard et al., 2008) with more than 90 per cent of evaluation respondents being aware of the campaign when prompted, significant increases in the proportion who knew the recommended servings and gave accurate perceptions of their own current intake, and increases in individual consumption, particularly for vegetables (Pollard et al., 2009).

QUESTION

Thinking about the elements of success of the 'Go for 2&5' campaign, how would you go about developing an approach to *reduce* the consumption of energy-dense and nutrient-poor foods (e.g. sugar-sweetened beverages, alcohol or foods containing added salt and/or sugar and saturated fat)?

Environmental determinants of health

When we talk about the environment in the context of human health, we are commonly referring to our surroundings and related external conditions, especially as they affect our lives. Access to clean water and air, safe food and a safe built environment are generally acknowledged as the most fundamental **environmental determinants** of health. These factors determine our likely exposure to potential hazards in our surroundings, and hence our very survival.

Environmental health determinants contribute to high morbidity and mortality across the globe, particularly in low and middle-income countries. The WHO (2020) estimates that 13 million deaths worldwide – one-quarter of the global burden of disease – could be prevented solely by making our environments healthier. The specific fraction of disease attributable to the environment varies widely across different disease conditions due to differences in environmental exposures across the regions. Generally, the per-capita disease burden from environmental factors is much higher in low-income countries; however,

Environmental determinant – an external factor or condition that affects human health, often beyond an individual's control.

for certain non-communicable diseases, such as cardiovascular diseases and cancers, the burden is greater in high-income countries.

Disproportionate effects

Vulnerability – the reduced capacity of an individual or group to withstand, adapt, respond and recover from the effects of natural or human-made hazards.

The effects of environmental hazards on human health are dependent on the **vulnerability** of the affected population. Environmental factors tend to disproportionately affect the impoverished and isolated. This includes those in low and middle-income countries as well as socially disadvantaged groups in high-income countries, such as Aboriginal and Torres Strait Islander communities in remote areas of Australia. These groups are less likely to have the adaptive capacity or resources to manipulate their environments to withstand hazards or to respond appropriately to minimising the continuing effects of environmental factors (Bertolatti et al., 2015).

The management of environmental factors that affect health has traditionally focused on areas of underdevelopment such as poor water and air quality, inadequate sanitation and waste disposal, unsafe food, presence of disease vectors, sub-standard housing and communicable diseases. While most of these factors have been managed with varying degrees of success in high-income countries, they continue to be major causes of morbidity and mortality in lower-income countries, where the WHO has estimated that up to one-third of death and disease is a direct result of environmental causes (Baum, 2016; WHO, 2020). Bertolatti and colleagues (2015) estimated that better environmental management could prevent 40 per cent of deaths from malaria by vector management; 41 per cent of deaths from lower respiratory infections by improving ambient air quality and phasing out the indoor use of unflued, solid fuel stoves; and 94 per cent of deaths from diarrhoeal disease by improvements in hygiene, sanitation and food and water quality. They also estimated that in children under the age of five, where almost one-third of all disease is attributable to environmental factors such as unsafe water and air pollution, the lives of 4 million children could be saved by preventing exposure to these environmental risks.

New hazards

While low and middle-income countries continue to struggle with fundamental environmental health problems, many countries, including high-income countries, are now faced with new and more complex hazards arising from the rapid development of new technologies, especially in the continuing search for new sources of energy (Baum, 2016). There is concern that technologies such as hydraulic fracturing (fracking), which is used to exploit sub-surface gas reserves, may potentially expose local communities to contaminated soil and groundwater. Overconsumption and unchecked exploitation of natural resources are also major concerns as the relevance of the environment to health appears to have become obscured, particularly regarding long-term integrity and sustainability (Baum, 2016).

Pruss-Unstan and colleagues (2017) note that, in addition to reducing the incidence of communicable disease, healthier environments could significantly reduce the incidence of non-communicable conditions such as cancers, cardiovascular diseases, asthma, musculoskeletal diseases and injuries. Increasing communally available greenspace in urban areas by the inclusion of parks, gardens and playgrounds has been shown to not only help reduce exposure to excessive heat, noise and air pollutants, but also to contribute towards improved mental and physical health by relieving stress and encouraging physical exercise (WHO, 2016).

A changing climate

Many countries are now affected by direct and indirect consequences of climate change. Environmental impacts range from mild fluctuations in weather patterns to potentially catastrophic extreme weather events that have the potential for significant health and social effects (National Climate Change Adaptation Research Facility [NCCARF], 2019). Increases in ambient temperature can lead directly to dehydration and heat stress, and indirectly to increased air pollution, thereby adversely affecting respiratory and cardiovascular health. Changes in local weather patterns, including temperature and rainfall, may alter the temporal and spatial distribution of mosquito breeding and hence mosquito-borne disease. The severity of the effects depends on a country's adaptive capacity, which is directly related to financial security, placing poorer countries in an even more vulnerable position. In places that already have unsafe water and air quality, a further loss of quality due to limited resources to prepare and respond could have devastating consequences (NCCARF, 2019). The challenge for the future is to reduce the unnecessarily high morbidity and mortality associated with both traditional and emerging environmental exposures.

REFLECTION QUESTION

Have you considered that climate change may have implications for public health? What are some of these implications in the Australian context? How does this differ from the global context?

SPOTLIGHT 8.3

Accessing essential services in remote Aboriginal communities to prevent environmental health related diseases

Dr Mel Stoneham and Scott MacKenzie - #endingtrachoma team, Public Health Advocacy Institute (Curtin University)

In 2013, the Australian Department of Health (2013) estimated that up to half of the health inequalities experienced by Aboriginal and Torres Strait Islander peoples can be attributed to poor environmental health (Department of Health, 2013). The burden of disease in these groups is estimated as 2.3 times that of the broader Australian population (Al-Yaman, 2017).

Many of these diseases are preventable and are related to poor environmental health conditions, particularly in remote communities. Living conditions such as overcrowding, inadequate facilities or equipment and poor hygiene all lead to a higher rate of hygiene-related diseases than in the wider Australian population (Foster & Dance, 2012). For example, trachoma is endemic in Australia and almost all cases occur within Aboriginal and Torres Strait Islander populations. Trachoma is caused by a bacterium, and is completely preventable, yet is it the world's leading cause of infectious blindness (WHO, 2006).

A Western Australian project, #endingtrachoma, aims to reduce the incidence of trachoma and environmental health-related infections in remote Aboriginal communities by building capacity in these communities and bringing services to the people. This is achieved by training and mentoring local Aboriginal Environmental Health Practitioners to conduct healthy home assessments and perform maintenance inside houses.

Like many environmental health-related diseases, trachoma arises from the inability to wash one's body and clothes. Consequently, the #endingtrachoma project focuses on safe and functional bathrooms and laundries. Aboriginal Environmental Health Professionals determine the effectiveness and safety of bathroom and laundry plumbing (health hardware). The assessment includes installation of mirrors at child height, coloured towels to reduce sharing, towel hooks, soap, light bulbs, hygiene packs and conversations with household members about the importance of how and when to wash their hands and faces. Minor plumbing fixes such as replacing shower heads, unblocking drains and replacing tap spindles are conducted. An important component of the healthy homes program is coordination with government to ensure that more serious plumbing issues are identified and reported.

QUESTION

Suggest reasons Indigenous people in remote communities may experience the same or similar health outcomes as populations in low and middle-income countries.

SUMMARY

In this chapter you have learnt about behavioural, nutritional and environmental determinants of health. Important issues regarding these determinants of health are summarised here.

Learning objective 1: Describe key concepts informing health behavioural change and the strengths and limitations of behavioural approaches in public health.

Behavioural change is complex and influenced by environmental, social, cultural and individual factors. Public policy plays a role in providing environments that are both health-enhancing and supportive of positive changes in health behaviours. Additionally, understanding the motivation to undertake a particular behaviour is important. Risk perception will vary depending on life experiences and also social contexts. Blaming or crediting individuals for their health status is unhelpful as many of these factors are outside an individual's control and work in combination to determine whether someone is healthy or not.

Learning objective 2: Identify the major nutritional determinants of health and discuss how they affect populations in low, middle and high-income countries.

Food is a basic human need and should be safe, nutritious and affordable. Nutritional requirements vary over the course of a person's lifetime, and there is considerable evidence that links diet to health. Regular consumption of a poor diet can lead to malnutrition or overweight and obesity, and diet-related health problems. The increasing wealth of countries also leads to the double burden of malnutrition involving growth stunting and deficiencies, along with increasing non-communicable disease such as diabetes, heart disease and some cancers. It is important to understand the influences on dietary behaviour at all levels, from the individual level (e.g. knowledge, attitudes and beliefs) to the food environment context (e.g. physical, economic, policy and sociocultural) when developing health-promotion interventions.

Learning objective 3: Identify the major environmental determinants of health and discuss how they affect populations in low, middle and high-income countries.

The fundamental environmental factors that determine our health are access to clean water and air, safe food and a safe built environment. When any of these factors are compromised, our very survival may be at risk. Environmental factors disproportionately affect those who are most vulnerable, particularly in low and middle-income countries, and marginalised groups in high-income countries. These groups are less likely to have the social or financial resources to modify or adapt their environment. Globally, we are now faced with environmental challenges arising from overconsumption and exploitation of environmental resources.

TUTORIAL EXERCISES

1   *Healthier choice, the harder choice*. Pick two health issues. List examples in which the environment has reinforced a health-damaging behaviour or might discourage people from even trying to engage in healthy behaviours. *Making healthier choices easier choices*. Pick two health issues. List examples in which the environment has encouraged people to engage in healthy behaviours.

2   Visit the NOURISHING policy framework (http://www.wcrf.org/int/policy/nourishing-framework) and read more about how to promote healthy diets and reduce obesity. Select one of the example policy actions listed and describe how this may lead to changes in health behaviours.

3   Discuss the following statement from Jackson (2017): 'If health promotion is a key strategy to address the Sustainable Development Goals, including the ones related to the ecological determinants of health, what are the actions that local health promotion practitioners can take?'

FURTHER READING

Australian Indigenous HealthInfoNet. (2021). (Website.) http://www.healthinfonet.ecu.edu.au

Australian Institute of Health and Welfare (AIHW). (2020). Australia's health 2020: In brief. *Australia's Health Series No. 17*. (Cat. No. AUS 232). AIHW.

Egger, G., Spark, R., & Donovan, R. (2013). *Health promotion strategies and methods*. McGraw-Hill.

Hawkes, C., Jewell, J., & Allen, K. (2013). A food policy package for healthy diets and the prevention of obesity and diet-related non-communicable diseases: The NOURISHING framework. *Obesity Reviews, 14* (Suppl. 2), 159–68.

Karr, S., Interlandi, J., & Houtman, A. (2015). *Environmental science for a changing world* (2nd ed.). Macmillan Education & Scientific American.

REFERENCES

Al-Yaman, F. (2017). The Australian burden of disease study: Impact and causes of illness and death in Aboriginal and Torres Strait Islander people, 2011. *Public Health Research and Practice, 27*(4), e2741732.

Allman-Farinell, M., Byron, A., Collins, C., Gifford, J. ,& Williams, P. (2014). Challenges and lessons from systematic literature reviews for the Australian dietary guidelines. *Australian Journal of Primary Health, 20*, 236–40.

Australian Institute of Health and Welfare (AIHW). (2014). *Australia's health 2014. Australia's Health Series No. 14* (Cat. No. AUS 178). AIHW.

Barton, H. (2005). A health map for urban planners: Towards a conceptual model for healthy, sustainable settlements. *Built Environment, 31*(4), 339–55.

Baum, F. (2016). *The new public health* (4th ed.). Oxford University Press.

Baum, F., & Fisher, M. (2014). Why behavioural health promotion endures despite its failure to reduce health inequities. *Sociology of Health and Illness, 36*(2), 213–25.

Bertolatti, D., Hannelly, T., & Jansz, J. (2015). Environmental health and safety: Social aspects. In J. Wright (Ed.), *International encyclopedia of the social and behavioral sciences*. Elsevier Science & Technology Books.

Black, R., Victora, C., Walker, S., A Bhutta, Z., Christian, P., de Onis, M., . . . Maternal and Child Nutrition Study Group. (2013). Maternal and child undernutrition and overweight in low-income and middle-income countries. *The Lancet, 382*(9890), 427–51.

Brown, G., Ellard, J., Mooney-Somers, J., Prestage, G., Crawford, G., & Langdon, T. (2014). 'Living a life less ordinary': Exploring the experiences of Australian men who have acquired HIV overseas. *Sexual Health, 11*(6), 547–55.

Coulston, A. M., Boushey, C. J., Ferruzzi, M. & Delahanty, L. (2017). *Nutrition in the prevention and treatment of disease* (4th ed.). Academic Press, Elsevier.

Crawford, G., Lobo, R., Brown, G. & Maycock, B. (2016). The influence of population mobility on changing patterns of HIV acquisition: Lessons for and from Australia. *Health Promotion Journal of Australia, 27*(2), 153–4.

Department of Health. (2013). *National Aboriginal and Torres Strait Islander Health Plan 2013–2023*. Australian Government.

D'Innocenzo, S., Biagi, C., & Lanari, M. (2019). Obesity and the Mediterranean diet: A review of evidence of the role and sustainability of the Mediterranean diet. *Nutrients, 11*(6), 1306.

Egger, G., Spark, R., & Donovan, R. (2013). *Health promotion strategies and methods*. McGraw-Hill.

FAO, IFAD, UNICEF, WFP and WHO. (2020). *The state of food security and nutrition in the world 2020: Transforming food systems for affordable healthy diets.* Retrieved https://doi.org/10.4060/ca9692en

Fisher, M., Baum, F. E., MacDougall, C., Newman, L., McDermott, D., & Phillips, C. (2017) Intersectoral action on SDH and equity in Australian health policy. *Health Promotion International, 32*(6), 953–63.

Foster, T. & Dance, B. (2012). Water washed diseases and access to infrastructure in remote Indigenous communities in the Northern Territory. *Water, 39*(4), 72–8.

Glanz, K., Rimer, B.K., & K. Viswanath. (2015). *Health behavior: Theory, research, and practice* (5th ed.). Jossey-Bass.

Hallett, J., Maycock, B., Kypri, K., Howat, P., & McManus, A. (2009). Development of a web-based alcohol intervention for university students: Processes and challenges. *Drug and Alcohol Review, 28*(1), 31–9.

Hallett, J., McManus, A., Maycock, B., Smith, J., & Howat, P. (2014). 'Excessive drinking – an inescapable part of university life?' A focus group study of Australian undergraduates. *Open Journal of Preventive Medicine, 4*, 616–29.

Hawkes, C., Jewell, J., & Allen, K. (2013). A food policy package for healthy diets and the prevention of obesity and diet-related non-communicable diseases: The NOURISHING framework. *Obesity Reviews, 14* (Suppl.2), 159–68.

Jackson, S. F. (2017). How can health promotion address the ecological determinants of health? *Global Health Promotion, 24*(4), 3–4.

Kindig, D. A., & Stoddart, G. (2003). What is population health? *American Journal of Public Health, 93*(3), 380.

Kypri, K., Hallett, J., Howat, P., McManus, A., Maycock, B., Bowe, S., & Horton, N. J. (2009). Randomized controlled trial of proactive web-based alcohol screening and brief intervention for university students. *Archives of Internal Medicine, 169*(16), 1508–14.

Lang, T., & Rayner, G. (2007). Overcoming policy cacophony on obesity: An ecological public health framework for policymakers. *Obesity Reviews, 8*(S1), 165–81.

Laverack, G. (2017). The challenge of behaviour change and health promotion. *Challenges, 8*(2), 25.

Lawrence, M, Baker, P., Pulker, CE, Pollard, C.M. (2019) Sustainable, resilient food systems for healthy diets: the transformation agenda. *Public Health Nutrition, 22*(16), 2916-20.

Lobo, R., Rayson, J., Hallett, J., & Mak, D. B. (2020). Risk perceptions, misperceptions and sexual behaviours among young heterosexual people with gonorrhoea in Perth, Western Australia. *Communicable Diseases Intelligence, 44*.

Lorenc, T., Petticrew, M., Welch, V. & Tugwell, P. (2012). What types of interventions generate inequalities? Evidence from systematic reviews. *Journal of Epidemiology & Community Health, 7*(2), 190–3.

Mason-D'Croz, D., Bogard, J. R., Sulser, T. B., Cenacchi, N., Dunston, S., Herrero, M., & Wiebe, K. (2019). Gaps between fruit and vegetable production, demand, and recommended consumption at global and national levels: An integrated modelling study. *The Lancet Planetary Health, 3*(7), e318–29.

Miller, V., Mente, A., Dehghan, M., Rangarajan, S., Zhang, X., Swaminathan, S., . . . Lopez, P. C. (2017). Fruit, vegetable, and legume intake, and cardiovascular disease and deaths in 18 countries (PURE): A prospective cohort study. *The Lancet, 390*(10107), 2037–49.

Murray, C. J., Aravkin, A. Y., Zheng, P., Abbafati, C., Abbas, K. M., Abbasi-Kangevari, M., . . . Borzouei, S. (2020). Global burden of 87 risk factors in 204 countries and territories, 1990–2019: a systematic analysis for the Global Burden of Disease Study 2019. *The Lancet, 396*(10258), 1223–49.

Nanri, A., Mizoue, T., Shimazu, T., Ishihara, J., Takachi, R., Noda, M., . . . Japan Public Health Center-Based Prospective Study Group. (2017). Dietary patterns and all-cause, cancer, and cardiovascular disease mortality in Japanese men and women: The Japan public health center-based prospective study. *PloS One, 12*(4), e0174848.

National Climate Change Adaptation Research Facility. (2019). Retrieved http://www.nccarf.edu.au

National Institute for Health and Care Excellence (NICE). (2014). Behaviour change: Individual approaches. *NICE Public Health Guideline PH49*. NICE.

NSW Department of Health. (2010). *Public health classifications project: Determinants of health. Phase Two: Final Report*. Retrieved http://www.health.nsw.gov.au/hsnsw/Publications/classifications-project.pdf

Pollard, C., Miller, M., Woodman, R. J., Meng, R., & Binns, C. (2009). Changes in knowledge, beliefs, and behaviors related to fruit and vegetable consumption among Western Australian adults from 1995 to 2004. *American Journal of Public Health*, *99*(2), 355–61.

Pollard, C. M., Miller, M. R., Daly, A. M., Crouchley, K. E., O'Donoghue, K. J., Lang, A. J., & Binns, C. W. (2008). Increasing fruit and vegetable consumption: Success of the Western Australian Go for 2&5 campaign. *Public Health Nutrition*, *11*(3), 314–20.

Prestage, G., Brown, G., Down, I., Jin, F., & Hurley, M. (2013). It's hard to know what is a risky or not a risky decision. Gay men's beliefs about risk during sex. *AIDS Behavior*, *17*, 1352–61.

Pretorius, C., Chambers, D., & Coyle, D. (2019). Young people's online help-seeking and mental health difficulties: Systematic narrative review. *Journal of medical Internet research*, *21*(11), e13873.

Pruss-Ustun, A., Wolf, J. Corvalan, C., Neville, T., Bos, R., & Neira, M. (2017). Diseases due to unhealthy environments: an updated estimate of the global burden of disease attributable to environmental determinants of health. *Journal of Public Health*, *39*(3), 464–75.

Raza, A., Fox, E. L., Morris, S. S., Kupka, R., Timmer, A., Dalmiya, N., & Fanzo, J. (2020). Conceptual framework of food systems for children and adolescents. *Global Food Security*, *27*, 100436.

Shi, Y., & Zhong, S. (2014). From genomes to societies: A holistic view of determinants of human health. *Current Opinion in Biotechnology*, *28*, 134–12.

Smith, J., Griffiths, K., Judd, J., Crawford, G., D'Antoine, H., Fisher, M., Bainbridge, R., & Harris, P. (2018). Ten years on from the World Health Organization Commission of Social Determinants of Health: Progress or procrastination? *Health Promotion Journal of Australia*, *29*(1), 3–7.

Sundmacher, L., Scheller-Kreinsen, D., & Busse, R. (2010). The wider determinants of inequalities in health: A decomposition analysis. *International Journal for Equity in Health*, *10*(30), 1–13.

Swinburn, B., Kraak, V., Rutter, H., Vandevijvere, S., Lobstein, T., Sacks, G., ... & Magnusson, R. (2015). Strengthening of accountability systems to create healthy food environments and reduce global obesity. *The Lancet*, *385*(9986), 2534–2545.

Tanudjaja, S. A., H. J. Chih, S. Burns, G. Crawford, J. Hallett, and J. Jancey. (2021). Alcohol consumption and associated harms among university students in Australia: Findings from a cross-sectional study. *Health Promotion Journal of Australia*, *32*(2), 258–63.

Watt, R. (2007). From victim blaming to upstream action: Tackling the social determinants of oral health inequalities. *Community Dentistry and Oral Epidemiology*, *35*, 1–11.

Watt, R., & Sheihan, A. (2012). Integrating the common risk factor approach into a social determinants framework. *Community Dentistry and Oral Epidemiology*, *40*(4), 289–96.

Whitehead, M., & Dahlgren, G. (1991). *Policies and strategies to promote social equity in health. Background document to WHO – Strategy paper for Europe*. Institute for Future Studies.

World Cancer Research Fund International (2018). *Diet, nutrition, physical activity, and cancer: A global perspective: A summary of the third expert report*. Retrieved https://www.wcrf.org/wp-content/uploads/2021/02/Summary-of-Third-Expert-Report-2018.pdf

World Health Organization (WHO). (2020). *WHO global strategy on health, environment and climate change: the transformation needed to improve lives and well-being sustainably through healthy environments*. WHO. Retrieved https://apps.who.int/iris/bitstream/handle/10665/331959/9789240000377-eng.pdf?sequence=1&isAllowed=y

——(2006). *WHO Alliance for the Global Elimination of Blinding Trachoma by 2020. Making progress toward the global elimination of blinding trachoma.* WHO.

——(2004). *Global strategy on diet. Physical activity and health World Health Assembly 2002 (Resolution WHA55.23).* WHO.

——(2016) Urban green spaces and health: A review of evidence. Retrieved https://www.euro.who.int/__data/assets/pdf_file/0005/321971/Urban-green-spaces-and-health-review-evidence.pdf

9

Individual decision-making in public health

John Bidewell

LEARNING OBJECTIVES

After studying this chapter, you should be able to:

1 distinguish between social and individual determinants of health
2 explain how perceptions, emotions and thoughts contribute to personal decisions influencing health
3 describe major theories of individual behaviour and choice
4 explain how theories of individual behaviour and choice can inform public health campaigns
5 identify limitations to targeting personal choice as a means to improving public health.

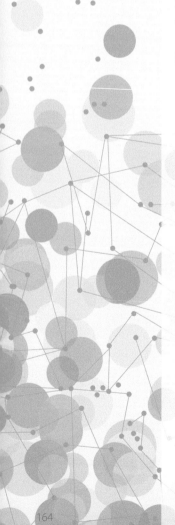

VIGNETTE

Individual behaviour during epidemics and pandemics

On 5 June 1981, the first case of AIDS was identified (HIV.gov, 2021). Since then, almost 35 million people have died of HIV/AIDS. In 2020, more than 30 million people were living with HIV (UNAIDS, 2021). The HIV/AIDS epidemic saw public health become politically important and a focus of media attention, everyday conversation and personal relevance. Public health initiatives to combat HIV/AIDs included media messages to modify perceptions of risk and to change individuals' behaviours (BFI.org, 2016).

On 31 December 2019, the World Health Organization (WHO) became aware of pneumonia cases in Wuhan province, China, now known as COVID-19 and eventually classed as a global pandemic (WHO, 2020a). By mid-June 2021, more than 177 million cases of COVID-19 were confirmed worldwide, along with 4 million deaths (WHO, 2021). Public health again became politically, socially and personally important.

Both HIV/AIDs and COVID-19 are contagious viral diseases. Decisions made by individuals affect the spread of both diseases and, therefore, public health. Unlike HIV/AIDS, transmission of the COVID-19 can occur from a distance, through aerosol spray droplets dispersed by infected persons, or through contact with contaminated surfaces (WHO, 2020b). While public cooperation is essential to preventing both HIV/AIDS and COVID-19, preventing COVID-19 imposes more compromises on everyday life and, in this regard, presents an even more difficult problem than HIV/AIDS. To reduce the toll from these diseases, public health policy must aim to reduce incidence (i.e. new cases) by modifying individual behaviours.

People's choices and actions remain crucial to controlling a great many infectious diseases and numerous other illnesses, including common non-infectious chronic conditions associated with life-style choices. The challenge for public health to enable people to change their habits and adopt new behaviours to protect their own and others' health. Effective public health practice therefore requires an understanding of how individuals make decisions affecting their health.

Introduction

A person's geographic, social and economic circumstances affect their health and life expectancy. These factors are referred to as 'social determinants'. Social determinants are difficult for individuals to change. Not everyone can move to an affluent, well-serviced area. Nor can everyone work under ideal conditions or spend large amounts on health care. Many social determinants of health can be addressed only through collective action, such as by governments.

This chapter looks at another influence on public health: the choices each of us makes. While we cannot personally improve the quality of air we breathe in our neighbourhood, we can choose whether to smoke. Office workers may spend their working lives in sedentary jobs, but they can choose to exercise in their spare time. The choices people make influence their health and the health of others.

Public health interventions such as campaigns asking people to eat better, exercise more, quit smoking and take care on the roads assume that people will modify their behaviour in response to warnings and advice. This assumption is questionable. People routinely ignore health messages. Despite warnings on cigarette packets, many people continue to smoke. Poor dietary choices are plainly visible every day in shopping trolleys passing through supermarket checkouts.

To change people's behaviour we need to understand how and why people make choices that may be good or bad for their health. That is why models of individual behavioural choice are described in this chapter. The chapter also considers whether people are truly free to make their own choices, or whether individual decisions are at least partly determined socially.

Social and individual determinants of health

Enjoying a long and healthy life requires more than luck. Social determinants and biological factors do not account for all inequalities in health. McGinnis and colleagues (2002) write that 'The daily choices we make with respect to diet, physical activity, and sex; the substance abuse and addictions to which we fall prey; our approach to safety; and our coping strategies in confronting stress are all important determinants of health' (p. 82). Distinguishing between social and individual determinants does not mean that one is more important than the other. Instead, we should think of individual behaviours as occurring within a wider social and physical environment (Bronfenbrenner, 1992). The individual has choices, although these choices may be influenced or constrained by the person's social and physical environments and their financial situation.

SPOTLIGHT 9.1

Valentina wears a face mask to protect others

Valentina, aged in her 20s, volunteers to deliver groceries to elderly residents in her neighbourhood. Valentina has seen media information showing COVID-19 as a disease mostly contracted by young people and especially young females (highest incidence), while being most dangerous for old people and especially older males (highest case-fatality rate). Valentina considers herself to be at increased risk of COVID-19, yet she regards her risk of serious illness to be low. Despite the low perceived risk to herself, and the cost, inconvenience and unattractiveness of face masks, Valentina wears a mask to protect herself and the older persons whose homes she visits on her delivery rounds.

QUESTIONS

1   If Valentina chooses to wear a face mask to protect herself and others, why do so many other people choose not to wear a face mask in public? Rather than answer simply by labelling people according to their choices – for example, describing some people as 'selfish' – try instead to explain the different decisions.

2 What public health message, if any, could encourage more people to follow expert advice and recommendations to protect their health?

3 What other challenges, beyond COVID-19, require decisions by individuals to improve public health?

Perceptions, cognition, affect and choice

To understand personal choices related to health we should start by examining how individuals make decisions. Figure 9.1 shows how various factors combine to influence people's voluntary choices. Three influences on behaviour are:

1 *Perceptions* – what we see, hear and touch; information about the world. Perceptions include observations of society: what family, friends and influential people are saying and doing, and what happens to them; also, what is expected behaviour according to law and social convention.

2 *Affect* – the emotional reactions a person experiences. Emotions are internally generated in response to perceptions, experiences, cognitions and other emotions.

3 *Cognitions* – the thoughts, knowledge, ideas and beliefs a person holds. Cognitions are internally generated in response to experiences, emotions and other cognitions.

The arrows in Figure 9.1 show how perceptions, thoughts and emotions affect each other. Choices arise from the way our perceptions are processed and acted upon through our thoughts and emotions.

Perception – becoming aware of the external world through the senses. Can also mean awareness of one's own thoughts, emotions or internal states such as pain.

Affect – a person's emotional response; feelings in response to an event. Similarly, affective, meaning emotional. Not to be confused with the verb *to affect*, which means to influence something.

Cognition – thinking; gaining knowledge or understanding from thought processes.

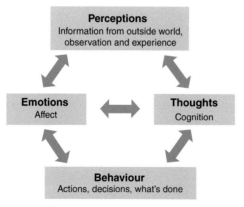

Figure 9.1 Psychological influences on behaviour.

Figure 9.1 provides basic ideas supporting the more elaborate theories of individual behaviour discussed in this chapter. When learning about theories of individual behaviour, you will see (with a single exception: behaviourism) how perceptions, thoughts and emotion influence choices that, in turn, lead to better or worse health outcomes.

REFLECTION QUESTION

In making decisions affecting health, such as what to eat, how much exercise to get and following other public health advice, do people rely more on their immediate, intuitive ideas that may be emotionally driven, or do they use careful reasoning and choose their actions based on predictions about the immediate and future consequences?

Theories of individual behaviour

Theory – an explanation, model, or system of ideas explaining how or why events happen. Scientific theories enable prediction or control of events.

A **theory** attempts to explain how and why events happen as they do. Good theories support accurate predictions about what will happen under known background conditions. This section introduces theories about why and how people choose between available options. Each theory offers insights into health-related decisions. When exploring these theories, consider how well each theory explains people's health-related behaviour, and how each theory could be applied to public health programs. If we understand how and why people choose healthy or unhealthy options, we as public health practitioners are better able to influence those choices, so people choose more for their long-term interests. It has been said that there is nothing more practical than a good theory.

Behaviourism

Behaviourism – a method of studying behaviour without reference to thoughts and emotions or unconscious processes; it looks at how experiences shape behaviour through associations between events that affect the person and the rewards and punishments resulting from personal actions.

Figure 9.1 shows that behaviour occurs through interactions between perceptions, affect and cognition. **Behaviourism** takes a more restricted view. Behaviourism (Watson, 2017) draws direct links between the environment and behaviour without intervening thoughts and emotions. Thoughts, emotions or other internal, invisible mental processes ('the mind') are excluded from the behaviourist model.

For the behaviourist, individual behaviour arises through learning from experience. Through experience we learn that some events happen together, often depending on what we do. These experiences and our responses can be rewarding or unrewarding, which influences how we respond to similar events in future. We learn from pleasant and unpleasant incidents, and from the consequences of our actions. Learning in this way is known as **conditioning**.

Conditioning – in behaviourism, learning or acquiring behaviours through observed connections between events, and rewards or punishments in response to actions.

The environment shapes behaviour through:

- *Classical conditioning.* The individual passively learns a response to a repeated experience. Smokers trying to quit may experience cravings in situations they associate with smoking, such as after meals or when drinking coffee, or in places matched to smoking such as public bars.
- *Operant conditioning.* The person responds to a signal from the environment and receives rewarding or unrewarding feedback linked to their behaviour. Behaviours that are rewarded will be *reinforced* (encouraged), so they are repeated more often in future. Behaviours that go unrewarded are suppressed. Different types of operant conditioning are recognised:

- *Positive reinforcement*. The behaviour is followed by a positive experience. Foods high in fat, sugar and salt are often pleasurable to eat and reward increased consumption.
- *Negative reinforcement*. The behaviour is reinforced by removal of a disagreeable experience. Smoking reduces unpleasant nicotine cravings, so smoking is rewarded.
- *Punishment*. The behaviour is followed by an unpleasant experience, and discourages behaviour. Monetary fines and license suspensions for dangerous driving are examples. An exercise routine that makes a person feel mostly pain and exhaustion will likely be abandoned.

Consistent with behaviourism is the claim that unhealthy habits develop and persist because the habits are quickly rewarded; for example, the pleasant taste sensation experienced immediately from sugary foods and drinks. The health penalties, such as tooth decay and obesity, are delayed. Healthier habits are adopted only if they are rewarded more strongly or even more quickly than unhealthy habits.

Public health interventions aimed at modifying people's actions by altering the rewards and punishments associated with their behaviour are behaviourist. Thoughts or emotions that promote and maintain behaviours are not explicitly addressed. Examples of behaviourist approaches to public health practice include:

- Penalising individuals or organisations, including businesses, for failing to use distancing or personal protection such as face masks in accordance with regulations aimed at suppressing COVID-19.
- Removing tobacco products from display in public, thereby reducing visible information that encourages an unplanned purchase.
- High taxes on alcohol and tobacco products, making them more expensive, and thus encouraging people to reduce or stop consumption.
- Reducing vehicle insurance premiums to reward safe drivers.
- Requiring complete vaccination before access to child care is permitted (Fraser et al., 2016).

Behavioural methods are practical as public health interventions only when:

- The connection between events, actions and their consequences are obvious and meaningful to people.
- Rewards and punishments are experienced repeatedly, quickly and consistently.

Behaviourism argues that the environment shapes behaviour. However, behaviourism does not identify other specific reasons for healthy and unhealthy choices, such as social influences, cultural or economic context; indeed, many social determinants of health, and people's complex thinking and emotions.

Social learning theory

Bandura (1977) writes that 'Human functioning would be exceedingly inefficient, not to mention dangerous, if behaviour were controlled only by directly experienced consequences. Fortunately, people can profit greatly by the experiences of others' (p. 24). In these two sentences, Bandura contrasts **social learning** with behaviourism. Bandura argues that patterns of behaviour are acquired vicariously, through observation without involvement; that is, by seeing what other people do and noting what happens to them as a result of their actions.

Social learning – learning from observation or the experience of other people and what happens to them; includes passive learning through observation, followed by imitation.

Observational learning is central to social learning theory. Observational learning involves *modelling*, by which a person serves as a *role model* influencing other people's cognitions, emotions and actions (Bandura, 1996). If, upon entering a shopping centre, you put on your face mask only because most other people you see are also wearing face marks, you are conforming with other people through observation alone, consistent with social learning theory and not because of rewards, punishments or conditioning. Among the factors affecting observational learning are:

- People acting only upon what they observe.
- People acting only upon what they remember.
- People adopting only behaviours of which they are capable.
- People adopting behaviours only if those behaviours are perceived as personally cost-effective (Bandura, 2008; McLeod, 2016).

Self-efficacy – a person's belief in their ability to do something; confidence in the belief that one can perform an action.

The concept of **self-efficacy** ties in with social learning theory. Self-efficacy is about a person feeling able to perform a specific action. Persons high in self-efficacy feel more competent to perform a given task compared with others low in self-efficacy. Self-efficacy promotes action to protect or improve health. For example, Ahn and Oh (2018) found a positive association between self-efficacy and protective behaviours against falls among a sample of elderly women at high risk of falls and fracture due to osteoporosis.

Locus of control – belief that one's own behaviour and the results of that behaviour are within one's own control (internal locus), as opposed to control by outside agencies (external locus).

Locus of control is another aspect of social learning theory. A person with an *internal locus of control* towards health will perceive themselves as responsible for their own health. Someone with an *external locus of control* will consider luck, destiny or other outside forces beyond their control as determining their future health. Amit Aharon and colleagues (2018) found that internal locus of control, along with a belief in the importance of luck and the influence of powerful others, predicted parents' full compliance with childhood immunisation schedules.

Social learning theory is important for public health because it maintains that people will adopt healthy behaviours if they observe those behaviours being rewarded and valued among significant people, and if the observers believe themselves capable and responsible for maintaining or improving their own health. Role models for healthy choices can include family, friends and the wider community, as well as admired public figures: leaders, celebrities, sporting identities and fictional heroes.

Transtheoretical model – stages of change

Public health programs directed at individuals try to persuade people to change from unhealthy to healthy behaviours. The transtheoretical model of behaviour change (Prochaska & Velicer, 1997) argues that behavioural change occurs in stages rather than instantly. A sequence of six stages for health-related behavioural change is identified:

1 *Precontemplation* – before the person even considers changing their behaviour.
2 *Contemplation* – the person considers changing their behaviour but remains undecided because they know that not changing carries its own short-term benefits, whereas change may impose immediate costs and inconvenience.
3 *Preparation* – the person intends and plans to take action soon. They may have obtained information or are in other ways ready and willing to change.
4 *Action* – the person actually does something, such as acting to reduce a health risk.

5 *Maintenance* – after successful behavioural change, the person must work to prevent relapse into former preferences and habits.

6 *Termination* – the person has lost interest in reverting to earlier, undesirable behaviours. There is no temptation to relapse. Termination may be unachievable. Losing all interest in an earlier addiction could be unrealistic, with the person remaining always in maintenance.

Processes linked to these stages include:

- *Raising consciousness* of the possibility and reasons for change.
- *Emotional response* within the person, to heighten the intensity of the problem.
- *Self-evaluation*, as the person imagines themself with and without an unhealthy habit.
- *Environmental appraisal*, such as the person considering the effects of their behaviour on others.
- *Self-liberation*, where the person realises that they can change. Self-liberation resembles self-efficacy.
- *Social liberation*, where society provides opportunities for positive alternatives to current behaviours.
- *Counterconditioning*, the substitution of new, positive behaviours to replace undesirable habits.
- *Stimulus control*, removing environmental signals that promote unhealthy behaviours.

The transtheoretical model shows how change entails more than a single or simple process of acting. Furthermore, changes in behaviour require attention and effort to maintain. People who lose weight through improved diet and exercise need to persist with their healthy lifestyle to avoid regaining weight.

The stages of change model provides a framework for public health practitioners assisting individuals to adopt healthy behaviours. Stages of change begin with initial reflection, followed by a decision to act. Realistic goals for change are decided. Obstacles to change are identified in advance so they can be overcome. Small gains can be celebrated to enhance self-efficacy. Maintenance of new behaviours becomes part of the process.

Theory of planned behaviour

The theory of planned behaviour, illustrated in Figure 9.2, is most commonly associated with the psychologist Icek Ajzen (1991).

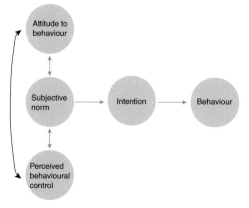

Figure 9.2 Theory of planned behaviour.
Source: Ajzen (1991), p. 182.

Subjective norm – what a
person believes they are expected
to do; what someone believes is
approved behaviour without
regard to whether the person
wants to do it.

Central to the theory of planned behaviour is *intention*. Intentions come about because of attitudes, subjective norms and perceived behavioural control:

• *Attitude* refers to the person's appraisal of the behaviour, whether favourable or unfavourable.
• *Subjective norms* refer to perceptions of social pressure to perform the behaviour, conformity with what other people do and their expectations.
• *Perceived behavioural control* refers to individuals' beliefs about their ability to perform an action. This concept aligns with self-efficacy, introduced earlier in this chapter.

The three factors of personal attitude, wider subjective norms and the individual's perception of behavioural control contribute, through intentions, to a decision about whether to do something. The theory of planned behaviour relates to public health by proposing conditions necessary for someone to adopt a healthier lifestyle. If an individual views an option favourably, believes that other people are doing it while encouraging more people to do the same, and the individual considers themself capable of that behaviour, then that behaviour becomes an intention leading to action. Among numerous examples of the theory of planned behaviour applied to health, Lin and colleagues (2020) describe the theory to predict self-care behaviours among persons with diabetes.

Health belief model

The health belief model originated in the 1950s in response to concerns that public health programs had limited effect (Rosenstock, 1974, 2000). According to the model, people mentally compare costs and benefits of preventative action before choosing an action. Five prior conditions are necessary for people to protect or improve their health (Janz & Becker, 1984; Rosenstock, 2000):

1 *Perceived susceptibility*. The person considers there is a threat to their health.
2 *Perceived severity*. The threat to health is considered serious. Susceptibility and severity combine to heighten a perception of threat.
3 *Perceived benefits* from acting, considering the imagined effectiveness of the action, which could include personal satisfaction, social approval and cost savings as well as better health.
4 *Perceived barriers* to action, which could include financial costs, time, inconvenience, access difficulties, lack of support, personal effort, pain or discomfort and adverse effects. While perceived threat stimulates action, perceived barriers hinder or prevent action. Self-efficacy, the belief in one's own capability, can determine whether a person will overcome perceived barriers.
5 *Cues to action*, which provide external information, can push a person towards initiating a health-promoting action. A cue could be an incidental observation of someone else's experience or a healthy lifestyle message that converts a person's readiness or willingness to act into real action (Green & Murphy, 2014).

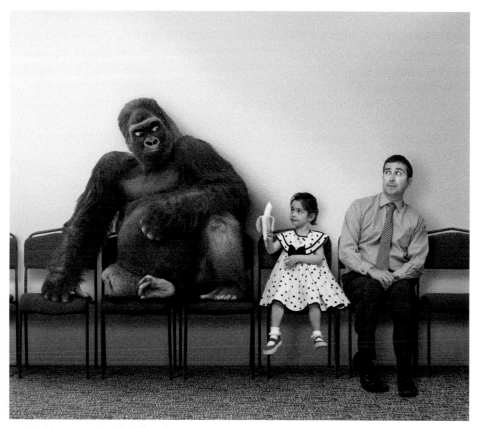

Figure 9.3   We all perceive risks differently.

The health belief model explains why people act to protect their health and why they may not act. Smokers (a) who consider themselves at high risk of serious illness related to smoking (perceived threat), and (b) who believe that quitting smoking will reduce that risk, save money and earn social approval (perceived benefits), and (c) who are prepared to withstand nicotine cravings (perceived barrier), and (d) who notice health warnings and advertising of quit-smoking programs (cues to action), are more likely to quit than other smokers who (i) downplay the risks and severity of smoking-related health disorders, (ii) underestimate the benefits from quitting, (iii) regard quitting as too hard, and (iv) are less exposed to messages prompting action. Research over many years has used the health belief model to explain and predict people's decisions relating to personal health. Al-Metwali and colleagues (2021) used the health belief model to develop a survey of healthcare workers and the general population about the acceptability of vaccination against COVID-19.

SPOTLIGHT 9.2

Mobile phone use and pedestrian safety

Pedestrians' use of mobile phones while crossing roads is a known safety hazard (Simmons et al., 2020). Pedestrians may neglect to check for oncoming traffic before crossing roads, sometimes with tragic results. Engineering countermeasures have been suggested, such as the strategic placement of warning lights in kerbside pavements, at road crossings, in the hope that pedestrians looking downwards may notice the lights, but this solution is impractical for all streets. To reduce the risk, behavioural change among pedestrians is needed.

QUESTIONS

1 Why would public education campaigns based on social learning theory, stages of change and the theory of planned behaviour be more effective than behavioural-only strategies for encouraging users of mobile phones to show more care when crossing roads?

2 What theories of individual behaviour described above are the most useful for informing a public education campaign?

Nudging people towards better decisions

Nudge – what a person believes they are expected to do; what someone believes is approved behaviour without regard to whether the person wants to do it.

Choice architecture – the physical environment that influences people's choices, often without them realising it.

Thaler and Sunstein (2009) use the term **nudge** to describe ways to encourage people towards better choices. Nudging is about making better choices easier than less-beneficial alternatives. The approach is behaviourist. Nudging works through small, often hardly noticeable, modifications to the environment; the **choice architecture**, specifically, being 'any small feature of the environment that attracts our attention and influences the behaviour' (Thaler, 2011, p. 39). If you have noticed a checkbox, or options button, already selected for you on a website or online form, so you opt in if you do nothing (but you if want to opt out you must actively deselect it), then you have experienced a nudge.

Nudging offers an alternative to coercive methods such as banning so-called junk-food or other ways to enforce people's choices. Thaler and Sunstein (2009) argue that environmental designers should make it easier for people to choose wisely without having their choices reduced. Instead, we modify the choice architecture to encourage better choices. Choice architecture refers to an environment that is designed to promote choice, such as the urban environment in which most people in developed countries live. Thaler (2011) uses the example of the university cafeteria in which people have to pass the salad bar to get to the burgers. Locating the salad bar to maximise its exposure while making the fried and fatty food options less conspicuous increases the chances of people making a healthy purchase. Strategic placement of products in supermarkets, such as in aisle bins, is widely used to influence people's purchases, often for commercial reasons rather than to improve public health. On a larger scale, town planners might design new suburbs with off-road paths to encourage walking and cycling while separated from motorised transport.

Immediate versus delayed consequences

The section on behaviourism introduced the timing of rewards and punishments for modifying behaviour. Extending the concept of time, many of the daily choices we make involve trade-offs between immediate rewards and later rewards or adverse events. How outcomes are perceived over time greatly affects decisions related to health. A universal tendency known as **delay discounting** or **time discounting** sees sooner or immediate rewards valued more highly, or even over-valued, when compared with delayed rewards or adverse consequences (punishments) in the distant future. Smaller, sooner rewards may be more influential than more important but delayed events. Few people want to become obese, but many people want to unwrap just one more chocolate.

Time or delay discounting – the psychological tendency to subjectively value immediate or sooner outcomes over delayed, later outcomes.

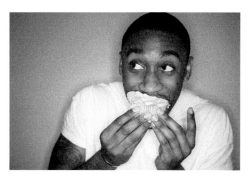

Figure 9.4 Immediate pleasures are often valued much more highly than their long-delayed consequences.

Using delay discounting as a model, Ainslie (2001) argues that many of us do in the short term what we know goes against our long-term interests. Immediate priorities conflict with our welfare in the remote future. A young person can choose between:

- Playing music loudly through headphones and having more fun now while risking hearing loss that later diminishes quality of life.
   OR
   Playing music at moderate volume now and later in life enjoying better hearing.
- Partying more, studying less and having more fun now.
   OR
   Partying less, studying more now and earning higher grades to secure a future career or lifestyle.

Since unhealthy behaviours such as smoking, poor diet and a sedentary lifestyle may bring immediate pleasures or avoidance of pain while increasing the risk of future ill health through chronic, incurable diseases, choice over time is crucial to public health. The teenager who takes up smoking because their friends smoke (social learning) fails accurately to assess the risk of serious illness decades hence, because middle age lies far beyond the adolescent's time horizon.

Preventing people from discounting at all is not possible, as the tendency to prefer the immediate over the future is psychologically entrenched. Nor is it reasonable always to deny immediate gratification, else we could never enjoy the present, and not all pleasures are harmful. There are situations in which people happily make immediate sacrifices so they can safeguard or improve their future; for example, the university student who foregoes immediate income and incurs a course-fees debt so they can earn more money from a better job after graduating.

Problems with conflicting motives arise when current action leads to future regret. People become more future-oriented when they learn to evaluate and plan their immediate and future options so that the two are less in competition. Choosing a delicious healthy snack over a snack loaded with fat, salt and sugar aligns a person's immediate and future interests. Encouraging people to harmonise their immediate and future interests is potentially an effective strategy for public health promotion.

Health as chosen or determined

Models of behaviour described in this chapter allow for environmental and social influences on individual decision-making. People's health-related decisions partly depend on their geographical, social and economic contexts. Behaviourism emphasises how people learn from experiences meted out by their environment. Social learning theory is about social influences on behaviour. For the theory of planned behaviour, subjective norms affect intentions which, in turn, drive behaviour. The health belief model incorporates perceptions informed by observation and experience, along with external cues to action. The transtheoretical model holds that social influences trigger contemplation for change, with social influences affected by geographical and economic factors.

Clearly, people do not make health decisions separately from outside influence. The question arises as to a person's capacity for choice. If people's decisions are mostly dictated by their circumstances, there is little point in asking people to improve their choices without first addressing the social determinants that largely govern those choices (Baum & Fisher, 2014; Stuhlberg, 2014).

SPOTLIGHT 9.3

Does life allow us to live healthily?

Social learning theory, the transtheoretical model and the theory of planned behaviour look at whether people consider themselves in charge of their own life (locus of control) and able to take alternative actions, such as healthier lifestyles (self-efficacy). However, the choices available to people depend also on their physical, social and economic environments. Long commutes to places of employment and long working hours reduce the time available for exercise and to prepare healthy meals from fresh ingredients. Parenting, other relationship and domestic responsibilities further intrude on available time for personal care. The COVID-19 pandemic, starting in 2020, and the associated community lockdowns, have made it more complicated for many people to live healthily. For many workers, long commutes were replaced by working from home in unfavourable conditions. Educating children at home placed parents and carers under further pressure. Loss of employment through reduced economic activity posed another threat to wellbeing. Evidence is accumulating that COVID-19 lockdowns have affected mental health (e.g. O'Connor et al., 2021) and choices about daily living that affect physical health (e.g. Robinson et al., 2021). People may know they can benefit by improving their diet, exercising more, attending more to family and friends, and more community participation, yet they are convinced that unavoidable aspects of their lifestyle prevent them from living better.

QUESTIONS

1   What is the value of public health campaigns telling people to eat better, exercise more and look after their physical and mental health when people see themselves as trapped in an unhealthy lifestyle that society forces them to live?

2   How can public health interventions encourage people to adopt the healthy lifestyle they may prefer but feel unable to attain?

REFLECTION QUESTION

If public health is socially determined, with people's choices limited by their physical environment and their social and economic circumstances, why do so many public health interventions target individual behaviours, such as quit smoking, road safety and education about diet and exercise?

SUMMARY

Learning objective 1: Distinguish between social and individual determinants of health.

Individual choices are contrasted with social and biological determinants of health. Whereas social determinants, such as a person's social, environmental and economic contexts, along with biological factors, are largely beyond a person's control, personally initiated decisions also affect our own and others' health. Many public health campaigns aim to improve people's health by targeting individuals' personal choices.

Learning objective 2: Explain how perceptions, emotions and thoughts contribute to personal decisions influencing health.

A general model for psychological influences on behaviour illustrates the relationship between perceived experiences, thoughts (cognitions), emotions (affect) and actions (behaviours). This general model provides a foundation for more detailed models of individual behaviour.

Learning objective 3: Describe major theories of individual behaviour and choice.

The major theories of individual behaviour and choice include behaviourism, social learning theory, transtheoretical model, theory of planned behaviour and the health belief model. Behaviourism explains how people learn from associations between events and from the results of their actions. Social learning theory adds the modelling of behaviour from vicarious observations of others, and belief in our own ability and responsibility to act. The transtheoretical model describes how behavioural change happens through stages. The theory of planned behaviour and the health belief model reveal how perceptions, attitudes and evaluations contribute to action or inaction. Discounting can overly diminish the perceived importance of risk to health in the distant future. These models identify within-person factors that explain why people act to protect or improve their health, or why they may not.

Learning objective 4: Explain how theories of individual behaviour and choice can inform public health campaigns.

The theories show how public health interventions can target psychological processes that drive individual choice and action while acknowledging that decisions result also from external influences. Without accounting for both the environmental (external) and psychological (internal) forces that affect behaviour, public health campaigns may naively rely on simply telling people what to do, which is long known to have limited effectiveness (e.g. Eakin et al., 1996). Nudging is a strategy that assists in modifying the designed environment so that people are prompted towards better choices without coercion.

Learning objective 5: Identify limitations to targeting personal choice as a means to improving public health.

Due to personal beliefs, and for practical reasons, people may resist lifestyle changes to improve their health. Events beyond people's control also affect their health-related decisions. Targeting individual choices without reference to wider – including social – determinants of those choices could have limited practical value. The chapter concludes by questioning whether health behaviours are ever truly chosen independently and individually.

TUTORIAL EXERCISES

1   Choose one model of individual decision-making from those described in this chapter. Show how that model explains the change in people's behaviour in response to the COVID-19 pandemic. Examples of

behavioural change may include wearing masks, distancing in public, following other public health orders, accepting or rejecting vaccination, and panic-buying during lockdowns.

2 Zlatevska, Dubelaar and Holden (2014) report how food consumption increases with portion size. Reducing the size of food packages, plates and bowls should nudge people towards eating less without dietary experts telling them what to do. Think of other ways to nudge people (Thaler & Sunstein, 2009) towards better choices by slightly adjusting their environment. Road safety offers many possibilities because transport environments are modifiable. You could also list ways in which people are nudged towards *unhealthy* choices, such as in supermarkets.

3 Pleasurable experiences are preferred now rather than later. Unpleasant experiences matter less when they are delayed. The prospect of HIV/AIDS in the distant future may not deter a person from having unsafe sex now. Moreover, people change their intentions and plans. They break promises they have made to themselves, such as New Year's resolutions. They exhibit temporary preferences (Ainslie, 2001) and maintain habits they know are unhealthy, such as consumption of high-energy, salt-laden foods or tobacco, alcohol and recreational drugs, participating in unsafe sex, leading sedentary lifestyles and other behaviours with long-delayed ill consequences. Think of one personal habit that you are willing to tell others about where you have knowingly acted against your own best interests. You may have attended a party when you knew you should instead have studied for an exam. What would it take for you to choose the higher-value, later reward over the lower-value, sooner reward? List examples from everyday life where immediate temptation jeopardises future health. How can public health practitioners encourage people to adopt long-term perspectives in relation to their health?

4 For discussion: 'The unresponsiveness of young people to expert anti-smoking exhortation and to health promotion programming is seen as resistance to "reasoned action"' (Eakin et al., 1996, p. 162). Why do people not change their behaviours in response to health messages and warnings? Using what we have learned from this chapter, what can public health professionals do to promote healthy lifestyles and overcome people's resistance to advice?

5 For discussion: Is each of us truly in charge of our own health? How much is our health chosen *by* us, or instead chosen *for* us by society? What determinants of our health are within our personal control? How much of our personal health destiny lies beyond our control, so that there is nothing we can do to improve it?

FURTHER READING

de Vries, H. (2017). An integrated approach for understanding health behavior: The I-Change model as an example. *Psychology and Behavioral Science International Journal, 2*(2), 555585.

Han, M., & Lee, E. (2018). Effectiveness of mobile health application use to improve health behavior changes: A systematic review of randomized controlled trials. *Healthcare Informatics Research, 24*(3), 207–26.

Nutbeam, D., Harris, E., & Wise, M. (2010). *Theory in a nutshell: A practical guide to health promotion theories* (3rd ed.). McGraw-Hill.

Prestwich, A. J., Kenworthy, J., & Conner, M. (2017). *Health behavior change: Theories, methods and interventions*. Routledge.

Revenson, T. A., & Gurung, R. A. R. (2018). (Eds.), *Handbook of heath psychology*. Routledge.

REFERENCES

Ahn, S., & Oh, J. (2018). Relationships among knowledge, self-efficacy, and health behavior of osteoporosis and fall prevention in old aged women. *Korean Journal of Women Health Nursing, 24*(2), 209–18.

Ainslie, G. (2001). *Breakdown of will.* Cambridge University Press.

Ajzen, I. (1991). The theory of planned behavior. *Organizational Behavior and Human Decision Processes, 50,* 179–211.

Al-Metwali, B. Z., Al-Jumaili, A. A., Al-Alag, Z. A., & Sorofman, B. (2021). Exploring the acceptance of COVID-19 vaccine among healthcare workers and general population using health belief model. *Journal of Evaluation in Clinical Practice, 27*(5), 1112–22.

Amit Aharon, A., Nehama, H., Rishpon, S., & Baron-Epel, O. (2018). A path analysis model suggesting the association between health locus of control and compliance with childhood vaccinations. *Human Vaccines & Immunotherapeutics, 14*(7), 1618–25.

Bandura, A. (1977). *Social learning theory.* Retrieved http://www.asecib.ase.ro/mps/bandura_ sociallearningtheory.pdf

——(1996). Modelling. In A. S. R. Manstead & M. Hewstone (Eds.), *The Blackwell encyclopedia of social psychology.* Blackwell Publishing.

——(2008). Observational learning. In W. Donsbach (Ed.), *The international encyclopedia of communication.* Wiley Blackwell.

Baum, F., & Fisher, M. (2014). Why behavioural health promotion endures despite its failure to reduce health inequities. *Sociology of Health & Illness, 36*(2), 213–25.

BFI.org.uk (2016). AIDS: Monolith (1987). Retrieved https://www.youtube.com/watch?v=iroty5zwOVw

Bronfenbrenner, U. (1992). Ecological systems theory. In R. Vasta (Ed.), *Six theories of child development: Revised formulations and current issues* (pp. 187–249). Jessica Kingsley Publishers.

Eakin, J., Robertson, A., Poland, B., Coburn, D., & Edwards, R. (1996). Towards a critical social science perspective on health promotion research. *Health Promotion International, 2*(1), 157–65.

Fraser, A. C., Williams, S. E., Kong, S. X., Wells, L. E., Goodall, L. S., Pit, S., Hansen, V., & Trent, M. (2016). *Public Health Amendment (Vaccination of Children Attending Child Care Facilities) Act 2013*: Its impact in the Northern Rivers, NSW. *Public Health Research and Practice, 26*(2), e2621620.

Green, E. G., & Murphy, E. (2014). Health belief model. In W. C. Cockerham, R. Dingwall & S. R. Quah (Eds.), *The Wiley Blackwell encyclopedia of health, illness, behavior, and society* (1st ed.). John Wiley & Sons, Inc.

HIV.gov (2021). *40 years of progress - it's time to end the HIV epidemic.* Retrieved https://www.hiv.gov/events/ 40-years-of-hiv

Janz, N. K. & Becker, M. H. (1984). The health belief model: A decade later. *Health Education Quarterly, 11*(1), 1–47.

Lin, C.-Y., Cheung, M. K. T., Hung, A. T. F., Poon, P. K. K., Chan, S. C. C., & Chetwyn, C. H. C. (2020). Can a modified theory of planned behavior explain the effects of empowerment education for people with type 2 diabetes? *Therapeutic Advances in Endocrinology and Metabolism, 11,* 1–12.

McGinnis, J. M., Williams-Russo, P. & Knickman, J. R. (2002). The case for more active policy attention to health promotion. *Health Affairs, 21*(2), 78–93.

McLeod, S. A. (2016). Bandura – social learning theory. Retrieved www.simplypsychology.org/bandura.html

O'Connor, R. C., Wetherall, K., McClelland, H., Melson, A J., Niedzwiedz, C. L., O'Carroll, R. E., . . . Robb, K. A. (2021). Mental health and well-being during the COVID-19 pandemic: Longitudinal analyses of adults in the UK COVID-19 Mental Health & Wellbeing study. *The British Journal of Psychiatry, 218*(6), 326–33.

Prochaska, J. O., & Velicer, W. F. (1997). The transtheoretical model of health behavior change. *American Journal of Health Promotion, 12*(1), 38–48.

Robinson, E., Boyland, E., Chisholm, A., Harrold, J., Maloney, N. G., Marty, L., . . . Hardman, C. A. (2021). Obesity, eating behavior and physical activity during COVID-19 lockdown: A study of UK adults. *Appetite, 156* (104853), 1–7.

Rosenstock, I. M. (1974). Historical origins of the health belief model. *Health Education Monographs*, *2*(4), 328–35.

——(2000). Health belief model. In A. E. Kazdin (Ed.), *Encyclopedia of psychology* (vol. 4, pp. 78–80). Oxford University Press.

Simmons, S. M., Caird, J. K., Ta, A., Sterzer, F., & Hagel, B. E. (2020). Plight of the distracted pedestrian: A research synthesis and meta-analysis of mobile phone use on crossing behaviour. *Injury Prevention*, *26*(2), 170–6.

Stuhlberg, B. (2014). The key to changing individual health behaviors: Change the environments that give rise to them. *Harvard Public Health Review*, *2*, 1–6.

Thaler, R. H. (2011, July 30). *Richard Thaler – Nudge: An overview*. (Video). YouTube. Retrieved https://www.youtube.com/watch?v=xoA8N6nJMRs

Thaler, R. H., & Sunstein, C. R. (2009). *Nudge* (Revised ed.). Penguin.

UNAIDS (2021, June 5). Global HIV & AIDS statistics – Fact sheet. Retrieved https://www.unaids.org/en/resources/fact-sheet

Watson, J. B. (2017). *Behaviorism*. Routledge.

World Health Organization (WHO). (2020a). *Listings of WHO's response to COVID-19*. Retrieved https://www.who.int/news/item/29-06-2020-covidtimeline

——(2020b). *Coronavirus disease (COVID-19): How is it transmitted?* Retrieved https://www.who.int/news-room/q-a-detail/coronavirus-disease-covid-19-how-is-it-transmitted

——(2021). *WHO Coronavirus (COVID-19) Dashboard*. Retrieved https://covid19.who.int/

Zlatevska, N., Dubelaar, C., & Holden, S. S. (2014). Sizing up the effect of portion size on consumption: A meta-analytic review. *Journal of Marketing*, *78*(3), 140–54.

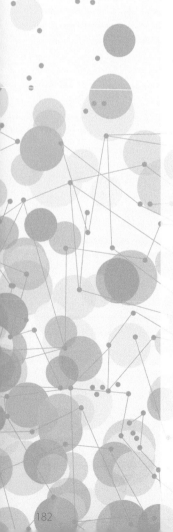

10

Political determinants of public health

Marguerite C. Sendall

LEARNING OBJECTIVES

After studying this chapter, you should be able to:

1 understand the balance between governments' responsibility and people's rights, and the influence of political will in public health
2 understand the distinctive features of the Australian healthcare system and political susceptibility in public health
3 comprehend the influence of cost-effectiveness and cost–benefit ratios, and the economic and social contexts of policy in public health
4 analyse levels of evidence and the gap between policy and practice in public health
5 analyse the role of advocacy and the use of evidence in advocacy in public health.

VIGNETTE

Health as a political football

In 2007, the Australian Labor Party, led by Kevin Rudd MP, won the federal election. This election, for the first time ever, saw public health 'up front' on the political agenda. The Australian Greens, led by former general practitioner (GP) Senator Bob Brown, promoted public health as a policy platform on its campaign flyers. After the successful 'Kevin07' campaign, Prime Minister Rudd proposed to reform the national health agenda through the Health and Hospital Reform package. The final report, released in 2009, proposed more than 100 reforms. The most significant of these was to funding arrangements whereby the federal government, rather than the states and territories, would fund 60 per cent of public hospitals and the newly created Local Hospital Networks, primary healthcare interfaces, known as Medicare Locals, and 28 GP 'super clinics'. Effectively, the federal government was planning to pay for 60 per cent of health and hospital costs, and would continue to pay 60 per cent as the costs increased. Furthermore, the government set up the National Preventive Health Taskforce. Recommendations from the taskforce led to the establishment of the Australian National Preventive Health Agency (ANPHA), auspiced to address three recommended priority areas: tobacco, alcohol and obesity.

The Liberal–National Coalition, led by Tony Abbott MP, won the following federal election in early 2014. Claiming a budget crisis, the Abbott Government proposed a number of policy initiatives, including a $7 GP co-payment. The GP co-payment was not supported by the Palmer United Party, the Australian Greens nor the independent cross-benchers who held the balance of power in the Senate, and was abandoned in early 2015. The ANPHA was abolished and a new Medical Research Future Fund was established.

After a successful leadership challenge, the Coalition's new right-of-centre leader, Malcolm Turnbull MP, promised to appease his far-right party members with a plebiscite on the legalisation of same-sex marriage, despite reported high levels of community tolerance and calls for a conscience vote in Parliament. In late 2017, the Bill passed through the Australian Senate with minor amendments. It was among the most significant social reforms since the Whitlam years.

Action on climate change is a good example of a 'political football'. The Intergovernmental Panel on Climate Change (IPCC), auspiced by the United Nations, is accountable for progressing climate change knowledge. Evidence for climate change, and its effects on health, is irrefutable and action is urgent. Some gains have been made but progress is dangerously slow. The Paris Agreement (2016) is an international, legally binding treaty which sets emissions-reduction targets to limit global warming to less than 2 degrees Celsius (and preferably to 1.5 degrees) compared to pre-industrial levels. In March 2021, 190 (of 194) signatory countries ratified or acceded to the Paris Agreement, including China and India (the largest and third-largest carbon emitting countries, respectively), the European Union and Australia. The United States, under President Trump, withdrew from the Paris Agreement in late 2020, claiming it would undermine the American economy. By January 2021, President Biden had re-signed the Paris Agreement. Peak bodies in Australia, such as the Climate and Health Alliance (CAHA), consider the federal government is not acting urgently or decisively to meet and exceed targets set by the Paris Agreement. CAHA's current campaign, 'Real. Urgent. Now.' promulgates immediate action to mitigate catastrophic effects of climate change, such as recently witnessed bushfires and floods, and their health and other effects.

Introduction

As illustrated in the opening vignette, public health is vulnerable to political cycles. Politics and health are inextricably linked through the government's responsibility to provide health care, funded by taxation. It is this interwoven link between politics and health that directs the allocation of taxpayers' money and, ultimately, the distribution of resources to address issues of social justice, fairness and equity. The political determinants of health underpin, directly and indirectly, all other determinants of health. Therefore, public health is innately political by the very virtue of its existence and its vulnerability to political cycles, political agendas, political will and promises of change. Public health should consider three-term prime ministers and parties, like those of the Menzies and Howard eras, a phenomenon of the past. It should also consider the urgent need to develop an aggressive strategy to respond to the short and volatile political cycles seen in the past decade. Health, public health and health promotion are intensely political (Galea & Vaughan, 2019; Sundin, 2019; Lawson, 2020). Consequently, politics represents a determinant of health.

There are many examples of political decisions as determinants of health – food, work, leisure, parenting – which, like herd immunity, can only be understood at the population level. Other examples are mass killings in wartime (Mackenbach, 2014), trade agreements and, recently, the COVID-19 pandemic (Lawson, 2020). There are also social health examples. Think about this one. In 2017, a fire in the 24-storey Grenfell public housing block, located in a poor, multi-ethnic community in a rich London borough, claimed 71 lives. The fire trapped people inside as it spread upwards and sideways through exterior cladding panels (Australian Broadcasting Corporation, 2017). The subsequent inquest found renovations had included the removal of fire-retardant materials between flats and in corridors that were not reported by council safety inspectors (McKee, 2017). Media commentary suggested that the government had failed to act on the coroner's recommendations from previous residential tower fires and reports that indicated widespread safety breaches in the use of highly flammable materials and the absence of sprinkler systems (Wainwright & Walker, 2017).

This chapter introduces the fundamental concepts associated with political determinants of public health. To begin with, the chapter discusses government responsibility for providing health services and people's right to access health care. Government responsibility and people's rights are underpinned by political ideologies such as political will, and this idea is also discussed. Australia's healthcare system is distinctive, and this is explored in the next section of the chapter. To appreciate the complexities of Australia's healthcare system within the political context, the chapter considers political susceptibility and presents the state of Queensland as an example. In particular, it looks at public health as vulnerable to the political cycle. Next, the chapter considers healthcare costs in the political context. Public health has strong arguments for good returns on dollars spent, but the problem lies in the political context, where vote-winning is linked to funding support for acute care services, such as the reduction of waiting lists for elective surgery. This is compounded by having to demonstrate evidence for short-term health outcomes, since most public health advances are gained over the long term. Tobacco smoking is a good example.

The next section covers ideas about evidence-based policy and what counts as 'evidence'. The chapter discusses underpinning epistemological debates as well as the hierarchy of

Social justice – the equitable distribution of benefits and burdens among populations.

evidence, which needs to be interpreted and translated in a meaningful way. Systematic reviews, considered the highest level, may not offer the best evidence. Most experts agree that there is a practice–policy gap, and there is a new focus on **translational research**. The last section covers **advocacy** and ethics; in particular the role of advocacy for better health outcomes (especially for at-risk groups), ethics as underpinning advocacy and coercive policies, people's rights and population outcomes.

Translational research – the meaningful translation of research evidence to policy and practice.

Advocacy – acting on behalf of others who have less capacity and power for change.

Government's role in health

Governments have always played a role in health and public health. You may have heard about some of these examples already (e.g. Edwin Chadwick's campaign to bring about the *Public Health Act* (1848) in Great Britain), and of seminal documents that have influenced the political nature of public health. In the new public health phase, the *Ottawa Charter for Health Promotion* (World Health Organization, 1986) and Canada's *Lalonde Report* (1974) have been influential politically and have brought about change. There are other benchmark documents from the current ecological phase of public health, such as the World Health Organization's (WHO) *Health 2020: The European policy for health and well-being* (WHO, 2018), which underpins the political agenda and acts as a beacon to guide ecological public health momentum.

Responsibility and rights

Governments enact polices about how society should be organised, based on their philosophical and social ideologies, and how desired outcomes should be achieved. These policies, which may restrict people's behaviours to reduce health risk, can be seen as paternalistic or 'nanny-like'. But people and populations are the centrepiece. All governments must balance their responsibility to provide equitable and cost-effective health services and maintain population health with respect for the rights of individuals to access appropriate and timely health care. Governments have a spectrum of approaches available, from education to legislation, but the legitimacy of interventions depends on social and cultural tolerance and acceptance. Legislation is a useful tool to expedite the pace of change, but it is just one mechanism. Governments should strive for the right approach to ensure organised efforts of all those working towards the common goal of public health balance; for example, access and equity of resources, the distribution of power and the relationship between individuals and the state (Bekker et al., 2018). Essentially, there is a delicate balance of power between political will and people's willingness for change.

REFLECTION QUESTION

During the COVID-19 pandemic, state and territory governments in Australia enacted measures such as lockdowns and border closures. What were the health consequences of these political decisions? How well do you think these and other measures were tolerated by specific population groups?

Political will

There is some contention about the concept of political will. The term assumes a centrality to policy change. In particular, 'the lack of political will' has become a catch phrase overused in the popular media and, although it has essentially lost its effect, it has become a dominant focus of discourse in the political narrative of current affairs in health. The idea of political will emerged alongside the health promotion movement, which burgeoned in the early 1980s. 'Political will' assumed currency because health promotion is underpinned by ideologies of social justice and human rights. Thus, there is a logical link to advocacy, one of health promotion's strongest weapons. The juxtaposition of political will and health promotion is highlighted in the editorial of the first edition of the journal *Health Promotion International*. Dr Halfdan Mahler, the Director-General of the WHO, wrote:

> The political will and the intersectoral action necessary to create the healthy environments which favour the development of healthy lifestyles and secure basic health protection are sadly lacking in many countries (Mahler, 1986, p. 1).

How do we create political will? Galea and Vaughan (2019) suggest that, given the term 'political' is so entwined with public health, a new and meaningful narrative within political science needs to be created to inform political action, and to drive political will. However, creating political will is time-consuming and costly, complicated by political cycles and politicians' desire for short-term outcomes, and compounded by the desire in the media for newsworthy headlines. Beyond these ideological sentiments, the reality of operationalising political will is much more complex than the rhetoric. Advocacy, underpinned by a much better understanding of how politics works and what can be achieved (Kickbusch, 2015), offers some hope as a lever to shift political will for public health. But there is a long way to go before public health is embedded in the political psyche. Public health needs to mobilise power, have a voice and do more than promise change – it needs to enact it.

SPOTLIGHT 10.1

Climate change: Real, urgent and now

Think back to the opening vignette. Countries such as Canada, Japan and South Korea made bigger commitments to the Paris Agreement (2016) than they had done previously, and promised to cut net emissions to zero by 2050. Globally, Australia was seen as a laggard. This sentiment was similar at home because the federal government was challenged by lack of agreement within and between parties, and seen to be procrastinating on a decision. For the most part, the federal government has focused on industry to implement energy-efficient and mitigation measures. However, households have a responsibility, too. The average Australian household generates over 7 tonnes of greenhouse gas emissions each year and accounts for about 20 per cent of Australia's total emissions. Nearly half of Australian household energy use is consumed by heating and cooling. About a third is used for refrigeration and appliances, a quarter is used for heating water and the remainder is used for lighting (Department of Industry, Science, Energy and Resources, 2021). Household gains are offset by population growth and increasing uptake of affordable electrical appliances. However, households could reduce their emissions significantly by conserving energy, using energy-efficient technologies and using renewable energy sources.

QUESTION

What strategies do you think local, state and federal governments should consider to encourage households to reduce their greenhouse gas emissions?

Australia's healthcare system

The strong labour movement in Australia, which reflects principles of social justice, has influenced public health. In particular, the social reform agenda of Labor Prime Minister Gough Whitlam in the early 1970s aligned with the principles of public health. For example, the single mother's pension was introduced, women were given the legal right to access a termination of pregnancy, the number of sexual health clinics grew and, in 1972, the first Aboriginal Medical Service was set up in Redfern, New South Wales. This era saw the advent of a universal health insurance scheme in the form of Medibank, now Medicare, and the Pharmaceutical Benefits Scheme.

Uniquely, the Australian healthcare system is managed at three levels of government. The federal government is responsible for collecting taxes to fund the healthcare system, including Medicare. There have been several significant milestones in the federal healthcare system. For example, in 1986 the Better Health Commission was established to address the national health agenda, and in 1990 the National Goals and Targets were established. In 1996, four National Health Priority Areas (NHPA) were identified: cardiovascular health, cancer control, injury prevention and control, and mental health. From 1997 to 2012, a further five NHPA were added: diabetes, asthma, musculoskeletal disorders, obesity and dementia. State and territory governments fund the healthcare system – in particular, hospitals – and implement strategies to meet the national agenda. Local governments are responsible for prevention of infection, and for monitoring and surveillance. However, the relationship between levels of government varies across states and territories. For example, the South Australian *Public Health Act 2011* devolved responsibilities so local government in that state has a broader mandate for public health.

Another distinctive feature of the Australian healthcare system is the relationship between public and private health care. The government offers tax incentives to encourage people to purchase private health insurance. Initially, in 1997, the tax rebate on private health premiums was 30 per cent. In 2005, this was increased to 35 per cent for those aged between 65 and 69 years and 40 per cent for those aged over 70 years. People who earn over $76 000 per annum and do not take out private health insurance are required to pay a 2 per cent Medicare surcharge (usually 1 per cent). In 2005, there was public debate about a proposal to introduce means-testing for the private health insurance rebate. Proponents claimed that means testing would see only 70 000 people leave private health insurance. Opponents claimed it would simply clog up the public health system.

The relationship between public and private health care is further complicated by the growing number of private patients being treated in the public health system because of rising private health premiums and perceived benefits. In late 2017, the Turnbull Government announced a private health insurance package to address this problem, by instructing insurers to give up to 10 per cent discount on premiums for 18 to 29-year-olds until they are 40 years old, to increase the maximum excess payable to reduce premiums and to simplify private health insurance by categorising products and standard definitions (Commonwealth of Australia, 2017).

Political susceptibility

To gain a deeper understanding of the Australian healthcare system in the political context, and political susceptibility, we examine Queensland as an example. In March 2012, the Liberal National Party (LNP) won power with a majority (up from 34) of 78 from a possible 89 seats, the largest majority in Queensland history (Green, 2012, para. 1). The LNP was led by Campbell Newman who, as presiding mayor of Brisbane and an outsider, won the seat of Ashgrove (Australian Broadcasting Corporation, 2012). The Senate, or upper house, in the Queensland Parliament had been abolished in 1922 (Queensland Parliament, 2010). With control of the lower house, Premier Newman repealed legislation protecting jobs and passed a new award (*Queensland Public Service Award – State 2012*). As a consequence, reported whole-of-government job losses were between 1000 and 16 000. Approximately 6200 jobs were lost across the health sector. As an example, in the Office of Health and Medical Research, responsible for administering federal and state research monies, staff numbers were reduced from 26 to 7. Initially, public health employees holding temporary positions were not offered another contract. Then, permanent employees were required to apply for half the existing positions. There were approximately 1700 job losses (personal communication, December 2012).

SPOTLIGHT 10.2

The strategy: Better, more and money

Again, think back to the opening vignette, and the establishment and abolishment of the ANPHA. Since then, the prevention agenda has not received much greater attention on the national stage and remains politically susceptible. Over recent decades, the preventive health budget in Australia has hovered as low as 1.5 per cent of total health expenditure. In 2019–20, the federal government consulted with the preventive health workforce through several roundtables and a consultation paper. In 2021, a draft National Preventive Health Strategy 2021–2030 (NPHS) was released. The draft acknowledged that most of the health budget is spent on treatment and that a better balance could be achieved by more investment in prevention. The draft proposed to increase prevention investment to 5 per cent of total health expenditure by 2030. Peak bodies such Australian Health Promotion Association (APHA), Climate and Health Alliance (CAHA) and Public Health Association of Australia (PHAA) coordinated a response. Broadly, these peak bodies supported the draft because it reflected, more than ever, a greater understanding of preventive health. The peak bodies congratulated the authors of the draft for addressing previous exclusions such as the social determinants of health and the effects of climate change, but felt these fundamental issues should be front and centre of the strategy. Despite a shift in the government's position towards preventive health, the subsequent federal budget did not allocate any funding to the NPHS.

QUESTION
If investment in prevention is politically vulnerable, how do you think public health can advocate for investment security?

The policy environment

Governments, through policy settings, influence the allocation of limited resources that shape the determinants of health, the economy and environment, and our culture and society, with the potential to maximise population health outcomes. Political determinants of health are futuristic because policy settings are about enacting a vision. Planning can be viewed in four domains: constant and stable leadership, prudent investment, evidence-based policy and practice, and fruitful and enduring partnerships. Additionally, there is a range of policy options available to governments, such as legislation, which escalate change for priority areas at a faster rate than might otherwise happen if behavioural change was left to take a natural course (Eaton & Kalichman, 2020; Navarro & Markel, 2021). Consider as examples legislation on the wearing of seatbelts in vehicles, and travel restrictions during COVID-19 lockdowns. Governments have a range of options on a continuum of intervention, such as education, curriculum development, professional development, organisational change, environmental change, welfare policy, budget allocations, research funding and taxation.

Healthcare costs

Traditionally, the gross domestic product (GDP) and the gross national income (GNI) of a country have been recognised as indicators of the standard of living and have been used as frameworks for human development. Economic development equals economic growth, which is ultimately intertwined with human development and the growth of communities, populations and societies. Thanks to the work of the United Nations, human development is now seen as distinct from economic prosperity. Nonetheless, their relationship is interdependent and complex. Small investments in health in low-income countries can have a significant effect on life expectancy. In high-income countries, there is a law of diminishing returns on investment because treatment is favoured over prevention. Take, for example, type 2 diabetes. As healthcare costs rise, the cost–benefit and cost-effectiveness ratios of dollars invested influence how the health dollar is spent. Another example is population screening. Scoliosis, hearing and vison screening in Queensland lost funding in the early 2000s because the cost of the screening program was not considered justifiable for identifying a small number of at-risk children. The **health economics** of screening this population were simply not justified, and targeted screening was introduced. Other well-established programs, such as breast cancer screening, are provided free of charge to the consumer, are

Health economics – cost–benefit and cost-effectiveness analyses of health interventions.

well-utilised by the 'worried well' but poorly utilised by those at risk and are costly to deliver to most at-risk populations.

Policy economics

The integrity of political and economic systems may be more powerful than government's commitment to policy change, which could be considered fickle. A recent study looked at the type of government and their commitment to providing the 10 prerequisites for health identified in the Ottawa Charter. There is a scale, from rhetoric to action. Liberal governments, including those of Canada, Australia and the United Kingdom, and social democratic welfare governments, such as those of Norway, Sweden and Finland, are more likely to make 'explicit rhetorical commitments' to address **prerequisites for health** than conservative governments, such as those of France, Belgium and Germany, and Latin welfare governments, such as those of Italy and Spain. The evidence suggests that liberal welfare governments, despite the rhetoric, are less likely to implement public policies that address the prerequisites for health. And conservative and Latin welfare governments, which do not make explicit commitments, do quite well at providing the prerequisites for health. This suggests that the political economy (i.e. the overall organisation of economic and political mechanisms) is more likely to shape public policies for prerequisites for health than 'explicit rhetorical commitments' (Raphael, 2014; Greer, 2018). A systems perspective may offer hope to public health: it suggests there are existing systems that could be adopted to support the public health agenda. Examples are incentives for population-level public health, where funds can be redirected from medical care premiums to community wide interventions that address air quality, urban design and outlet-zoning.

Prerequisites for health – eight states that must exist for health attainment, outlined in the *Ottawa Charter for Health Promotion.*

Context of policy

Governments might consider policy change in view of the prevailing and shifting social context by asking: what will the population tolerate? Progressive legislation across Australia on smoking in schools and universities, restaurants, pubs, clubs and public spaces was enacted without much debate because the social change had already occurred. The Nuffield Ladder of Intervention (Nuffield Council on Bioethics, 2014–15) is a tool that offers governments guidance about policy interventions (Figure 10.1). It has been successfully used in the United Kingdom by the House of Lords' Science and Technology Committee and the Department of Transport, and as a cornerstone of the Healthy Lives Healthy People strategy. There is strong evidence that other sectors can positively influence health outcomes by implementing health-promoting policies, which should be core business for, and across, all levels of government and departments (Nuffield Council on Bioethics, 2014–15). This approach to policy may affect people's behaviour in a non-corrosive manner and could result in improved population health outcomes.

REFLECTION QUESTION

Let's reflect on the COVID-19 pandemic and Australia's approach to lockdowns and border closures. Using the Nuffield Ladder of Intervention in Figure 10.1, how well do you think these measures were tolerated by specific population groups?

| Eliminate choice |
| Restrict choice |
| Guide choice by disincentives |
| Guide choice by incentives |
| Guide choice by changing the default policy |
| Enable choice |
| Provide information |
| Do nothing |

Figure 10.1   Nuffield Ladder of Intervention.
Source: Nuffield Council on Bioethics (2014–15).

SPOTLIGHT 10.3

COVID-19 vaccine: Nationalism, altruism and globalisation

Let's explore Australia's policy efforts in vaccine nationalism during the COVID-19 pandemic. Globally, many advocacy organisations campaigned for greater access and equity to COVID-19 medical products, including vaccines. Essentially, more vaccines needed to be produced and distributed in developing countries as quickly as possible. Organisations such as Médecins Sans Frontières called for all legal and technical barriers to be temporarily removed. This would enable developing countries such as India and Brazil to enhance their manufacturing capacity to increase vaccine production. However, a rise in nationalism saw wealthy nations monopolise vaccine supplies and meant countries with more vulnerable populations and fewer resources and capacity had less access to vaccine supplies than their wealthy counterparts (Cole & Dodds, 2021). Wealthy nations were accused of failing to be altruistic towards the distribution of health care and costs. However, in May 2021, the United States temporary waived the international law of intellectual property rules governing vaccine patents (PHAA, 2021). This international law, known as TRIPS (or the Agreement on Trade-Related Aspects of Intellectual Property Rights) is a legal agreement between all member nations of the World Trade Organization. Experts called for the Australian government to follow suit and consider other strategies like technology transfer and raw material supply.

QUESTION
What legislative and policy directions do you think Australia should adopt to reduce nationalism and contribute to greater global health equity?

Evidence for policy

The notion of evidence-based policy is widely accepted, but what counts as evidence for policy? There are epistemological arguments such as 'If science (and therefore evidence) is considered not to be absolute (there is no single truth), what does it take to change policy?' Or, if the social context of health behaviours is dynamic (i.e. they are always changing), how can health policy-makers ensure the correct setting? There is a hierarchy of evidence, but evidence needs to be interpreted and translated in a meaningful way (see also Chapter 12). So, what is the evidence for the effectiveness of an intervention, and how can this be used to influence population health outcomes? The results of one study, however good it might be, does not provide sufficient evidence to underpin public health policy. There are few, although increasing, empirical studies across a range of topics that address the influence of politics on population health (Mackenbach, 2014). A body of evidence is required to enact policy change and influence the political determinants of health.

Evidence for effectiveness

A body of evidence can be found in systematic reviews, meta-analyses and meta-ethnographies. These meta-syntheses can be found in databases such as the Cochrane Collection, but there is contention about their inclusion criteria. A new wave of thought about what constitutes evidence and how it should be used is known as translational research: how policy-makers (and practitioners) translate evidence to policy and practice (Kemp, 2019). Ironically, one use for evidence is that it can offer justification for economic rationalisation, which may influence funding for public health. Again, public health is vulnerable because it is difficult to provide outcomes in short political cycles. For example, in Australia in the early 1990s, harm-minimisation policy frameworks were implemented in drug and alcohol services. One of the most notable of these was the needle-exchange programs and services. More recently, controversial 'lockout laws' have been designed, along with other measures such as the 'One punch can kill' campaign, to address alcohol-fuelled violence. While there have been claims of success, there is significant debate about the evidence for their effectiveness in reducing the incidence of alcohol-fuelled violence.

Policy–practice gap

There is a sufficient body of evidence to suggest that a gap, or lag, exists between the development of policy and their implementation into practice. This can be attributed to the time taken from the publication of evidence to the translation of this evidence into policy and the implementation of these policies. This lag is often attributed to a lack of political will or politicians' apathy. Think back to the idea of political will discussed earlier in this chapter. Perhaps public health and health promotion are not important enough to politicians? Several factors could play a role in influencing politicians to give precedence to health promotion. These include a prioritised public health agenda, the realisation of tangible health outcomes that are grounded in political action and the absence of political costs, such as losing their seat. More than ever before, the COVID-19 pandemic compelled politicians to actively participate in, and to prioritise, public health measures (Webster & Neal, 2021). In Australia, this level of investment by politicians saw the successful implementation of strategies to contain the spread of the virus and to support the economy while doing so. However, the vaccine rollout provides a stark example of the complexity of the practice–policy gap, despite the strength of existing systems. The gap between policy and practice may be reduced if public health improves its relationship with politicians and the political cycle.

SPOTLIGHT 10.4

Black Lives Matter: Equity, fairness and justice

Now, let's think about the policy–practice gap in the association between race and health inequities. Globally, there is unequivocal evidence to indicate significant health and other disparities in certain populations groups, such as Aboriginal and Torres Strait Islander peoples in Australia and African-Americans in the United States. In May 2020, these racial disparities were played out on the international stage when George Floyd, an African-American man, died in police custody in Minneapolis. Police Officer Chauvin was captured on video, kneeling on Floyd's neck for 9 minutes and 29 seconds despite cries from Floyd that he could not breathe. Chauvin was later convicted of two counts of murder. In response to the public outcry in the United States, the Black Lives Matter (BLM) movement spearheaded protest rallies in many states and galvanised support from communities around the world. In Australia, BLM rallies took place in most states and territories during the COVID-19 pandemic lockdown. Rally organisers were criticised for risking another outbreak of the virus and endangering lives. Rally supporters responded that seizing the moment was important to highlight injustices in health, economic, social and political disparities on the basis of race. In Australia, this moment in recent history highlights the disproportionate rates of incarceration, deaths in custody, life expectancy and mortality and morbidity among Aboriginal and Torres Strait Islander peoples. It is a stark reminder that not much has changed from the report of the Royal Commission into Aboriginal Deaths in Custody 30 years ago (National Archives of Australia, 2021).

QUESTION

What do you think it will take for evidence-based policy to be adopted to address health inequity among Aboriginal and Torres Strait Islander peoples in Australia?

Ethical advocacy

Advocacy is identified in global documents such as the Ottawa Charter and the Galway Consensus (Barry et al., 2019) as a core competency for public health practitioners. Public health has a vital role in advocating for change in the political determinants of health and to reduce **health inequities** in vulnerable and marginalised populations (see also Chapter 5). Advocacy is driven by professionals, consumer groups, communities and populations, and is underpinned by four ethical principles: autonomy, beneficence, non-maleficence and justice. It is a political process about challenging those who hold power to force action for change. It is underpinned by coalitions, collective action and evidence. Community-based, *bottom-up* advocacy is about community connectedness, **social capacity building** and empowering communities and populations to engage with the political process to enact change. A great example of people power in the glocal (local + global) environment (Milne, 2015) was seen in Newcastle-upon-Tyne in the United Kingdom. Fast-food giant McDonald's submitted a planning application to the city's council to build a two-story restaurant and drive-through facility. The council rejected the application, partly due to an opposition campaign organised spontaneously by the local community.

Health inequity – the disparity between health resources and outcomes across populations.

Social capacity building – the use of human skills and resources to build strong communities.

McDonald's appealed the decision, but, following community backlash, withdrew its appeal (Kelly, 2015).

Political advocacy

Advocacy can influence broader societal reform; for example, sexual health promotion in the early 1970s. A series of 'Grim Reaper' advertisements supported an intense sexual health-promotion campaign to address the HIV/AIDS epidemic. The resulting political and social change was supported by several public health initiatives, such as installation of condom-vending machines in nightclubs and testing for people working in the sex industry. Despite, or maybe because of, the evidence for success across several social and health outcome indicators, the campaign eventually lost its public funding. Another example is when the 'morning-after pill' was made available over the counter in pharmacies to girls over 14 years of age. Today, new technologies offer advocacy an efficient means of mobilising sentiment. Social media platforms are effective mechanisms to harness the collective power of those with shared beliefs and values though forming coalitions and alliances (e.g. the not-for-profit organisations GetUp! and Crikey).

Seminal health-promotion documents, such as the *Lalonde Report* (1974), the *Declaration of Alma-Ata* (1978) and the Ottawa Charter (1986) implicitly and explicitly highlight the political determinants of health: power and control, governance and resource distribution, systems and decision-making, and inequities and empowerment. Change needs to be motivated through more explicit political and moral perspectives than health as an investment, a global public good or a human right, health and human security and development, or health and global justice (McNeil & Ottersen, 2015). And health promotion practitioners working passionately at the grassroots level are political advocates by the nature of their work, in that they form alliances to enact change. But advocacy is compromised because many public health practitioners work for the government, lack confidence to be politically active or feel they have little power to influence policy. Consequently, they risk being 'engaged followers' who acquiesce to the authority of government (Galea & Vaughan, 2019; Peplow & Augustine, 2020). This may be an underlying problem for advocacy in public health (see also Chapter 6).

REFLECTION QUESTION

As a starting point, think about the Black Lives Matter movement or climate change action. What strategies could mobilise advocacy efforts underpinned by explicit moral and political perspectives? How can the power of these perspectives be harnessed to ensure change?

Ethics-based advocacy

Ethics underpins advocacy. Ethics in public health advocacy is about action and inaction, rights and liberties, power and inequalities. Public health ethics are grounded in consequentialism, whereby ethics are determined by the outcome of an action (see also Chapter 5). Population-based polices are created for the social or collective good so that most people can have better health outcomes. These policies may affect people's rights by restricting behaviour and infringing on civil liberties. Think back to our discussion about the Nuffield Ladder of Intervention. In developing this model, the Nuffield Council on Bioethics (2014–15) explored the ethical issues related to public health interventions, and proposed a stewardship model to balance liberty and collectivism underpinned by principles related to harm, vulnerability, autonomy and consent. Other examples are vaccinations for children to achieve 90 per cent 'herd immunity' and thereby protect the 10 per cent who are not immunised; and the addition of fluoride into the drinking-water supply. International bodies such as the United Nations and the WHO have been instrumental in implementing global policies (e.g. the 1948 *Universal Declaration of Human Rights*) for the right of all people to health.

But are coercive policies always universally beneficial, and do they justify the overriding of values such as personal freedom? Legislation relating to, for example, alcohol licensing, food labelling and junk-food advertising provokes debate. Opponents argue on a civil-rights platform that people should have the freedom to make their own choices about what they eat and drink. Proponents of public health argue the government can, and should, alter environments to influence the behavioural determinants of health (see Chapter 7). Internationally, there is strong evidence to suggest government policy on taxation (e.g. increasing the tax excise on alcohol), access (e.g. smoke-free workplaces), advertising (e.g. comprehensive bans on tobacco) and behaviour (e.g. seatbelts and drink-driving) affect population health outcomes. The evidence suggests that population-based health outcomes outweigh small limitations on freedom of choice (Mykhalovskiy & French, 2020).

SPOTLIGHT 10.5

Advocacy in action: Commitment, activism and change.

Let's consider the ethical dilemma associated with the density of alcohol outlets in low socio-economic areas. Unsurprisingly, it is not accidental that alcohol (and fast-food) outlets are built where people have lower educational attainment, low-paying jobs, are more likely to be welfare recipients and suffer domestic violence. This is where ethico-political advocacy can make difference. In 2015, the Woolworths supermarket chain proposed to build a new Dan Murphy's alcohol outlet in Darwin, in the Northern Territory (NT). To avoid the NT government's five-year freeze on new liquor licenses, Woolworth's applied to transfer the license of a small Dan Murphy's alcohol outlet near the town centre to a proposed megastore (48 times the size), within walking distance of three 'dry' Aboriginal communities. When the NT Liquor Commission refused Woolworths' application, the company appealed to the NT Civil and Administrative Tribunal. Despite the loss of the Woolworths appeal, the NT government introduced special legislation to fast-track the proposal. Community leaders and organisations, such as the Foundation for Alcohol Research & Education (FARE), joined forces to oppose the development. Aboriginal Elders led advocacy efforts, including shared social media content and an open letter published in the *Financial Review*, and challenged Woolworths in the NT Supreme Court. Designed to coincide with Woolworths' annual general meeting of shareholders, an open letter signed by more than 100 000 Australians through a change.org petition called on Woolworths to abandon its plans (Gibson, 2021). After nearly five years, Woolworths decided not to proceed with the development proposal.

QUESTION

What other advocacy efforts do you think could support more political wins for communities such as this one?

SUMMARY

In this chapter you have learnt about issues relating to the political and organisational determinants of health, from both the Australian and international perspectives. The salient issues covered in the chapter are summarised here.

Learning objective 1: Understand the balance between governments' responsibility and people's rights, and the influence of political will in public health.

The chapter provided several historical examples of governments' role in public health. Then it considered people as central to health care and how governments balance their responsibilities with people's rights. The chapter introduced a range of tools available to governments and how these should be viewed in the context of people's willingness to change. Next, political will and the nexus between health promotion and advocacy were discussed. This discussion considered the dilemma of creating and operationalising political will for change and better health outcomes.

Learning objective 2: Understand the distinctive features of the Australian healthcare system and political susceptibility in public health.

Australia's healthcare system today was propelled by the social reform, and underpinning principles of social justice, of the 1970s. Australians pay taxes to the government, which in turn provides a healthcare system. The chapter described distinctive features of the Australian healthcare system, such as the relationship between the local, state and federal governments. It also discussed the relationship between the public and private sector, where there are incentives and penalties for purchasing private health insurance. The chapter considered political susceptibility due to the effects of the political cycle and changes in government by considering Queensland as an example.

Learning objective 3: Comprehend the influence of cost-effectiveness and cost–benefit ratios, and the economic and social contexts of policy in public health.

Policy involves having a vision for change, and underpins the distribution of health resources. The chapter described the complex and interwoven relationship between health and economics, and considered population screening as an example. It discussed political economics and the use of existing health systems as more influential than the political ideologies that underpin them. The chapter also considered the population's tolerance to interventions and the context of social change, and the Nuffield Ladder of Intervention.

Learning objective 4: Analyse levels of evidence and the gap between policy and practice in public health.

Policies are underpinned by evidence. The chapter described the hierarchy of evidence, and how evidence might influence policy. It introduced the idea of a body of evidence, and where it might be accessed. The chapter discussed translational research and how this is affected by political cycles. It also considered the policy–practice gap and what could be done to ensure politicians actively pursue good public health policy.

Learning objective 5: Analyse the role of advocacy and the use of evidence in advocacy in public health.

Advocacy is a tool to address health inequities in vulnerable populations. The chapter described how advocacy can bring about broader societal reforms and how technology can be used to support the formation of coalitions and to mobilise power for change. It discussed the concept of consequential ethics and collective good, and how coercive policies, which restrict individual freedom, are universally good.

TUTORIAL EXERCISES

1 Source a current local newspaper, either in print or online. First, from the front to the back, count the number of articles about health. This will give you an idea of role of popular media in reporting health and how the media cycle is linked to health politics. Now, select one of these articles to discuss in your tutorial group. In particular, you should think about how health is reported in the popular media within the prevailing social context of health. That is, do the policy issues reflect the social norms of the communities and populations for whom they are designed?

2 Think back to the question in Spotlight 10.3, which asked you to consider potential policy directions to address the global supply and distribution of COVID-19 vaccines. In your tutorial groups, first discuss the population's tolerance to your policy ideas. Then, using Nuffield's Ladder of Intervention, think about other interventions that might affect the global supply and distribution of vaccines in view of the population's tolerance.

3 Go to the website of the not-for-profit organisation GetUp! (https://www.getup.org.au/). Go to the campaigns tab and select a campaign, related to health, which interests you. Gather more information from other reliable sources. Now, go to the suggestions tab on the GetUp! home page and think about what you could do to support your chosen campaign. You should discuss, and refine, your suggestion with your tutorial group. Consider posting your suggestion on the website. Or why not volunteer as a group? Just go to the volunteer tab and sign up. You might prefer the Crikey site (https://www.crikey.com.au/) instead.

FURTHER READING

Climate and Health Alliance (CAHA). Retrieved https://www.caha.org.au/ Read the news and look at current campaigns and projects about climate change. Then go to the Resources/Reports by CAHA and read *Australia in 2030: Possible alternative futures*. Sign up for the newsletter, make a donation, decide to volunteer and take action by emailing your local MP.

The Conversation. Retrieved https://theconversation.com/au This is a free, collaborative electronic forum that offers informed analytical comment about current issues. You will find relevant conversations on the *Health + Medicine* and *Politics + Society* pages. And have a look at the *Business + Economy* and *Education* pages. Why not follow a topic?

United Nations Climate Change (Website). The Paris Agreement. Retrieved https://unfccc.int/process-and-meetings/the-paris-agreement/the-paris-agreement Read about climate change from an international perspective. Scroll towards the bottom of the homepage and watch the short YouTube clip called *What is the Paris Agreement? And how does it work?* Then go to the Climate Action page and review the *Climate Action Blog*.

Read local and national newspapers regularly so you are well informed about current political health issues.

REFERENCES

Australian Broadcasting Corporation. (2012). As it happened: LNP pulls off crushing win. *ABC News*. Retrieved http://www.abc.net.au/news/2012-03-24/live-blog3a-queensland-votes/3910364

——(2017). Grenfell Tower fire: Survivors, Royal family attend memorial service for victims. *ABC News*. Retrieved http://www.abc.net.au/news/2017-12-15/grenfell-fire-royal-family-attends-memorial-service/9260634

Barry, M. M., Allegrante, J. P., Lamarre, M-C., Auld, M. E., & Taub, A. (2009). The Galway Consensus Conference: International collaboration on the development of core competencies for health promotion and health education. *Global Health Promotion*, *16*(2), 5–11.

Bekker, M. P. M., Greer, S. L., Azzopardi-Muscat, N., & McKee, M. (2018). Public health and politics: How political science can help us move forward. *European Journal of Public Health*, *28*(Suppl 3), 1–2.

Cole, J., & Dodds, K. (2021). Unhealthy geopolitics? Bordering disease in the time of coronavirus *Geographical Research*, *59*, 169–81.

Commonwealth of Australia. (2017). The Hon Greg Hunt MP Minister for Health Care and Ageing. Retrieved http://www.health.gov.au/internet/ministers/publishing.nsf/Content/health-mediarel-yr2017-hunt106.htm

Department of Industry, Science, Energy and Resources. (2021). Households – quick wins (Webpage). Retrieved https://www.energy.gov.au/households/quick-wins

Eaton, L. A., & Kalichman, S. C. (2020). Social and behavioral health responses to COVID-19: Lessons learned from four decades of an HIV pandemic. *Journal of Behavioural Medicine*, *43*, 341–5.

Galea, S., & Vaughan, R. D. (2019). Public health, politics, and the creation of meaning: A public health of consequence. *American Journal of Public Health*, *109*(7), 966–8.

Gibson, J. (2021). Woolworths and NT government blasted in damning review of Darwin Dan Murphy's proposal. *ABC News*. Retrieved https://www.abc.net.au/news/2021-06-09/nt-woolworths-releases-independent-darwin-dan-murphys/100200942

Green, A. (2012). Post-election pendulum for 2012 Queensland election (Blog post). Retrieved http://blogs.abc.net.au/antonygreen/2012/05/post-election-pendulum-for-2012-queensland-election.html

Greer, S. L. (2018). Labour politics as public health: How the politics of industrial relations and workplace regulation affect health. *European Journal of Public Health*, *28*(Suppl 3), 34–7.

Kelly, M. (2015). *Kenton Lane McDonald's 'drive thru': Fast food giant to appeal planning decision*. Retrieved http://www.chroniclelive.co.uk/news/north-east-news/kenton-lane-mcdonalds-drive-thru-8771295

Kemp, L. (2019). Translational research: Bridging the chasm between new knowledge and useful knowledge. In P. Liamputtong (Ed.), *Handbook of research methods in health social sciences*. Springer Nature.

Kickbusch, I. (2015). The political determinants of health – 10 years on. *British Medical Journal*, *350*, h81.

Lawson, E. (2020). The political determinants of health. *British Journal of General Practice*, *701*, 569–616.

Lalonde, M. (1974). *A new perspective on the health of Canadians*. Minister of Supply and Services Canada. Retrieved http://www.phac-aspc.gc.ca/ph-sp/pdf/perspect-eng.pdf

Mackenbach, J. (2014). Political determinants of health. *Health European Journal of Public Health*, *24*(1), 2.

Mahler, H. (1986). Towards a new public health. *Health Promotion*, *1*(1), 1.

McKee, M. (2017). Grenfell Tower fire: Why we cannot ignore the political determinants of health. *British Medical Journal*, *357*, j2966.

McNeil, D., & Ottersen, O. P. (2015). Global governance for health: How to motivate political change? *Public Health*, *129*, 833–7.

Milne, E. M. G. (2015). Governance for health – grasping at the levers of glocal health. *Public Health*, *129*, 870–1.

Mykhalovskiy, E., & French, M. (2020). COVID-19, public health, and the politics of prevention. *Sociology of Health and Illness*, *42*(8), 4–15.

National Archives of Australia. (2021). *Royal Commission into Aboriginal Deaths in Custody*. Retrieved https://www.naa.gov.au/explore-collection/first-australians/royal-commission-aboriginal-deaths-custody

Navarro, J. A., & Markel, H. (2021). Politics, pushback, and pandemics: Challenges to public health orders in the 1918 influenza pandemic. *American Journal of Public Health*, *111*, 416–22.

Nuffield Council on Bioethics. (2014–15). The intervention ladder. Retrieved http://nuff-ieldbioethics.org/report/public-health-2/policy-process-practice

Peplow, D., & Augustine, S. (2020). The submissive relationship of public health to government, politics, and economics: How global health diplomacy and engaged followership compromise humanitarian relief. *International Journal of Environmental Research and Public Health*, *17*, 1420.

Public Health Association of Australia (PHAA). 2021. Australia should follow US decision on COVID-19 vaccine patents (Media Release, 6 May). Retrieved https://www.phaa.net.au/documents/item/5141

Queensland Parliament. (2010). Everyone's Parliament Factsheet 3.20 Abolition of the Legislative Council. Retrieved https://www.parliament.qld.gov.au/documents/explore/education/factsheets/Factsheet_ 3.20_AbolitionOfTheLegislativeCouncil.pdf

Queensland Public Service Award – State. 2012. Repeal and New Award (A/2010/145). Retrieved http://www .qirc.qld.gov.au/resources/pdf/awards/q/q0350_q0110_ar10.pdf

Raphael, D. (2014). Beyond policy analysis: The raw politics behind opposition to healthy public policy. *Health Promotion International*, *30*(2), 380–96.

Sundin, J. (2019). Public health is politics. *Interchange*, 50, 129–36.

Wainwright, O., & Walker, P. (2017). 'Disaster waiting to happen': Fire expert slams UK tower blocks. *The Guardian*. Retrieved https://www.theguardian.com/uk-news/2017/jun/14/disaster-waiting-to-happen-fire-expert-slams-uk-tower-blocks

Webster, P., & Neal, K. (2021). Covid reflections: Let us talk of politicians and professors. *Journal of Public Health*, *43*(1), 1–2.

World Health Organization (WHO). (1978). Declaration of Alma-Ata. International Conference on Primary Health Care, Alma-Ata, USSR. Retrieved https://www.who.int/publications/almaata_ declaration_en.pdf

——(1986). *The Ottawa Charter for Health Promotion*. Retrieved https://www.euro.who.int/__data/assets/ pdf_file/0004/129532/Ottawa_Charter.pdf

——(2018). *Health 2020: The European policy for health and well-being*. WHO. Retrieved http://www.euro.who .int/en/health-topics/health-policy/health-2020-the-european-policy-for-health-and-well-being

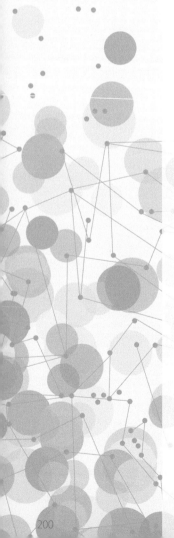

11

Human rights, social justice and public health

Ann Taket

LEARNING OBJECTIVES

After studying this chapter, you should be able to:

1   describe human rights and the various global, regional and national systems that exist to support their achievement
2   describe the ways in which human rights are important in public health
3   understand the different ways that governments can be held to account for their human rights performance
4   understand the links between human rights and empowerment.

VIGNETTE

Brazil's 'María da Penha Law'

One significant example of the use of global human rights systems to secure progress in addressing an important public health issue is provided by the case of Brazil's 'María da Penha Law'. In 1983, María da Penha, a Brazilian bio-pharmacist, was the victim of two homicide attempts by her then-husband and father of her three daughters, inside their house, in Fortaleza, a city in northeastern Brazil (CLADEM, n.d.). The first of these attempts left María with irreversible paraplegia (CLADEM, n.d.). María pursued a case against her husband through the legal system in Brazil, but 15 years later there was still no definitive decision and her husband remained at liberty (Inter-American Commission on Human Rights, 2001). María, working with two non-governmental organisations (NGOs), the Center for Justice and International Law (CEJIL) and the Latin American and Caribbean Committee for the Defense of Women's Rights (CLADEM), then submitted a case to the Inter-American Commission on Human Rights, Organization of American States (CEJIL, n.d.).

María's case was that the Federative Republic of Brazil had for years condoned domestic violence perpetrated in the city of Fortaleza, Ceará State by Marco Antônio Heredia Viveiros against his wife at the time, culminating in attempted murder and further aggression in May and June 1983 (Inter-American Commission on Human Rights, 2001). They argued that the state had condoned this situation since, for more than 15 years, it failed to take effective measures required to prosecute and punish the aggressor, despite repeated complaints, which constituted a violation of several articles of the Organization of American States' American Convention on Human Rights; namely, Obligation to Respect Rights, and to ensure a Fair Trial, Equal Protection, and Judicial Protection (Inter-American Commission on Human Rights, 2001). The commission found the case proven, in its judgment dated 16 April 2001, and made recommendations to Brazil (Inter-American Commission on Human Rights, 2001).

In response, working together with NGOs (Special Secretariat for Women's Policies, 2006) the Brazilian government formulated and then in 2006 enacted a law, Law 11.340 (CEJIL, n.d.), under the symbolic name 'María da Penha Law on Domestic and Family Violence', which created a range of mechanisms to restrain domestic and family violence (UN Women, 2011).

In July 2008, María received a formal apology and financial compensation from the government (CLADEM, n.d.). On the fifth anniversary of the enactment of the law, in August 2011, the National Council of Justice of Brazil collected data showing positive results: more than 331 000 prosecutions and 110 000 final judgments, and nearly 2 million calls to the Service Center for Women (UN Women, 2011).

Introduction

The vignette of María da Penha, based on a major public health issue, demonstrates that the achievement of **social justice** goes hand in hand with progress in tackling public health issues. Social justice is so central to the new public health model that it has been described as the field's core value or principle. The achievement of social justice is closely connected with

Social justice – the equitable distribution of benefits and burdens among populations.

progress on the achievement of human rights and the reduction of health inequities. The member states of the United Nations (UN) have ratified the *Universal Declaration on Human Rights* and a range of other covenants and conventions covering human rights, thereby acquiring obligations to respect, protect and fulfil human rights. This represents a significant political agreement, and this chapter is concerned with exploring the instrumental value of this in relation to the new public health model.

The sections that follow in this chapter introduce human rights and the various global, regional and national systems that exist to support their achievement, discussing the different ways in which human rights are important in public health. Human rights-based approaches are of great potential importance in providing grounding for public health policy and practice that seeks social justice in the health arena. There are considerable overlaps between the social determinants of health and human rights, and consequently inextricable links between the achievement of social justice, **health equity** and human rights. An understanding of the UN human rights system, the various human rights instruments, and the monitoring and reporting system is thus of great relevance to public health professionals.

Health equity – a situation in which groups with different levels of underlying social advantage or disadvantage (wealth, power or prestige) do not experience health inequalities associated solely with their social positioning.

Global, regional and national systems for human rights monitoring and accountability are introduced, and the chapter explores how progress towards meeting obligations to respect, protect and fulfil rights relates to progress towards achieving the social determinants of health and progress towards health equity. There are different routes by which governments can be held accountable for their achievements or lack of them, and action to address social injustice and health inequities supported. Three main routes are through the UN system, through national or regional legislation, and through the policy and programming processes. Advocacy by concerned actors such as NGOs can play an important role in each of these three routes. The final section in the chapter explores the links between human rights and empowerment.

What are human rights?

Human right – a right held to justifiably belong to any person or group of people.

Human rights are the rights and freedoms that belong to all people. These include the right to life, the right to liberty, the right to be free from slavery and inhuman and degrading treatment, and the right to respect for private and family life. Rights cannot be taken away, but some can be restricted in specific circumstances. A public authority can restrict rights if they have a legitimate aim (e.g. if they are concerned about someone's safety, or to protect the wider community from harm), so public health practitioners may limit freedom of movement or association for particular groups in order to protect public health.

> Alongside securing peace and security and working to realize development throughout the world, promoting and protecting all human rights for all people is one of the three pillars of the UN. This is established in the UN Charter and international human rights law ... The Office of the United Nations High Commissioner for Human Rights (OHCHR) is a lead organization within the UN working for human rights promotion and protection. It works closely with UN specialized agencies, funds and programmes ... to maximize the impact of human rights work ... International human rights treaties (covenants and conventions) establish panels of independent experts, or treaty bodies, to regularly and periodically consider countries' implementation of human rights obligations. Inter-governmental bodies, or assemblies, composed of Member States of the UN are established to discuss human rights issues and situations (Office of the United Nations High Commissioner for Human Rights, 2014, p. 5).

The Office of the United Nations High Commissioner for Human Rights (OHCHR) also works to protect and support human rights defenders – those individuals or groups who work to promote and protect human rights.

In 1948, the *Universal Declaration of Human Rights* (UDHR) was adopted (UN, 1948); the content of its 30 articles is summarised in Figure 11.1. One article in the UDHR has particular relevance to public health: Article 25, which states, in part: 'Everyone has the right to a standard of living adequate for the health and well-being of himself and his family, including food, clothing, housing and medical care and necessary social services.' Since 1948, more than 20 multilateral human rights treaties have been adopted, creating legally binding obligations on the countries that have ratified them. Particularly significant treaties are the two covenants: *International Covenant on Civil and Political Rights* (ICCPR) and the *International Covenant*

1 We are all free and equal	2 No discrimination	3 Right to live in freedom and safety
4 No slavery	5 No torture	6 You have rights no matter where you go
7 We are all equal before the law	8 Your human rights are protected by law	9 No unfair detainment
10 Right to public trial	11 We are always innocent until proven guilty	12 Right to privacy and no defamation
13 Freedom of movement	14 Right to asylum	15 Right to nationality
16 Right to marriage and family of own choosing	17 Right to your own things	18 Freedom of thought and religion
19 Freedom of expression	20 Right to public assembly	21 Right to democracy and participation
22 Social security	23 Right to work and income	24 Right to rest and leisure
25 Standard of living adequate for health and wellbeing	26 Right to education	27 Right to share in arts and science
28 A fair and free world	29 Responsibility	30 No one can take away your human rights

Notes: Background shading indicates rights that are covered in detail in:

International Covenant on Civil and Political Rights (ICCPR)

International Covenant on Economics, Social and Cultural Rights (ICESCR)

Figure 11.1 Summary content of the articles of the *Universal Declaration of Human Rights*.
Source: Based on United Nations (1948).

on Economic, Social and Cultural Rights (ICESCR). Both were adopted by the UN General Assembly on 16 December 1966. The ICCPR and ICESCR, plus the UDHR and the *Charter of the United Nations*, are often referred to as the 'International Bill of Human Rights'.

REFLECTION QUESTION

Considering your own experience in your personal, student or professional life, what human rights infringements have you seen or experienced?

Universality and other key features

Perhaps the most important feature of human rights is their universality: the understanding that human rights are rights belonging to *all* human beings and are fundamental to every type of society. Each person has the same basic human rights, regardless of gender, age, culture, ethnicity, religion, sexuality and (dis)ability.

Individual human rights do not exist in isolation of each other; they are indivisible, interrelated and interdependent. This does not, however, mean that all rights reinforce one each other. Rights can affect each other adversely. For example, the right to freedom of expression may interfere with the right to privacy or with the right to freedom from discrimination. In situations of resource scarcity, many rights, such as to a healthy environ-ment, education, health care and social security, may be in competition with each other.

The distinction between absolute and relative rights is important. Absolute rights are those where restrictions may not be placed on them in any circumstances. These include the rights to be free from torture, slavery or servitude; to a fair trial; and to freedom of thought. The right to life is not absolute; what is forbidden is arbitrary deprivation of life. The right to freedom of thought or opinion and the right to hold any opinion do not include unlimited rights to free expression of opinion; this is qualified by restrictions relating to the protection of the rights of others, or in certain specific circumstances. This illustrates the complex interdependence that exists between the achievement of rights of different groups within the same community. Some of the articles in the conventions and covenants provide guidance on when rights can justifiably be restricted; this is discussed further in the next section.

Regional human rights systems

Established regional human rights systems, based on a human rights charter, together with some regional enforcement mechanisms, exist in Africa, the Americas and Europe. In the Asia-Pacific region and the Middle East, more limited regional developments have taken place. The 10 countries of ASEAN (Association of Southeast Asian Nations) do have a Human Rights Declaration, adopted in November 2012; however, the associated monitoring body has been heavily criticised for its weak record in comparison to other regional and international systems (Hanung et al., 2018). The vignette that begins this chapter shows how the regional system in the Americas was used to secure an important legal change in Brazil of public health importance.

In Africa, the basic regional human rights instrument is the *African Charter on Human and Peoples' Rights*. Human and peoples' rights are set out in articles 1 to 26 of that charter.

The particular formulation used in the charter, as well as within the title of the associated commission and court, of 'human and peoples' rights' rather than simply 'human rights' can be seen as a move to include explicitly the notion of 'collective rights' held by a group as well as 'individual rights' held by every person.

There are two overlapping regional systems in Europe. The first is based on the *European Convention on Human Rights*, associated with the Council of Europe, which was signed in 1950 and entered into force in 1953; its original title was the *Convention for the Protection of Human Rights and Fundamental Freedoms*. The European Court of Human Rights covers the Council of Europe member states that have ratified the convention. The second European system is associated with the European Union (EU) and is based on the *Charter of Fundamental Rights of the European Union* (EU, 2000). An analysis by McHale (2010) concludes that, although the charter potentially has considerable implications for health law and health policy throughout the EU, its long-term effects are uncertain.

National human rights institutions

In the time since the establishment of the UN, national systems for supporting human rights have developed in terms of different types of national human rights institutions (NHRIs). Pohjolainen (2006) distinguishes four different functions that NHRIs may have: (1) monitoring of observance of human rights, sometimes including complaint investigation; (2) advisory, providing advice to government and sometimes to other relevant actors; (3) education and information, including awareness-raising, education and training; and (4) research, undertaking specific investigations, studies and sometimes public inquiries.

At the national level, possibilities depend on the position of human rights within the country concerned and the nature of the country – leading in some cases to more than one NHRI. The World Conference on Human Rights in 1993 endorsed the establishment of national institutions (UN General Assembly, 1993) and the use of the 'Principles relating to the status of national institutions' that had been formulated in 1991 and are generally known as the 'Paris Principles', after the city in which they were formulated. The main features of the Paris Principles are (1) a mandate with emphasis on the national implementation of international human rights standards; (2) independent of the state; (3) a pluralist representation of civil society and vulnerable groups in governance mechanisms; and (4) handling of complaints from individuals (derived from Lindsnaes, Lindholt & Yigen, 2000). At January 2021, there were 117 NHRIs wholly or partially in compliance with the Paris Principles listed on the website of the International Coordinating Committee of National Institutions for the Promotion and Protection of Human Rights (OHCHR, n.d.), and a further 10 institutions that are non-compliant.

SPOTLIGHT 11.1

Improving the lives of women and children

The *Convention on the Elimination of All Forms of Discrimination against Women* and the *Convention on the Rights of the Child* came into force in 1979 and 1990, respectively. The World Health Organization

(WHO) took the lead in carrying out a wide-ranging investigation to look at the extent to which measures to improve human rights move beyond laws and institutions to actually improve the lives and wellbeing of women and children. Bustreo and Hunt (2013) summarised evidence from four diverse countries: Brazil, Italy, Malawi and Nepal. They concluded that applying human rights to women's and children's health policies, programs and interventions not only helps governments to comply with international and national obligations, but also contributes to improving the health of women and children (Bustreo & Hunt, 2013). Yamin (2013) traced the influence of rights-based approaches in women's health from the 1990s onwards, providing examples of successful influence around the globe.

QUESTION
Why do you think that the formulation of specific human rights instruments for different population groups has proved helpful?

Why are human rights important to public health practitioners?

Human rights are of great importance in public health practice for several reasons. First, there are extensive and close links between specific human rights and the social determinants of health, so that action to support human rights is at the same time supporting the reduction of health **inequity,** and action to reduce health inequity often also has positive consequences for human rights; this is considered further in this section.

Inequity – inequality as a consequence of unfairness or bias.

Human rights also provide a very powerful basis for public health advocacy, based on the understanding of the right to health, also discussed in this section. Since the 1990s, public health practitioners have been heavily involved in the development and use of rights-based approaches to support their work. The earliest work was carried out in the field of HIV/AIDS in order to counter the abuses of human rights suffered by those living with HIV/AIDS, and to respond to the evidence that discrimination was resulting in low uptake of HIV/AIDS prevention and care programs (Mann & Tarantola, 1998). The reports cited in Spotlight 11.1 (Bustreo & Hunt, 2013; Yamin, 2013) provide a wealth of examples in terms of the importance of rights-based approaches in women's and children's health. For a more detailed review of different types of approaches and their application to other health topics, see McKay and Taket (2020).

A final reason human rights are of importance to public health practitioners is that rights can legitimately be restricted to protect the health of the public (e.g. in infectious disease control). Conditions in which rights can be restricted are described later in this section.

Human rights and the social determinants of health

Human rights are closely linked to the social determinants of health. This can be seen through a few key documents. The *Ottawa Charter for Health Promotion* (the Ottawa

Charter) (WHO, 1986) lists social justice and equity as two of the prerequisites for health, along with peace, shelter, education, food, income, a stable ecosystem and sustainable resources. The report of the Commission on the Social Determinants of Health fore-grounds social justice and broad political and economic determinants in the world's health agenda (Muntaner et al., 2009). More recently, the debate on the post-2015 development agenda has emphasised that, in order to be truly transformative in tackling inequity, human rights must be recognised as its foundation (Pillay, 2013; Pomi, 2015; see chapters 1, 7 and 10).

Equity – fairness, to each according to their need.

The 'right to health'

One particularly important right for public health practitioners is the right to health. This is directly stated in the preamble to the WHO's constitution; article 25 of the UDHR mentions health and article 12 of the ICESCR makes it explicit. This explicit recognition of the highest attainable standard of health as a human right, as opposed to a good or commodity with a charitable construct, provides a very powerful basis for public health advocacy (McKay & Taket, 2020). It is important to note that the ICESCR mentions explicitly both mental health and physical health. Other international human rights instruments also address the right to health, both generally and in relation to specific groups.

To help move towards attainment of the right to health, the committee responsible for the ICESCR formulated General Comment 14, and the OHCHR and WHO have produced a fact sheet on the right to health (OHCHR and WHO, 2008). One of the key normative points about the right to health is that it extends to the underlying determinants of health (General Comment 14, paragraphs 4, 10, 11). Also important is the participation of population in all health-related decision-making at community, national, and international levels (General Comment 14, paragraphs 11, 17, 34, 54).

Justifiable restrictions on rights: The Siracusa principles and their public health equivalent

Here, we look at valid or justifiable limitations on human rights. The UDHR and the two covenants all discuss the issue, setting out circumstances in which limitation of rights can be justified. They do this in two different ways: first in general articles, and then specifically in relation to particular rights. The form of the limitation varies; of particular interest are limitations on public health grounds, applying to rights such as freedom of movement and association, freedom of expression and freedom to manifest one's religion or beliefs. Infectious diseases present one clear public health example in which restrictions of human rights may need to be enacted, as can clearly be seen in a variety of measures adopted during the COVID-19 pandemic.

Recognising the difficulty of the judgements that need to be exercised in deciding whether a specific limitation of rights is justified, a series of principles was formulated to assist such decisions: the Siracusa principles, which provide general criteria for rights limitation to be regarded as legitimate. In the case of restriction on the specific ground of protection of public health, Gostin (cited in Coker, 2001) has formulated some specific criteria; these are presented in Table 11.1.

Table 11.1   Criteria to assess whether rights can justifiably be limited

Siracusa principles – general	Restriction on the grounds of protection of public health
When a government limits the exercise of enjoyment of a right, this action must be taken as a last resort and will only be considered legitimate if the following criteria are met: • The restriction is provided for and carried out in accordance with the law. • The restriction is in the interest of a legitimate objective of general interest. • The restriction is strictly necessary in the democratic society to achieve this objective. • There are no less-intrusive and restrictive means available to reach the same goal. • The restriction is not imposed arbitrarily (i.e. in an unreasonable or otherwise discriminatory manner).	Gostin (quoted in Coker (2001)) suggests the following specific criteria for use where restriction is proposed on grounds of public health: • The proposal should be demonstrable and significant. • Proposed interventions should be demonstrably effective. • The approach should be cost-effective. • Sanctions should be least restrictive necessary. • Policy should be fair and non-discriminatory.

SPOTLIGHT 11.2

'To end AIDS, we must fight injustice'

The title for this spotlight comes from a video, called *I'll Walk with You*, which was released in late 2013 and describes how a network of paralegal professionals is working to ensure people living with HIV have access to law and **justice** in Uganda. The video explains that, in 2011, 8 people out of every 100 in Uganda were living with HIV/AIDS, and facing considerable stigmatisation, including through aspects of the law and property rights. Paralegals, many of whom are living with HIV/AIDS themselves and who are drawn from the communities they work within, help those living with HIV/AIDS to protect their rights. The video is available at https://vimeo.com/93595012.

Justice – fairness

QUESTION
What are the public health implications of the rights violations discussed in Spotlight 11.2?

REFLECTION QUESTION

Considering your own experience during the COVID-19 pandemic, which of your human rights were limited? Did these limitations fulfil the Siracusa criteria?

Holding governments to account

The various human rights instruments make clear that the role of governments in respect of human rights can be understood in terms of respecting, protecting and fulfilling rights.

Governments must not infringe people's human rights without justification, and must also go beyond this, protecting rights from infringement by others and taking action to promote fulfilment of rights. Two subsections here consider systems for monitoring and accountability: first at the global level, and second at regional and national levels.

Global systems for monitoring and accountability

Corresponding to the nine core human rights treaties, there are nine bodies or committees that monitor countries' performance. Each country is required to submit an initial report on the extent of its compliance with the treaty in question *at the time of the country becoming a party to the treaty*. Subsequently, further reports are submitted at four or five-yearly intervals. Committees also conduct hearings with government representatives to examine progress. NGOs can submit 'alternative' reports to the relevant committees; these may be used during the hearings. The Universal Periodic Review is an additional process that involves a review of the human rights record of each UN member state once every four years.

As well as being responsible for monitoring country progress, some of the committees may receive complaints (usually called 'communications') that human rights violations have occurred. Communications may be from states – but this is rare (Gruskin & Tarantola, 2005) – or from individuals. Five of the human rights treaty bodies may, under particular circumstances, consider complaints from individuals (details can be found on the OHCHR website https://www.ohchr.org). A committee's opinions or 'views' relating to individual complaints are not binding in any legal sense, but changes in laws or policies may result.

The work of special rapporteurs provides another means of supporting accountability and action. Mandates for special rapporteurs are based on topic and/or situation; they can make country and other visits, send communications to states regarding alleged human rights violations and submit annual reports on the activities carried out under the mandate to the commission and the General Assembly. Since 2002, there has been a special rapporteur on the right to health.

Regional and national-level possibilities for human rights-based accountability and action

The chapter's opening vignette has provided one example of the successful use of regional systems – namely the Inter-American Commission on Human Rights – to achieve progress on public health problems. The website of the Inter-American Commission on Human Rights (http://www.oas.org/en/iachr/mandate/what.asp) documents the activities of this regional system in a series of reports (annual, by country and by topic) as well as extensive details on cases, both completed and in progress.

In Europe, individuals or states can apply to the European Court of Human Rights to allege violation of the *European Convention on Human Rights*; judgments made by this court are binding on countries concerned (Goldhaber, 2007). National laws in Europe have been overturned on the grounds that they contravene the *European Convention on Human Rights* (Neuwahl & Rosas, 1995); for example, the Court ruled in 1981 that the criminalisation of homosexuality in Northern Ireland was illegal (*Dudgeon v UK*; see http://hudoc.echr.coe.int and search for Dudgeon). The Court's jurisdiction in relation to health is limited, since the *European Convention on Human Rights* does not contain a specific article on the right to health or the right to health care; however, cases have successfully been brought to support access to health care for marginalised groups. The website of the Court (http://www.echr.coe .int) contains country profiles as well as factsheets by topic.

In Africa, the system includes reports submitted every two years to the African Commission on Human and Peoples' Rights by countries on measures taken to support the rights and freedoms set out in the African charter. Country reports are published on the Commission's website (http://www.achpr.org), where judgments on complaints (communi-cations) can also be found.

At the national level, possibilities depend on the position of human rights within the country concerned. In some countries, the right to health or similar rights have been established in national constitutions; others have utilised non-binding policies instead, limiting recourse to courts. As examples of what can be achieved, Singh, Govender and Mills (2007) highlight the health reforms that have been achieved in Argentina, Ecuador, South Africa and India. Hogerzeil and colleagues (2006) examined completed court cases in low-income and middle-income countries where individuals or groups had sought access to essential medicines, with reference to the right to health. This review identified successful cases in 10 countries: eight countries in Central and Latin America, plus India and South Africa. Their interpretation of their findings is that litigation can help ensure governments fulfil their human rights obligations, but they suggest that courts should only be used as a last resort and it is better to ensure that human rights considerations are written into policy and programs.

Brennan and colleagues (2013) compare the effectiveness of four different routes in improving access to essential medicines by reducing the barriers that intellectual property laws create:

> (1) the use of human rights arguments in domestic court cases that deal with intellectual property laws, (2) the articulation of norms in the United Nations (UN) human rights system, (3) the use of human rights arguments and frameworks to secure greater pharmaceutical corporate accountability, and (4) the use of health-related rights to build multilateral and regional alliances that can more effectively oppose free trade agreements (FTAs) with TRIPS-plus provisions (TRIPS being Trade-Related Aspects of Intellectual Property Rights) (Brennan et al., 2013).

They found the first of these the most promising but demonstrate potential for each of the other three routes.

What about the accountability of non-state actors like multinational corporations?

Given increasing globalisation, and the associated development of multinational corporations whose activities affect health and the determinants of health on a widespread scale, since the 1970s countries and civil society groups have been calling for stronger accountability for such corporations. One possibility is through the development of a human rights treaty to prevent and address corporate human rights violations. Human Rights Council Resolution 26/9, adopted in June 2014, established a UN Working Group to develop a treaty to prevent and address human rights violations by transnational corporations and all business enterprises that have a transnational character in their operational activities.

How well is Australia doing in relation to its Indigenous peoples?

By 2021, the most recent report to the Human Rights Council concerning Australia's Indigenous peoples was the Report of the Special Rapporteur on the rights of Indigenous peoples, on her visit to Australia that took place between 20 March and 2 April 2017 (UN, 2017). The note by the Secretariat, published on the first page of the report, summarises:

> In the report, the Special Rapporteur observes that the policies of the Government do not duly respect the rights to self-determination and effective participation; contribute to the failure to deliver on the targets in the areas of health, education and employment; and fuel the escalating and critical incarceration and child removal rates of Aboriginal and Torres Strait Islanders.
>
> A comprehensive revision of those policies needs to be a national priority, and the consequences and prevalence of intergenerational trauma and racism must be acknowledged and addressed.

The body of the report contains detailed recommendations on the institutional and legal framework, self-determination and participation, health services, education, employment, housing, incarceration and the administration of justice, the removal of children, Stolen Generations and reparation, violence against women, political participation, and land rights and native title.

QUESTION

What implications about the performance of successive Australian governments can you draw from the contents of the report referred to above?

Human rights and empowerment

One important type of rights-based approach focuses on human rights education, empowering and building the capacity of people with the tools to take control of their own lives and to participate in the different sectors of society – an important contribution to the third and fourth action areas in the Ottawa Charter (WHO, 1986). This approach is concerned with making rights accessible to all, and concentrates on work with individuals or groups, often networked into and through different NGOs. Human rights education is an important component of the right to education (UDHR, article 26), and is important in supporting individuals and groups in achieving their right to participation in civil society (UDHR, article 21), and more specifically, participation in health-related decision-making that forms part of the right to health.

Empowerment can be understood as 'the process of increasing capacity of individuals or groups to make choices and to transform those choices into desired actions and outcomes' (Alsop, 2004, p. 120). Evidence for the importance of empowerment for health outcomes comes from the review conducted by Wallerstein (2006), which demonstrates that empowering initiatives can lead to improved health outcomes (both directly and indirectly); participation alone is insufficient without capacity building; and successful empowering interventions must be created or adapted to local contexts (e.g. gender and cultural appropriateness);

further discussion can be found in Taket (2013). Leavy and Howard (2013) demonstrated the importance of human rights education in the development context.

There is a growing number of examples in which human rights education has had direct consequences in terms of successful public health activism (see McKay & Taket, 2020). To give just a few examples from two countries. In India, Kapoor (2007) discusses the local level improvements gained for the Dalit community, and Dalit women in particular; while Bajaj (2012) and Kaushik and colleagues (2006) document the positive effects of human rights education in schools and tertiary education, respectively, in terms of growth in agency and actions within educational institutions, at home and in the wider community.

Taket (2013) discusses an example in South Africa, of the Soul City Institute for Health and Development Communication, an NGO which specialises in 'edutainment' designed to convey health information and prompt behavioural change. Soul Buddyz is a multimedia intervention targeting children aged 8 to 15 years. It has several components: a TV drama, *Soul Buddyz*, a lifeskills booklet for Grade 7 school students and Soul Buddyz clubs in primary schools for 8 to 12-year-olds, created after the response to the TV drama of children wanting to be Soul Buddyz. Complementary materials and messaging for parents and caregivers of children are also part of the intervention.

Soul Buddyz clubs were established in 2002, aiming to help children learn and develop skills that would facilitate mobilisation around issues affecting them, their schools and community. By 2004, there were 1900 clubs nationally. Club activities include weekly club meetings; discussions and debates on issues from the Soul Buddyz club monthly newsletter; projects relating to health and development issues like HIV and AIDS; doing research within communities about issues affecting children; preparing dramas and presenting these within their schools; and monthly and quarterly competitions. As Goldstein and colleagues (2001) identify, the rights in the *Convention on the Rights of the Child* are actively used in the program and each topic covered in the TV drama relates to a specific right.

The clubs provide their members with the opportunity to work on local issues in school or community. A wide range of successful activities is reported, including action on litter, development of vegetable gardens and action on bullying and abuse. Improvements in student discipline are also reported (Soul City, 2005). Evaluation (Soul City, 2005) demonstrates that the clubs are attractive to all cultural groups and are successful in skilling students to plan and take action: 'Soul Buddyz is different from other clubs because it teaches learners to become leaders. These kids are not afraid of anything, they are very articulate' (educator, quoted in Soul City, 2005, p. 36).

To support human rights education, there are growing sections of the OHCHR website. There is also an ever-increasing number of guides and resource books for use by concerned individuals, human rights defenders or activists. For example, at the global level, the Australian Human Rights Commission (AHRC, 2011) provides a guide to using the optional protocol to the *Convention on the Elimination of All Forms of Discrimination against Women* and other international complaint mechanisms; and OHCHR (2008) provides a handbook for civil society on working with the UN Human Rights Programme. The Organization for Security and Co-operation in Europe/Office for Democratic Institutions and Human Rights (2013b) presents guidelines on human rights education for human rights activists and the Organization for Security and Co-operation in Europe/Office for Democratic Institutions and Human Rights (2013a) offers the same for health workers. Asher (2004) provides a resource manual for NGOs on the right to health, and Asher and colleagues (2007) provide a tool kit for health professionals on the right to health and their day-to-day work.

SUMMARY

This chapter has discussed salient issues pertaining to human rights and health. These are summarised here.

Learning objective 1: Describe human rights and the various global, regional and national systems that exist to support their achievement.

The first section of the chapter examined the human rights contained in the UDHR and associated covenants and conventions. It discussed universality and other key features of human rights, and then presented an overview of the regional and national systems that work alongside the global system.

Learning objective 2: Describe the ways in which human rights are important in public health.

Human rights are of great importance in public health practice for several different reasons. First, there are extensive and close links between specific human rights and the social determinants of health. Second, they provide a very powerful basis for public health advocacy; rights-based approaches have proved extremely effect in supporting the development of public health practice and policy. Finally, human rights are of importance to public health practitioners as one of the reasons rights can legitimately be restricted is to protect the health of the public.

Learning objective 3: Understand the different ways that governments can be held to account for their human rights performance.

The third section looked at the variety of ways that governments can be held to account for their human rights records at global, regional and national levels, examining examples of where this has been at least partially successful, with important public health consequences. Recent moves to hold multinational corporations to account in relation to human rights were briefly overviewed.

Learning objective 4: Understand the links between human rights and empowerment.

The fourth section looked at the important links between human rights and empowerment, and between empowerment and health. Rights-based approaches incorporating human rights education have been particularly successful in empowering people to take positive action on their own and their family and community's behalf with consequent improvements in health.

TUTORIAL EXERCISES

1   As well as international human rights instruments, regions, countries, states and territories also have produced a variety of other human rights instruments. One such is the *European Convention on Human Rights* (https://www.echr.coe.int/Documents/Convention_ENG.pdf). Compare this to the UDHR (https://www.ohchr.org/EN/UDHR/Pages/Language.aspx?LangID=eng).
   a   Which is more comprehensive?
   b   What are the differences between them in their coverage of the social determinants of health?
   c   Which gives the strongest foundation for advocacy to ensure health equity?
2   Pick a country you are interested in and discuss what you think are its good and bad points in terms of protecting, promoting and fulfilling human rights. Make notes of your points.

      At the website of the OHCHR (https://www.ohchr.org/) locate the menu tab for 'Countries', use the search bar to select your country and then click >. In the centre of the screen, you will find links to the most recent reports on the country. Check them to see if your original assessment was accurate; update it where necessary.

      You can also explore the Universal Periodic Review for the country (https://www.ohchr.org/en/hr-bodies/upr/documentation); it is often very informative to compare the national report provided by the government with the compilation of UN information and the summary of information provided by other stakeholders, such as NHRIs and NGOs.

3   Human Rights Education Associates, Soka Gakkai International and the OHCHR have jointly produced a film. *A Path to Dignity: The Power of Human Rights Education* is a 28-minute movie based on three stories illustrating the effects of human rights education on school children (India), law-enforcement agencies (Australia) and women victims of violence (Turkey).

The film in English can be found at https://youtu.be/ahE0tJbvl78.

Watch the film and answer the following questions:

a   What were the most important messages you took from the introduction and conclusion to the film?

b   What are the key points from the Indian section?

c   What are the key points from the Australian section?

d   What are the key points from the Turkish section?

This can also be done as small group work: each group takes one of the questions above, watches the relevant section(s) of the film and then in a plenary session presents their findings to the group as a whole.

FURTHER READING

Chapman, A. R. (2010). The social determinants of health, health equity, and human rights. *Health and Human Rights*, *12*(2), 17–30.

Gruskin, S., Mills, E. J., & Tarantola, D. (2007). History, principles and practice of health and human rights. *The Lancet*, *370*, 449–55.

McKay F. H., & Taket, A. (2020). *Health equity, social justice and human rights* (2nd ed.). Routledge.

Office of the United Nations High Commissioner for Human Rights (OHCHR) and World Health Organization (WHO). (2008). The right to health, Fact sheet no. 31. Retrieved https://www.ohchr.org/sites/default/files/Documents/Publications/Factsheet31.pdf

World Health Organization (WHO). (2002). *25 questions and answers on health and human rights*. Retrieved https://apps.who.int/iris/handle/10665/42526

REFERENCES

Alsop, R. (Ed.) (2004). *Power, rights, and poverty: Concepts and connections, a working meeting sponsored by DFID and the World Bank*. World Bank/DFID.

Asher, J. (2004). *The right to health: A resource manual for NGOs*. Commonwealth Medical Trust.

Asher, J., Hamm, D., & Sheather, J. (2007). *The right to health: A toolkit for health professionals*. British Medical Association.

Australian Human Rights Commission (AHRC). (2011). *Mechanisms for advancing women's human rights: A guide to using the optional protocol to CEDAW and other international complaint mechanisms*. AHRC.

Bajaj, M. (2012). From 'time pass' to transformative force: School-based human rights education in Tamil Nadu, India. *International Journal of Educational Development*, *32*(1), 72–80.

Brennan, H., Distler, R., Hinman, M., & Rogers, A. (2013). *A human rights approach to intellectual property and access to medicines*. (Global Health Justice Partnership Policy Paper 1). Retrieved http://infojustice.org/archives/30664

Bustreo, F., & Hunt, P. (2013). *Women's and children's health: Evidence of impact of human rights*. WHO.

CEJIL (n.d.). *María da Penha/Brazil*. Retrieved https://www.cejil.org/en/maria-da-penha

CLADEM (n.d.). *María da Penha Case, Brazil (domestic violence against women)*. Retrieved http://www.cladem .org/en/our-programs/litigation/litigation-international/11-inter-american-commission-on-human-rights-oas/21-maria-da-penha-case-brazil-domestic-violence-against-women

Coker, R. (2001). Just coercion? Detention of nonadherent tuberculosis patients. *Annals of the New York Academy of Sciences, 953*, 216–23.

European Union (EU). (2000). Charter of fundamental rights of the European Union. *Official Journal of the European Communities, C364*, 1–22.

Goldhaber, M. D. (2007). *A people's history of the European Court of Human Rights*. Rutgers University Press.

Goldstein, S., Anderson, A., Usdin, U., & Japhet, G. (2001). Soul Buddyz: A children's rights mass media campaign in South Africa. *Health and Human Rights, 5*(2), 163–73.

Gruskin, S., & Tarantola, D. (2005). Health and human rights. In S. Gruskin, M. Grodin, S. Marks & G. Annas (Eds.), *Perspectives on health and human rights* (pp. 3–57). Routledge.

Hanung, C. D., Ginting, M. S., & Judhistari, R. A. (2018). Reasonable Doubt: The Journey within: A Report on the Annual Performance of the ASEAN Human Rights Mechanisms in 2017 [Online]. Asian Form for Human Rights and Development. Retrieved www.forum-asia.org/?p=27616

Hogerzeil, H. V., Samson, M., Casanovas, J. V. & Rahmani-Ocora, L. (2006). Is access to essential medicines as part of the fulfilment of the right to health enforceable through the courts? *The Lancet, 368*, 305–11.

Inter-American Commission on Human Rights (2001). *Report No 54/01* Case 12.051 Maria Da Penha Maia Fernandes BRAZIL April 16, 2001*. Retrieved http://www.cidh.org/women/brazil12.051.htm

Kapoor, D. (2007). Gendered-caste discrimination, human rights education, and the enforcement of the prevention of atrocities act in India. *Alberta Journal of Educational Research, 53*(3), 273–86.

Kaushik, S. K., Kaushik, S., & Kaushik, S. (2006). How higher education in rural India helps human rights and entrepreneurship. *Journal of Asian Economics, 17*(1), 29–34.

Leavy, J., & Howard, J. (2013). *What matters most? Evidence from 84 participatory studies with those living with extreme poverty and marginalisation, Participate*. IDS.

Lindsnaes, B., Lindholt, L., & Yigen, K. (Eds.) (2000). *National human rights institutions: Articles and working papers*. Danish Centre for Human Rights.

Mann, J., & Tarantola, D. (1998). Responding to HIV/AIDS: A historical perspective. *Health and Human Rights: An International Journal, 2*(4), 5–8.

McHale, J. (2010). Fundamental rights and health care. In E. Mossialos, G. Permanad, R. Baeten, & T. Hervey (Eds.), *Health systems governance in Europe: The role of European union law and policy* (pp. 282–314). Cambridge University Press.

McKay F. H. & Taket, A. (2020). *Health equity, social justice and human rights* (2nd ed.). Routledge.

Muntaner, C., Sridharan, S., Solar, O., & Benach, J. (2009). Commentary: Against unjust global distribution of power and money: The report of the WHO commission on the social determinants of health: Global inequality and the future of public health policy. *Journal of Public Health Policy, 30*(2), 163–75.

Neuwahl, N., & Rosas, A. (Eds.) (1995). *The European Union and human rights*. Kluwer Law International.

Office of the United Nations High Commissioner for Human Rights (OHCHR). (2008). *Working with the United Nations human rights programme: A handbook for Civil Society*. OHCHR.

——(2014). *Civil society space and the United Nations human rights system. A practical guide for civil society*.

——(n.d.). *The Global Alliance of National Human Rights Institutions (GANHRI)*. Retrieved https://www.ohchr .org/EN/Countries/NHRI/Pages/About-GANHRI.aspx

Office of the United Nations High Commissioner for Human Rights (OHCHR) and World Health Organization (WHO). (2008). The right to health, Fact sheet no 31. Retrieved https://www.ohchr.org/Documents/Publications/Factsheet31.pdf

Organization for Security and Co-operation in Europe and Office for Democratic Institutions and Human Rights. (2013a). *Guidelines on human rights education for health workers.* Author.

——(2013b). *Guidelines on human rights education for human rights activists* Author.

Pillay, N. (2013). Human rights in the post-2015 agenda: Open letter. Retrieved http://www.ohchr.org/Documents/Issues/MDGs/HCOpenLetterPost2015.pdf

Pohjolainen, A. (2006). *The evolution of national human rights institutions: The role of the United Nations.* Danish Institute for Human Rights.

Pomi, R. (2015). Joint statement (2013): Human rights for all post-2015. Retrieved https://sustainabledevelopment.un.org/content/documents/5123joint.statement.dec10.pdf

Singh, J. A., Govender, M., & Mills, (2007). Do human rights matter to health? *The Lancet, 370*, 521–7.

Soul City. (2005) *Soul Buddyz club evaluation report 2005.* Soul City Institute for Health and Development Communication. Retrieved http://www.soulcity.org.za/research/evaluations/series/soul-buddyz-series/soul-buddyz-clubs

Special Secretariat for Women's Policies. (2006). *Maria da Penha Law*, Law no 11.340 of August 7, 2006: Restrains domestic and family violence against women. Retrieved http://www.compromissoeatitude.org.br/wp-content/uploads/2012/08/SPMlawmariapenha2006.pdf

Taket, A, (2013). Using human rights-based approaches to support the engagement and empowerment of young people. *International journal of interdisciplinary social and community studies, 7*(1), 35–46.

United Nations. (1948). *Universal Declaration of Human Rights.* UN. Retrieved http://www.un.org/en/documents/udhr

——(2017). *Report of the Special Rapporteur on the rights of Indigenous peoples on her visit to Australia.* UN Document A/HRC/36/46/Add.2. Retrieved https://ap.ohchr.org/documents/dpage_e.aspx?si=A/HRC/36/46/Add.2

UN General Assembly. (1993). *Report of the World Conference on Human Rights: Report of the Secretary-General. A/CONF.157/24 (Part I).* New York: Author.

UN Women. (2011). *Maria da Penha Law: A Name that Changed Society.* Retrieved http://www.unwomen.org/en/news/stories/2011/8/maria-da-penha-law-a-name-that-changed-society

Wallerstein, N. (2006). *What is the evidence on effectiveness of empowerment to improve health?* WHO Regional Office for Europe. Retrieved www.euro.who.int/__data/assets/pdf_file/0010/74656/E88086.pdf

World Health Organization (WHO). (1986). *Ottawa Charter for Health Promotion.* WHO.

Yamin, A. E. (2013). From ideals to tools: Applying human rights to maternal health. *PLOS Medicine, 10*(11). Retrieved http://journals.plos.org/plosmedicine/article?id=10.1371/journal.pmed.1001546

PART 3

Public health and research

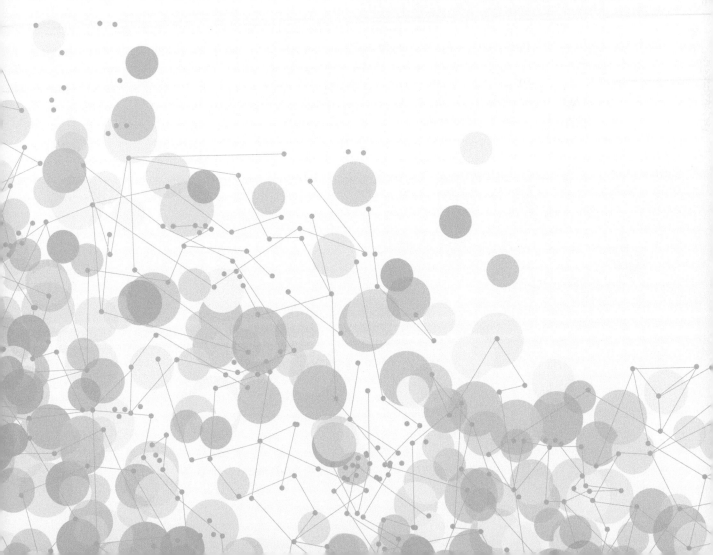

Qualitative research methodology and evidence-based practice in public health

12

Pranee Liamputtong and Zoe Sanipreeya Rice

LEARNING OBJECTIVES

After studying this chapter, you should be able to:

1   define and describe what qualitative research is and its importance for public health
2   understand the nature of the qualitative approach
3   describe the value of qualitative research in public health
4   describe the relevance of qualitative inquiry in evidence-based practice in health.

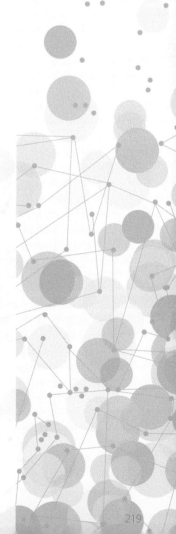

VIGNETTE

The 'Body and Soul' program in the Samoan community in Hawai'i

It is suggested that churches often have great capacity to promote health and to reach marginalised individuals and communities to reduce their health inequalities. Churches, for Samoan immigrants living in the United States, are established, trusted and well-attended organisations that have the ability to address the wellbeing of their communities. In this study, Cassell and colleagues (2014) qualitatively examined the adaption of 'Body and Soul', a faith-based, health promotion program, for use in Hawai'i's Samoan churches.

The findings from this study showed the value of qualitative research methods to inform the adaptation of evidence-based health promotion programs for communities experiencing health inequalities. Additionally, this research pinpointed possible intervention strategies that could work with other immigrants from Pacific Island jurisdictions who experience similarly poor health outcomes in the United States.

According to Cassell and colleagues (2014), interviews with Samoan community members helped to reveal 'underlying socioecological factors' that significantly contributed to obesogenic trends in Samoans living in Hawai'i. These factors included 'changes in the vocational structure of Samoan society, combined with influences because of migration and acculturation into Western societies, modified cultural norms surrounding the adoption of Westernised diets, and the prominence of Western foods within cultural practices' (p. 1668). The authors suggest that the qualitative approach was an 'efficient approach' that assisted in the implementation of health promotion interventions to suit a particular group of people (Cassell et al., 2014).

Introduction

Due to the shift to the social model of health care (see Chapter 1), public health researchers and practitioners have increasingly become interested in the insider perspectives and experiences of key players in health, including health consumers and healthcare providers (Olson, Young & Schultz, 2016). Thus, qualitative research has been adopted in public health in many ways and in numerous fields of health research (Padgett, 2012; Guest, Tolley & Wong, 2013; Tolley, 2016; Liamputtong, 2019a, 2020, 2022; Liamputtong & Rice, 2021a). The vignette above attests to the increasing adoption of qualitative inquiry in public health.

The focus of this chapter is on qualitative research. You will learn about the nature of qualitative inquiry and the need for qualitative research in public health. You will also gain a basic understanding of some philosophical assumptions about qualitative research that have led to different understandings about public health in different groups of people.

Attempts have been made in the past few decades to provide evidence-based public health care to individuals and communities. Thus, we have witnessed many research projects carried out in the public health arena, and often these have involvesdthe use of quantitative methodologies, including experimental design, epidemiology and systematic reviews of interventions (see Chapter 13). But will this research reflect the realities of the individual people? In particular, what does this mean for people who do not have opportunities to contribute to research that can be used as 'evidence' in health care? Evidence-based practice in public health and the need for qualitative inquiry are also discussed in this chapter.

Qualitative research

> The first contribution of qualitative inquiry is illuminating meanings and how humans engage in meaning making – in essence, making sense of the world.
>
> (Patton, 2015, p. 6)

Qualitative research is a form of social inquiry that attempts to understand how individuals construct meaning about the world in which they reside (Hesse-Biber, 2017; Rossman & Rallis, 2017; Denzin & Lincoln, 2018; Liamputtong, 2019a, 2020; Liamputtong & Rice, 2021a). Hence, qualitative research attempts to interpret the meaning-making process that people undertake in their everyday lives (Patton, 2015, p. 6), and this includes how people make sense of their health and illness (Liamputtong, 2019a, 2020, 2022; Liamputtong & Rice, 2021a). In the social world, we deal with the subjective experiences of human beings, and our 'understanding of reality can change over time and in different social contexts' (Dew, 2007, p. 434). Qualitative inquiry examines realities that influence the life, health and well-being of individuals or groups in a particular sociocultural context (Olson et al., 2016; Liamputtong, 2019a, 2020, 2022; Liamputtong & Rice, 2021a).

Qualitative research – a form of inquiry that attempts to understand how individuals construct meaning about the world in which they reside.

According to Denzin and Lincoln (2011), the term 'qualitative research' emphasises 'the qualities of entities and on processes and meanings that are not experimentally examined or measured in terms of quantity, amount, intensity, or frequency' (p. 8). Qualitative research aims to provide answers about the 'what', 'why' and 'how' of a reality, instead of questions about 'how many', 'how often', or 'how much' (Hesse-Biber, 2017; Creswell & Poth, 2018). Qualitative research relies heavily on words or stories that people tell us (Liamputtong 2019a, 2020, 2022; Liamputtong & Rice, 2021a). Typically, qualitative data is collected in the form of written or spoken language as well as images (Guest et al., 2013). Importantly, qualitative research is not used to test hypotheses, and it does not usually aim for generalisation and replication. Data generated from qualitative research can be only interpreted within the contexts in which the research is undertaken (Creswell & Poth, 2018). For most qualitative researchers, it is accepted that to understand people's behaviour we must first attempt to understand the meanings and interpretations that people give to their experiences. Because of the interpretive and flexible approach, qualitative research can provide answers to health problems that other methods cannot 'reach', particularly questions that are not responsive to quantitative measurement (Creswell & Poth, 2018).

SPOTLIGHT 12.1

Addiction and mental illness among young Russian immigrants in Germany

According to Flick (2015), young Russian-speaking immigrants in Germany have particularly strong patterns of alcohol and drug consumption. As such, they are at high risk of associated diseases.

However, they are also a group that tends to under-utilise existing health services. Flick (2015) and the research team wished to learn about how Russian-speaking immigrants saw their use of substances and their views about possible consequences, such as hepatitis infection, and how they deal with them. The researchers were also particularly interested in exploring conditions of the utilisation of health care, participants' expectations and experiences in those services, and where relevant why they did not utilise those services. Flick and his research team examined these issues by using a qualitative approach.

QUESTION
In your opinion, why should qualitative research be used in such a study?

The nature of qualitative research

Epistemology

Constructivism – an epistemology that suggests that 'reality' is socially constructed. It argues that there are multiple truths that are individually constructed, and rejects the ideal of a single truth.

Epistemology – the nature of knowledge and how knowledge is obtained.

Qualitative research is situated within the epistemology of **constructivism**. **Epistemology** focuses on the nature of knowledge and the way knowledge is obtained (Hathcoat & Nicholas, 2014; Bryman 2016; Hathcoat, Meixner & Nicholas, 2019). In public health, we ask what type of knowledge we need to have and whether our research can be conducted in the same way as those in the natural sciences (such as physics and chemistry).

Constructivism posits that 'reality' is socially constructed (Hershberg, 2014; Bryman, 2016; Liamputtong & Rice, 2022). According to Burr (2019), constructivism suggests that 'our knowledge of the world, including our understanding of human beings, is a product of human thought, language and interaction rather than grounded in an observable and definable external reality' (p. 2). Constructivism rejects the ideal of a single truth. Instead, it argues that there are multiple truths that are individually constructed (Lincoln, Lynham & Guba, 2011; Burr, 2019; Liamputtong & Rice, 2022). Reality is seen as being shaped by social factors such as social class, gender, age, ethnicity and culture (Grbich, 2007; Burr, 2019). Within this epistemology, it is accepted that research is a highly subjective process and that this is due to the active involvement of the researcher in the construction and conduct of the research (Lincoln et al., 2011; Hershberg, 2014; Bryman, 2016; Burr, 2019; Liamputtong & Rice, 2022). According to Grbich (2007), research situated within this epistemology emphasises 'exploration of the way people interpret and make sense of their experiences in the worlds in which they live, and how the contexts of events and situations and the placement of these within wider social environments have impacted on constructed understanding' (p. 8).

Constructivist researchers believe that when the social world is examined, it needs a different kind of research process than the processes used in the natural sciences (Burr, 2019; Liamputtong & Rice, 2022). Bryman (2016) contends that constructivist researchers need the kind of research 'that reflects the distinctiveness of humans as against the natural order' (p. 26). Within this constructivist paradigm, it requires the researchers to 'grasp the subjective meaning of social action' (p. 26). It is crucial, then, that a research approach that would enable people to articulate the meanings of their social realities is adopted. Essentially, this necessitates the use of a qualitative inquiry.

REFLECTION QUESTION

If we want to understand what global pandemics such as COVID-19 mean to Australian people, qualitative researchers argue that we need to adopt constructivism as our epistemology. What is your view about this? Why do you think such an epistemology will be useful for us to understand how Australian people think about the pandemic?

Methodological frameworks and qualitative methods

Qualitative research is also situated within several methodological frameworks (Flick, 2015; Hesse-Biber, 2017; Creswell & Poth, 2018; Liamputtong, 2019a, 2020). A **methodological framework** provides a means by which to view the conduct of qualitative research. In the first author's (PL) own writing about qualitative methodologies, she includes several salient frameworks, including ethnography, phenomenology, symbolic interactionism, hermeneutics, feminism and postmodernism (see Liamputtong, 2020). However, Creswell and Poth (2018) suggest five traditions, including narrative research, grounded theory, phenomenology, ethnography and case study as methodological frameworks in qualitative research. Each framework offers different understandings and assumptions about people's worldviews and behaviours. As such, each methodological framework advocates the use of different qualitative **methods** by which researchers might collect data (Flick, 2015; Taylor, Bogdan & DeVault, 2016; Hesse-Biber 2017; Silverman 2017). It must be noted that a particular methodological framework might be more appropriate in addressing some research questions than others. It is the task of qualitative researchers to consider carefully which methodology is more useful and suitable for their research projects.

Qualitative research uses several data collection methods. These include the in-depth interview, focus group interview, oral/life history interview, memory work, participatory action research and ethnographic methods. Among these, in-depth interviewing is the most commonly known and is widely employed by qualitative researchers (Brinkmann & Kvale 2015; Liamputtong, 2019a, 2020; Serry & Liamputtong, 2022). Recently, we have also witnessed the emergence of innovative and participatory qualitative methods such as drawing, photovoice, photo elicitation, diary, digital storytelling and online methods (Liamputtong, 2007, 2010, 2019b, 2020; Liamputtong & Rice, 2021b). Each method has its own salient features, advantages and limitations. Researchers need to select a method or procedure that suits their research, as well as the needs of research participants.

Despite differences in methodological framework and methods, Patton (2015, pp. 12–13) suggests that qualitative inquiry as a whole contributes to the generation of knowledge in several ways:

- It reveals meanings that people have.
- It captures stories so that individuals' perspectives and experiences can be understood.
- It examines how things work.
- It illuminates how systems work and their consequences for the lives of people.
- It often allows researchers to identify unanticipated consequences, which will help researchers to have a better understanding about the individuals.
- Contextual sensitivity is the essence of qualitative inquiry. It helps researchers to understand the context of those who participate in their research.

Methodological framework – a framework used to select suitable methods in qualitative research.

Method – a technique used in collecting data.

level and qualitative evidence (subjective data) is at the lower end (Liamputtong, 2022). The hierarchy of evidence-based public health suggests that 'subjective perceptions' are subordinated to 'objective quantification', and 'description' is less important than 'inferential testing' (Giacomini, 2001, p. 4). Within this model, the contribution to evidence-based practice of findings from qualitative research is undervalued and discounted (Grypdonck, 2006; Zuzelo, 2012; Olson et al., 2016; Liamputtong, 2022).

Evidence – information that public health practitioners can use to support and guide their practices to optimise the health and wellbeing of individuals and communities.

For public health practitioners, **evidence** is generated from research data (Brownson et al., 2011; Hess et al., 2014; Liamputtong, 2022). However, this data includes not only quantitative data but also qualitative data, which can be used in decision-making about public health programs and policies (White et al., 2014; Olson et al., 2016; Tolley, 2016; Liamputtong, 2022). Although evidence-based public health might have been claimed as stipulating clear responses to messy and difficult problems, and would provide 'certainty' in the uncertain world we are living in, dealing with people also needs 'a passion for humanity', as well as 'a belief in human potential' (McLoughlin, 2012, p. 97). This is what data from qualitative inquiry can indeed offer (Patton, 2015; Liamputtong, 2019a, 2020). McLoughlin (2012, p. 101) reminds us that 'not everything that is valuable is measurable and not everything that is measured is of value'.

Why use qualitative research in evidence-based practice in public health?

All too often, little is known about particular health problems of some population groups, or about intervention options that are not empirically based (Olson et al., 2016). Although there is research evidence that public health practitioners may find in the published literature, there are many health issues that remain unknown (Liamputtong, 2022). Additionally, efficacy research on health promotion and prevention is not readily available in public health (Asthana & Halliday, 2006). Therefore, it is often difficult to find a systematic review of public health interventions. Kirmayer (2012) states it clearly: 'Systematic literature reviews depend entirely on what evidence is available to critically evaluate and synthesize. Not everything gets studied and not every study that is completed gets published' (p. 250).

More importantly, public health practitioners may need evidence other than that which relates to the efficacy of interventions to inform their practice (Aoun & Kristjanson, 2005; MacLaughlin, 2012; Olson et al., 2016). Some health topics or issues in public health (such as the health effects of family or intimate partner violence, or the effects of smoking cessation on lung-cancer mortality) are not appropriate for an intervention (see Aoun & Kristjanson, 2005; Padgett, 2012; Zuzelo, 2012). Not all interventions can be delivered through randomised controlled trials (Hess et al., 2014). For example, interventions in psychological issues may be difficult to 'randomize (because they must be tailored to individuals), and blind (because psychosocial treatments may require explicit awareness, engagement, and commitment from patients for efficacy)' (Kirmeyer, 2012, p. 250). Evidence-based public health has also been criticised for its limited application for diverse cultural groups (Kirmayer, 2012; Maschi & Youdin, 2012). Currently, evidence-based public health does not apply to many of the health issues of certain population groups (e.g. certain ethnic minorities and Indigenous groups, recent immigrants and refugees, transgender individuals, gay men and lesbians, people living with disability, children, older people, rural people, and people with rare or particularly challenging health problems).

According to Layde and colleagues (2012), with the obsession of evidence-based public health, public health practitioners fail to consider the fundamental characteristics of a particular community and hence their needs tend to be ignored or not understood. When communities feel that they do not have ownership of health interventions, this can have detrimental consequences to the implementation and sustainability of the interventions (White et al., 2014). This leads Kohatsu, Robinson and Torner (2004) to provide an alternative definition of evidence-based public health: 'Evidence-based public health is the process of integrating science-based interventions with community preferences to improve the health of populations' (p. 419) Their definition includes 'the perspectives of community members', which promotes 'a more population-centered approach' (see also Brownson et al., 2011; White et al., 2014). This is in line with qualitative research inquiry discussed in this chapter.

Evidence obtained from qualitative research can assist public health practitioners to appreciate the issue and to utilise its findings in their practice. Qualitative research can offer evidence that may not be feasible from a quantitative approach or from a systematic review of quantitative studies (Olson et al., 2016; Liamputtong & Rice, 2022). The dominance of evidence-based practice in public health means that qualitative research can serve as a vehicle for practitioners to bring the consumers back to health care (Murray & Sargeant, 2011). Qualitative research enables public health practitioners to gain a better understanding about newly emerging as well as chronic illnesses. Qualitative research provides insights into barriers and facilitating factors that can influence the development and implementation of effective public health programs and policies (White et al., 2014; Tolley, 2016). Numerous researchers have argued that findings of qualitative research can enhance evidence-based practice (Grypdonck, 2006; White et al., 2014; Olson et al., 2016; Carpenter, 2017). Patton (2015) puts it clearly that 'qualitative evidence should be a part of evaluation's contribution to improving people's lives' (p. 178).

SPOTLIGHT 12.4

When battered women kill: The power of qualitative evidence

Angela Browne (1987) interviewed 42 women individually from 15 states in the United States who were charged with a crime that had resulted in the death or serious injury of their intimate partners. Often, through in-depth interviews, Browne was the first person to hear these women's stories. In order to reveal how an abusive relationship declines from a 'romantic courtship' to abuse, and how it eventually 'provoked a homicide', Browne used the history of one couple and nine case vignettes from other interviews to represent the women in her study. The findings of Browne's research led to legal recognition of the 'battered women's syndrome' as a 'legitimate defence' for women who commit crime against their violent partners. Her qualitative findings provided an in-depth understanding about violence in the women's lives and offered an answer to the common question, 'Why don't the women just leave?' This question is often asked by people who do not have any experience of family or intimate partner violence. According to Patton (2015, p. 17), 'the effectiveness of Browne's careful, detailed, and straightforward descriptions and quotations lies in their capacity to take us inside the abusive relationship'. Her qualitative evidence provides 'an insider perspective on the debilitating, destructive, and all-encompassing brutality of battering'. This is the power of qualitative evidence: 'Offering that inside perspective empowers' (Patton, 2015, p. 17).

QUESTIONS

1 What does evidence-based practice in public health mean to you?

2 Can you think of any research evidence you have heard or read about that you have used to inform your practice?

3 Would any of this evidence be better developed if a qualitative inquiry was used?

4 What would be your reasons for this view?

SUMMARY

In this chapter, the salient nature and value of qualitative inquiry in public health as well as a means for finding appropriate evidence in the era of evidence-based practice in public health have been discussed.

Learning objective 1: Define and describe what qualitative research is and its importance for public health.

Qualitative research is a form of 'social inquiry' that helps us to understand how individuals construct meaning about the world in which they reside. Thus, qualitative research attempts to interpret the 'meaning-making process' that people construct in their everyday lives, and this includes how people make sense of their health and illness

Learning objective 2: Understand the nature of the qualitative approach.

Qualitative research is situated within the epistemology of constructivism. Qualitative research is situated within several methodological frameworks and uses several data collection methods. These include the in-depth interview, focus group interview, oral or life history interview, memory work, participatory action research and ethnographic method. Among qualitative research methods, in-depth interviewing is the most widely known and is commonly employed by qualitative researchers.

Learning objective 3: Describe the value of qualitative research in public health.

Qualitative research has become an important and a crucial part of public health research. It has been witnessed that qualitative inquiry offers great insights into the perspectives of the service users. Not only have more public health researchers adopted the inquiry into their discipline, but a number of major health research funding bodies have advocated the need for qualitative research to 'give voice' to the experiences of service users (Gough & Deatrick, 2015, p. 289). The power and influence of qualitative research in public health and other health-related areas can be witnessed in many empirical studies (some examples have been given in this chapter).

Learning objective 4: Describe the relevance of qualitative inquiry in evidence-based practice in health.

Evidence-based public health has become a powerful model for determining public health issues and establishing the most effective health prevention and protection strategies (Hess et al., 2014; Olson et al., 2016; Tolley, 2016). As in the evidence-based practice in medicine, quantitative methods and systematic reviews of interventions are seen as scientific evidence that practitioners can use in their practice. This chapter has pointed to some pitfalls of this framework and advocates the use of qualitative approaches in evidence-based public health. Within public health, although qualitative inquiry has not been wholly recognised for its contribution, we have witnessed many examples of evidence-based practices that stem largely from the use of qualitative methodology (Olson et al., 2016). It is hoped that by now you can see the relevance and value of qualitative inquiry in public health and evidence-based public health.

TUTORIAL EXERCISES

1   Locate a qualitative study on any public health issue, read it and answer the following questions:
   a   How appropriate is the approach used in this study to the public health issue under study?
   b   Would the findings of this qualitative study contribute to evidence-based practice in public health? How?

2 Read the case example below and answer the questions that follow it.

> **Why eye injuries continue to persist**
>
> During his visit to an American medical facility in Iraq during the early part of the Iraq war, surgeon Gawande (2007) was impressed by the doctors' attention to eye-injury statistics among the young soldiers. Rather than feeling proud that they had saved some soldiers from blindness, the doctors asked a deeper and 'more unnerving question' about why so many injuries were occurring. They uncovered that the soldiers were not wearing their protective goggles, because they felt the goggles were 'too ugly'. Hence, the military changed the standard-issue goggles to 'cooler-looking Wiley X ballistic eyewear'. This encouraged the young soldiers to wear their eyewear more consistently and resulted in a significant reduction in the rate of eye injuries (Gawande, 2007).

    a What is your view about this case?

    b What type of knowledge do we need in public health?

    c In your view, should evidence-based practice in public health be based on the same hierarchy of evidence as in evidence-based medicine? Why or why not?

    d In your opinion, why is it important for public health researchers and practitioners to take into account the perspectives of service users and/or communities when developing a public health intervention? Discuss.

3 Find a quantitative research paper in public health. Read and critically examine what this study can offer in terms of evidence-based practice, and compare it to the qualitative paper that you have critiqued in Tutorial 1.

FURTHER READING

Brownson, R. C., Baker, E. A., Leet, T. L., Gillespie, K. N., & True, W. R. (2011). *Evidence-based public health* (2nd ed.). Oxford University Press.

Giacomini, M. K. (2001). The rocky road: Qualitative research as evidence. *Evidence-Based Medicine*, *6*(Jan–Feb), 4–5.

Grypdonck, M. H. F. (2006). Qualitative health research in the era of evidence-based practice. *Qualitative Health Research*, *16*(10), 1371–85.

Liamputtong, P. (2020). *Qualitative research methods* (5th ed.). Oxford University Press.

Olson, K., Young, R. A., & Schultz, I. Z. (2016). *Handbook of qualitative health research for evidence-based practice*. Springer.

REFERENCES

Aoun, S. M., & Kristjanson, L. J. (2005). Evidence in palliative care research: How should it be gathered? *Medical Journal of Australia*, *183*(5), 264–6.

Asthana, S., & Halliday, J. (2006). Developing an evidence base for policies and interventions to address health inequalities: The analysis of 'public health regimes'. *Milbank Quarterly*, *84*(3), 577–603.

Baker, E. A., Brownson, R. C., Dreisinger, M., McIntosh, L. D., & Karamehic-Muratovic, A. (2009). Examining the role of training in evidence-based public health: A qualitative study. *Health Promotion Practice*, *10*(3), 342–8.

Baum, F. (2016). *The new public health: An Australian perspective* (3rd ed.). Oxford University Press.

Brinkmann, S., & Kvale, S. (2015). *InterViews: Learning the craft of qualitative research interviewing* (3rd ed.). Sage Publications.

Browne, A. (1987). *When battered women kill.* The Free Press.

Brownson, R. C., Baker, E. A., Leet, T. L., Gillespie, K. N., & True, W. R. (2011). *Evidence-based public health* (2nd ed.). Oxford University Press.

Bryman, A. (2016). *Social research methods* (5th ed.). Oxford University Press.

Burr, V. (2019). Social constructionism. In P. Liamputtong (Ed.), *Handbook of research methods in health social sciences.* Springer Nature.

Carpenter, C. (2017). Phenomenology and rehabilitation research. In P. Liamputtong (Ed.), *Research methods in health: Foundations for evidence-based practice* (2nd ed.) (pp. 157–76). Oxford University Press.

Cassell, K. D., Braun, K., Ka'opua, L., Soa, F. & Nigg, C. (2014). Samoan Body and Soul: Adapting an evidence-based obesity and cancer prevention program. *Qualitative Health Research, 24*(12), 1658–72.

Creswell, J. W., & Poth, C. N. (2018). *Qualitative inquiry and research design: Choosing among five approaches* (5th ed.). Sage Publications.

de Visser, R. O., Graber, R., Hart, A., Abraham, C., Scanlon, T., Watten, P., & Memon, A. (2015). Using qualitative methods within a mixed-methods approach to developing and evaluating interventions to address harmful alcohol use among young people. *Health Psychology, 34*(4), 349–60.

Denzin, N. K. & Lincoln, Y. S. (Eds.) (2011). *Introduction: The discipline and practice of qualitative research. The Sage handbook of qualitative research* (4th ed.) (pp. 1–19). Sage Publications.

Denzin, N. K. & Lincoln, Y. S. (2018). Introduction: The discipline and practice of qualitative research. In N. K. Denzin & Y. S. Lincoln (Eds.), *The Sage handbook of qualitative research* (5th ed.) (pp. 1–26). Sage Publications.

Dew, K. (2007). A health researcher's guide to qualitative methodologies. *Australian and New Zealand Journal of Public Health, 31*(5), 433–7.

Flick, U. (2015). *An introduction to qualitative research* (5th ed.). Sage Publications.

——(2018). Triangulation. In N. K. Denzin & Y. S. Lincoln (Eds.), *The Sage handbook of qualitative research* (5th ed.) (pp. 444–61). Sage Publications.

Gawande, A. (2007). The power of negative thinking. *The New York Times*, 1 May. Retrieved http://www .nytimes.com/2007/05/01/opinion/01gawande.html?_r=0

Giacomini, M. K. (2001). The rocky road: Qualitative research as evidence. *ACP Journal Club, 134*, A11–12.

Gough, B., & Deatrick, J. A. (2015). Qualitative health psychology research: Diversity. power, and impact. *Health Psychology, 34*(4), 289–22.

Grbich, C. (2007). *Qualitative data analysis: An introduction.* Sage Publications.

Grypdonck, M. H. F. (2006). Qualitative health research in the era of evidenced-based practice. *Qualitative Health Research, 16*(10), 1371–85.

Guest, G., Tolley, E. E., & Wong, C. M. (2013). Qualitative research methods. In W. C. Cockerham, R. Dingwall, & S. R. Quah (Eds.), *The Wiley Blackwell encyclopedia of health, illness, behavior, and society.* John Wiley & Sons.

Hathcoat, J. D., Meixner, C., & Nicholas, M. C. (2019). Ontology and epistemology. In P. Liamputtong (Ed.), *Handbook of research methods in health social sciences.* Springer Nature.

Hathcoat, J. D., & Nicholas, M. C. (2014). *Epistemology.* In D. Coghlan, & M. Brydon-Miller (Eds), *The Sage encyclopedia of action research* (pp. 302–6). Sage Publications.

Hershberg, R. M. (2014). Constructivism. In D. Coghlan, & M. Brydon-Miller (Eds.), *The Sage encyclopedia of action research* (pp. 182–6). Sage Publications.

Hess, J. J., Eidson, M., Tlumak, J. E., Raab, K. K., & Luber, G. (2014). An evidence-based public health approach to climate change adaptation. *Environmental Health Perspectives, 122*(11), 1177–86.

Hesse-Biber, S. N. (2017). *The practice of qualitative research* (3rd ed.). Sage Publications.

Holloway, I., & Galvin, K. (2017). *Qualitative research in nursing and healthcare* (4th ed.). Wiley-Blackwell.

Kirmayer, L. J. (2012). Cultural competence and evidence-based practice in mental health: Epistemic communities and the politics of pluralism. *Social Science & Medicine, 75*, 249–56.

Kohatsu, N. D., Robinson, J. R., & Torner, J. C. (2004). Evidence-based public health: An evolving concept. *American Journal of Preventive Medicine, 27*(5), 417–41.

Layde, P. M., Christiansen, A. L., Peterson, D. J., Guse, C. E., Maurana, C. A., & Brandenburg, T. (2012). A model to translate evidence-based interventions into community practice. *American Journal of Public Health, 102*, 617–24.

Leko, M. M. (2014). The value of qualitative methods in social validity research. *Remedial and Special Education, 35*(5), 275–26.

Liamputtong, P. (2007). *Researching the vulnerable: A guide to sensitive research methods.* Sage Publications.

——(2010). *Performing qualitative cross-cultural research.* Cambridge University Press.

——(2019a). Qualitative inquiry. In P. Liamputtong (Ed.) *Handbook of research methods in health social sciences.* Springer Nature.

——(2019b). Innovative research methods in health social sciences: An introduction. In P. Liamputtong (Ed.), *Handbook of research methods in health social sciences.* Springer Nature.

——(2020). *Qualitative research methods* (5th ed.). Oxford University Press.

——(2022). Introducing evidence-based practice and health. In P. Liamputtong (Ed.), *Research methods in health* (4th ed.) (pp. 2–15). Oxford University Press.

Liamputtong, P., & Rice, Z.S. (2021a). Qualitative research in global health research. In R. Haring, I. Kickbusch, D. Ganten, & M. Moeti (Eds.), *Handbook of global health.* Springer Nature.

——(2021b). Qualitative inquiry and inclusive research methods. In P. Liamputtong (Ed.), *Handbook of social inclusion, research and practices in the health and social sciences.* Springer.

——(2022). The science of words and the science of numbers: Research methods in health. In P. Liamputtong (Ed.), *Research methods in health: Foundations for evidence-based practice* (4th ed.) (pp. 16–35). Oxford University Press.

Liamputtong, P., & Suwankhong, D. (2015). Biographical disruption, chaos and despair: Emotional experiences of women with breast cancer in southern Thailand. *Sociology of Health & Illness, 37*(7), 1086–1101.

Lincoln, Y. S., Lynham, S. A., & Guba, E. G. (2011). Paradigmatic controversies, contradictions and emerging confluences, revisited. In N. K. Denzin, & Y. S. Lincoln (Eds.), *The Sage handbook of qualitative research* (4th ed.) (pp. 99–128). Sage Publications.

Maschi, T., & Youdin, R. (2012). *Social worker as researcher: Integrating research with advocacy.* Pearson.

McLoughlin, H. (2012). *Understanding social work research: Evidence-based practice.* Sage Publications.

Murray, M. & Sargeant, S. (2011). Narrative psychology. In D. Harper & A. R. Thompson (Eds.), *Qualitative research methods in mental health and psychotherapy: A guide for students and practitioners* (pp. 163–75). Wiley-Blackwell.

Olson, K., Young, R. A., & Schultz, I. Z. (2016). *Handbook of qualitative health research for evidence-based practice.* Springer.

Packer, M. (2011). *The science of qualitative research.* Cambridge University Press.

Padgett, D. K. (2012). *Qualitative and mixed methods in public health.* Sage Publications.

Patton, M. Q. (2015). *Qualitative research and evaluation methods* (4th ed.). Sage Publications.

Rossman, G. B. & Rallis, S. F. (2017). *Learning in the field: An introduction to qualitative research* (4th ed.). Sage Publications.

Sandelowski, M. (2004). Using qualitative research. *Qualitative Health Research, 14*(10), 1366–86.

Serry, T., & Liamputtong, P. (2022). The in-depth interviewing method in health. In P. Liamputtong (Ed.), *Research methods in health: Foundations for evidence-based practice* (4th ed.) (pp. 76–92). Oxford University Press.

Silverman, D. (2017). *Doing qualitative research* (5th ed.). Sage Publications.

Sprague, C., Scanlon, M. L., & Pantalone, D. W. (2017). Qualitative research methods to advance research on health inequities among previously incarcerated women living with HIV in Alabama. *Health Education & Behavior*, *44*(5), 716–27.

Strauss, J., & Corbin, A. (2015). *Basics of qualitative research: Techniques and procedures for developing grounded theory* (4th ed.). Sage Publications.

Taylor, S. J., Bogdan, R., & DeVault, M. (2016). *Introduction to qualitative research methods: A guidebook and resource.* John Wiley & Sons.

Tolley, E. E. (2016). *Qualitative methods in public health: A field guide for applied research.* John Wiley & Sons.

White, F., Stallones, L., & Last, J. M. (2014). *Global public health: Ecological foundations.* Oxford University Press.

Zuzelo, P. R. (2012). Evidence-based nursing and qualitative research: A partnership imperative for real world practice. In P. L. Munhall (Ed.), *Nursing research: A qualitative perspective* (4th ed.) (pp. 481–500). Jones & Bartlett.

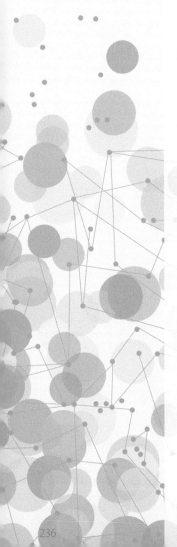

13

Assessing the health of populations: Epidemiology in public health

Patricia Lee

LEARNING OBJECTIVES

After studying this chapter, you should be able to:

1 understand the essence of epidemiology and outline the scope and purposes of epidemiology in public health
2 calculate measures of frequency of disease or health-related events and be able to compare the patterns of a health event with regard to time, place and personal characteristics in order to identify health issues or problems in the compared populations
3 be familiar with the major features of the commonly used epidemiological study designs and the use of epidemiological studies in relation to determining association between exposure and disease
4 apply appropriate quantitative measures of association to different study designs, in order to identify possible causes of a health outcome.

VIGNETTE

Global public health challenges and the importance of epidemiology

Global public health and health care are facing unprecedented challenges in the 21st century. The COVID-19 **pandemic** represents undoubtedly the greatest public health and humanitarian crises in modern history and has caused catastrophic effects on population health and profound disruptions to all aspects of human life. Since its emergence in late 2019, due to the high infectivity and a lack of immunity in the human population against this new virus, it was swiftly spread across the globe. In recognition of the potential large-scale effects of the disease, the World Health Organization (WHO) declared the outbreak a pandemic to activate the highest level of global response to the COVID-19 outbreak (WHO, 2021a). As the pandemic continues, public health measures such as travel restrictions, patient isolation, testing, contact-tracing, quarantines, social distancing and mask wearing will remain crucial in minimising illness and deaths associated with COVID-19 until a large proportion of vaccine roll-out in all countries is achieved (Wouters et al., 2021). In addition to health consequences such as illness and deaths directly associated with the exposure to the COVID-19 virus, the implications of the pandemic for health and wellbeing are substantial. International evidence shows an alarming increase in mental health problems and domestic violence since the pandemic began. The pandemic has also intensified health and social inequalities, food insecurity, refugee crises and forced displacement (Lambert et al., 2020; Pfefferbaum & North, 2020).

> **Pandemic** – an epidemic spreading across international borders or occurring worldwide, and usually affecting a large number of people.

Prior to the COVID-19 pandemic, there have been many large-scale infectious disease outbreaks since the beginning of the 21st century. The outbreak of SARS-CoV (severe acute respiratory syndrome) in 2003 overwhelmed the health service systems in many affected countries, and posed severe consequences on global economy, tourism and businesses (Lashley, 2006; WHO, 2007). Following the SARS-CoV outbreak, the swine 'flu (A(H1N1)pdn09) pandemic in 2009, the MERS-CoV (Middle Eastern respiratory syndrome) **epidemic**, the 2013–16 Ebola outbreak in West Africa and Zika infections in 2015–16 in South America were also recognised as public health emergencies at the international level. These infectious diseases have brought about a considerable burden on population health and pose a continuous threat to global healthcare systems. The burst in emerging and re-emerging infectious diseases, including COVID-19, in the past 20 years has highlighted the need for an improved global response and better preparedness for future outbreaks.

> **Epidemic** – the occurrence of a disease or a health-related event in a community that clearly exceeds the usual expected occurrence.

While the focus of global health is on containing the spread of COVID-19 and associated challenges, non-communicable or chronic diseases remain the major threats to population health. According to the recent WHO statistics (WHO, 2021b), non-communicable diseases (NCD) claim 71 per cent of global deaths (41 million deaths) and account for more than 15 million premature deaths (deaths in the ages 30–69 years). It is expected that the prevalence and overall burden of NCD will continue to rise. Importantly, 85 per cent of these premature deaths occur in low and middle-income countries. Given the context of the COVID-19 pandemic, people with chronic conditions are facing more complex health challenges. The double burdens of infectious diseases and NCD would have intensified, particularly in low and middle-income countries during the pandemic.

In response to this new era of health challenges, including new forms of infectious diseases and the increasing burden of NCD, public health practitioners and healthcare providers need to take timely action to address these health issues and protect the health of populations. There is no doubt that the visibility and importance of epidemiology (and epidemiologists) have heightened during the pandemic. Epidemiologists play an important role in public health and disease prevention. Their role is to investigate the occurrence of disease or other health-related events and contribute to the control of disease in specified populations (Last, Spasoff & Harris, 2000). Similarly, epidemiology is defined as 'the study of the distribution and determinants of health-related status or events in specified populations and application of this study to control of health problems' (Porta, 2008, p. 65). Its principles and evidence-based approach are essential to effective public health practice.

Introduction

The COVID-19 pandemic has highlighted the importance of epidemiology and public health. In addition to the intensified health challenges, along with the pandemic (as discussed above), the constantly changing environment, global warming, increased international travel and globalisation, and social, economic and political changes have all contributed to the fluctuating nature and patterns of disease and health issues. To better address the complex interrelationships of various determinants and health/illness outcomes, multidisciplinary efforts are required to protect and promote the population's health. Epidemiology is one such discipline in public health. No matter which specific career in public health a student eventually develops, the knowledge and skills involved in epidemiology will be useful. Its approach to critical thinking and problem-solving forms the basis for evidence-based decision-making in the health sciences as well as for health intervention research. Epidemiology uses quantitative methods to collect and analyse data to investigate disease occurrence and possible causes of disease, in order to find solutions to health problems in different populations. The definition of epidemiology (see Porta's 2008 definition) clearly outlines the purpose, the use and the applications of epidemiology. This chapter introduces the basic concepts in, and the use of, epidemiology, the common epidemiological study designs, and the quantitative measures used to describe the health status of populations and to identify potential determinants of ill health. It also draws on examples of international and Australian research and health data to strengthen the theoretical concepts and principles introduced in this chapter.

Highlights of the definition of epidemiology

Epidemiology – the study of the distribution and determinants of health-related events in specified populations and the application of this to the control of health problems.

An important role of epidemiology is to investigate the health status and health-related events in populations. Epidemiology is concerned with the health of populations rather than of individuals. A population can be specified as people living in a particular geographic area, such as a country, a city or a community, or as a group of people with specific characteristics (e.g. women aged 50 years and older, primary school children, or the Aboriginal population of Queensland). Health-related status or events cover anything that might directly and potentially affect health, regardless of whether it is good or bad, not limited to death, disease or disability. It is also important to understand the natural history of disease, which describes the process from healthy to diseased status.

REFLECTION QUESTION

1   What are the major public health challenges in the context of the COVID-19 pandemic?
2   In relation to the definition of epidemiology, which population groups should be prioritised when planning for the roll-out of COVID-19 vaccines? (List three population groups.)

Natural history of health or disease

A generic model for the development of a disease and the corresponding three levels of prevention are shown in Figure 13.1. The duration of the natural history may vary from disease to disease. For instance, the development of a seasonal 'flu takes only a few days, whereas it may take years for an individual to develop type 2 diabetes. The course of a disease often starts at the pathological onset. Primary prevention is implemented prior to the onset of a disease to prevent the disease from occurring. Immunisation and maintaining a healthy lifestyle (such as healthy eating and regular physical activity) are common examples of primary prevention. During the asymptomatic phase – from pathological onset to clinical diagnosis – the affected individual does not experience any symptoms, even though the disease already exists within their body. However, some subclinical signs of the disease can possibly be detected at an early stage.

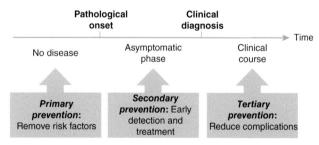

Figure 13.1   Natural history of disease and levels of prevention.
Source: Adapted from Gerstman (2013), Figure 2.1, p. 37.

Secondary prevention, such as screening for specific conditions, can be applied in the asymptomatic phase to achieve a better health outcome. For example, COVID-19 testing can be used to detect the virus in asymptomatic individuals who have contact with identified patients. As the disease progresses, the affected person begins to experience overt clinical symptoms and then seeks medical attention. At this stage, tertiary prevention (clinical treatment and care) needs to be administered to relieve the patient's symptoms and reduce the possibility of disability and death.

Traditionally, epidemiology was mainly concerned with epidemics of communicable disease. Nowadays, contemporary epidemiology has been extended to include NCD and chronic diseases, injuries, maternal and child health, environmental and occupational health, mental health and even a broad range of factors including social, economic, cultural, genetic, behavioural or lifestyle factors that contribute to the health and wellbeing of a population (see Part 2). Most importantly, epidemiology acknowledges the multi-causal nature of disease or health issues, and the fact that a disease is due to a complex interactive effect among the above-mentioned factors. A health promotion or prevention program (primary prevention; see Figure 13.1) addressing these 'upstream' factors is considered to be cost-effective to protect an individual from developing diseases (Webb, Bain & Page, 2019).

Descriptive and analytic studies

'The distribution and determinants of health-related status or events' in the definition of epidemiology refers to descriptive and analytic studies in epidemiology (Porta, 2008, p. 65). The details of these two broad categories of epidemiological study are discussed in later sections of this chapter. In descriptive epidemiology, researchers are interested in frequency and patterns of health events in a specified population. The frequency of health-related events involves a series of measures, including **prevalence** and **incidence**, to quantify the risk or rate of a health event in a population. These measures are introduced in the next section. The aim of descriptive epidemiology is to quantify the differences in disease occurrence in relation to time, place and personal characteristics, which indicate the patterns of disease or health-related events. Variations in disease patterns can be used to formulate hypotheses, and the hypotheses can be further tested in analytic investigations in order to identify possible causes of disease or health-related events. More specifically, analytic studies attempt to establish the associations between a disease or health outcome and the 'determinants' (or risk factors) of the health outcome in order to control and prevent the disease.

Prevalence (point prevalence) – the proportion of people with a disease in a specified population at one point in time.

Incidence – the number of new cases of a health-related event or disease in a specified population over a defined period.

SPOTLIGHT 13.1

Linking natural history of disease and disease prevention

As shown in Figure 13.1, the model of natural history of disease and the three levels of disease prevention can be applied to all kinds of disease. Understanding the natural course of a disease is essential to applying epidemiological principles for disease prevention.

QUESTION
What are the primary, secondary and tertiary prevention options in relation to different phases of disease development for the following interventions?

a　Breast cancer-screening in women aged 50 years and over
b　COVID-19 vaccination for healthcare workers.

Frequency of disease occurrence

Measures of disease occurrence form the basis of quantitative analysis in epidemiology. The measurement of disease frequencies enables epidemiologists or health practitioners to make meaningful comparisons between different populations or different geographic locations. In epidemiology, a 'proportion' or a 'rate' is preferred for the measure of disease frequency.

A simple count or the number of cases without a population reference is less useful than a proportion or a rate. A proportion describes the probability or the relative frequency of an event in a specified population, while a rate incorporates a time unit in the denominator. The most commonly used measures of disease frequency are prevalence and incidence. As they are the basic measures in descriptive epidemiology but very different in many ways, it is important to understand the definitions and purposes of these two measures.

Prevalence

The prevalence of a disease or health event expresses the number of existing cases in a population at a particular point in time. There are two common types of prevalence measures: period prevalence and point prevalence. Period prevalence measures the total number of existing cases of a disease during a particular period of time divided by the total number of people in the population during the same period of time. As students often confuse period prevalence with incidence, this chapter deals only with point prevalence. The formula for (point) prevalence calculation is:

$$\text{prevalence} = \frac{\text{number of existing cases}}{\text{total number of people in the population at a given point in time}}$$

The prevalence of a disease or a health event can be assessed in many ways, such as the baseline of a longitudinal study, disease screening or surveillance at a specific point in time (e.g. a cross-sectional survey). Data can also be collected from medical records, death registrations, routinely collected administrative data, disease surveillance (disease notification systems) and screening programs. Prevalence is a proportion, not a rate. It has no measurement unit but can be expressed in terms of *a population unit multiplier*, such as per 100 people (which can also be presented as a percentage, %), per 1000 people (10^3 people) or per 100 000 people (10^5 people) in relation to the size of the reference population (the population multiplier is denoted as 10^n). It does not involve a period of follow-up but changes from time to time, depending on the inflow of new cases and outflow of old cases (e.g. recoveries and deaths). Prevalence is a basic measure used to assess the burden of a disease in a population or community.

Incidence

Incidence measures the probability of developing a disease (or a health condition) over a given period of time. It takes into account the total new cases and the time of follow-up. There are two types of incidence, each represented as a proportion or rate. The choice of incidence measure depends on the data available and the purpose of calculation. In different forms of incidence, the numerator is always measuring the new events (e.g. total new cases over a specified time period) in different incidence measures.

Cumulative incidence (CI) is defined as the proportion of people in a population who develop a disease or a health-related event within a specific interval. It can be expressed as the following formula:

$$\text{cumulative incidence (CI)} = \frac{\text{number of new cases during the study period}}{\text{number of population at risk at the beginning of the study period}} \times 10^n$$

The denominator for CI is the total 'population at risk' (Webb, Bain & Page, 2019, p. 39) of developing the disease or health-related event at the beginning of the study. In other words, the candidate population should be composed of disease-free subjects at the starting point of the study (given a specific interval of observation). It assumes that all members in the population are followed up for the same period. It can be used to calculate the lifetime risk of an event.

In epidemiological practice, especially when the study involves a long period of observation, it is unrealistic to assume that all members in the population are followed up or stay in the study for the same amount of time. Participants leave a study for various reasons such as health conditions, death, losing contact or simply losing interest. To take into account the potential dropouts in a follow-up study as well as various lengths of observation, another form of incidence measure, incidence rate (IR), is often used. IR is defined as the number of new cases divided by the total person-time at risk in the study population. The formula is:

$$\text{incidence rate (IR)} = \frac{\text{number of new cases during the study period}}{\text{total person years (person-time at risk}} \times 10^{n}$$

The numerator in an IR calculation is total new cases in a specified period, which is the same as that in CI calculation. The denominator is the total person-time, which is the sum of each individual's time at risk. Person-time needs to be specified as person-days, months or years, depending on the unit of time measured in the observation. IR is a rate as it includes a time unit in the denominator.

SPOTLIGHT 13.2

Example of incidence rate

The following example (Figure 13.2) is a hypothetical follow-up study to measure the risk of disease X. It is assumed that the total observation period was 8 years. Of all 10 participants, some were followed up all the way through (for 8 years, participants 1, 6 and 9) but some left the study or developed the disease before the study ended.

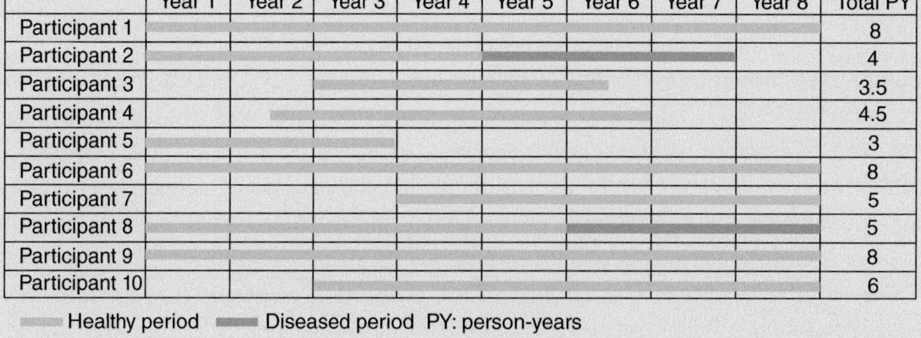

	Year 1	Year 2	Year 3	Year 4	Year 5	Year 6	Year 7	Year 8	Total PY
Participant 1									8
Participant 2									4
Participant 3									3.5
Participant 4									4.5
Participant 5									3
Participant 6									8
Participant 7									5
Participant 8									5
Participant 9									8
Participant 10									6

▬▬ Healthy period ▬▬ Diseased period PY: person-years

Figure 13.2 Example of an eight-year long follow-up study: IR calculation

QUESTION

What is the IR for disease X per 1000 person-years in this study sample?

Incidence and commonly used public health measures

'Incidence' refers to the risk of developing a disease. It can also be applied to measure the development of death or mortality. As population changes with time, in public health practice mid-interval population (as estimated average total person-time) is often used for population estimates. Other public health measures, such as maternal mortality rate and infant mortality rate, are common indicators used to compare the levels of public health status in different communities, countries or populations. They are two key indicators in the United Nation's Sustainable Development Goals (SDGs). In addition, attack rate and the case-fatality rate used in disease epidemic investigations are also extensive measures of incidence. The attack rate is the percentage of people at risk from an infectious agent who becomes sick, which is the most commonly used incidence measure for infectious disease. The case-fatality rate is the proportion of people with a specific disease who die from the disease in a given period of time, measuring the severity of a disease.

Descriptive epidemiology: Time, personal and place characteristics

With regard to patterns of health events in a population or populations, epidemiologists make comparisons of time, personal and place characteristics in order to find out the underlying causes of the events. Time characteristics are useful for assessing changes in the risks (such as prevalence and incidence) of disease or health-related events over time and identifying possible epidemics. For example, seasonal patterns have been noted in some disease occurrences, such as seasonal influenza – more prevalent during cool winters – and food poisoning, which is common during hot summers. Long-term monitoring of disease (disease surveillance) is crucial to identifying any unusual patterns or increase of disease rate, and thus helps public health authorities and practitioners to take timely action to control the disease and prevent large outbreaks. Figure 13.3 shows the changes of reported and accumulated COVID-19 cases over time in Australia (Australian Government, Department of Health, 2021). There were two distinct waves reflecting the large local epidemics across Australia (Wave 1) and concentration in Victoria and Melbourne (Wave 2) prior to the availability of COVID-19 vaccines. As the virus is highly infectious and can be transmitted from person to person, the case numbers rose dramatically at the early stage of each wave until aggressive control measures, such as lockdowns, travel restrictions, self-isolation and quarantine, started to take effect. The continuous monitoring of COVID-19 (temporal pattern) enables decision-making on the introduction of public health measures to contain the virus and protect the wider community, or to lift restrictions.

Descriptive comparisons regarding 'personal' characteristics include socio-demographic characteristics such as sex, age, race or ethnicity, marital status, education, employment status, socio-economic status and behavioural risk factors. Data from the Australian Institute of Health and Welfare (AIHW, 2014b) in Figure 13.4 shows that age-specific mortality rates appear to rise sharply in older age groups (e.g. those aged 50 years and older) for both males and females. Males seem to have higher mortality rates than females across different age groups. In addition, the figure also reveals an issue involving a sub-population, Aboriginal and Torres Strait Islander peoples in Australia. It is clear that the age-specific mortality rates in all age groups are double or even higher in Indigenous populations when compared with the general population, except the oldest group (75+ years). The figures can be used to address the issues of health inequality (see also chapters 1 and 7).

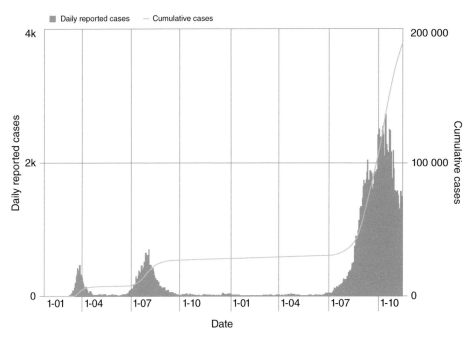

Figure 13.3   Daily new COVID-19 cases and accumulated cases from January 2020 to November 2021 in Australia
Source: Australian Government, Department of Health (2021).

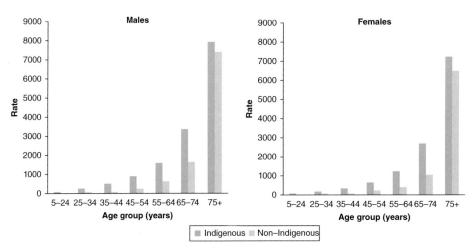

Figure 13.4   Age-specific mortality rates, by sex and Indigenous status, NSW, Qld, WA, SA and NT combined, 2008–12
(mortality: deaths per 100 000 population)
Source: Adapted from AIHW (2014a).

The characteristics of 'place' consider geographic variation, urban–rural differences, and locations of workplaces where the health issue or event occurs. Figure 13.5 shows the confirmed numbers of A(H1N1)pdn09 (swine 'flu) cases and deaths reported to the WHO in September 2009. Following the WHO's announcement of the start of pandemic swine 'flu on 11 June 2009, the disease spread across almost all continents within three months, including Australia. Scientists applied the Geographic Information System (GIS) to visualise geographic patterns of disease epidemics, so the comparison of the pandemic swine 'flu map at different points in time enabled epidemiologists to monitor how quickly the disease was spreading across countries and how severely the disease affected different regions or countries.

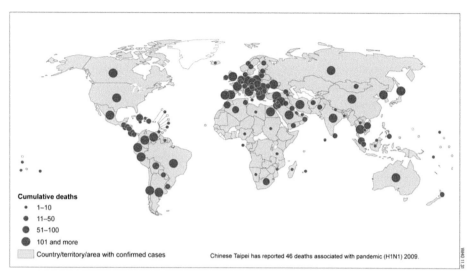

Figure 13.5   Pandemic (H1N1) in 2009: Countries, territories and areas with laboratory confirmed cases and the number of deaths as reported to the WHO.

Source: WHO (2011), p. 62.

SPOTLIGHT 13.3

Comparing mortality rates between populations

As mentioned in the section on incidence measures, mortality is a basic public health measure used to compare the public health status in different communities or populations. Figure 13.6 presents the gender-specific mortality rates between New South Wales and the Northern Territory from 2003 to 2013.

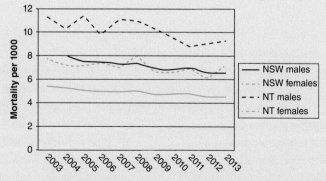

Figure 13.6   Standardised mortality rates between New South Wales and the Northern Territory, 2003–13

Note: The standardised mortality rate was used to adjust for differences in the age distribution of the states by applying the age distribution of total persons in the Australian population to both states.

Source: Australian Bureau of Statistics (2014).

QUESTION

How do the mortality rates vary in terms of time, personal and place characteristics between the populations in New South Wales and the Northern Territory? (See Figure 13.6.)

Epidemiological study designs

As discussed in the previous sections, epidemiological studies can be classified under two broad categories: descriptive and analytic approaches. Figure 13.7 illustrates the commonly used epidemiological study designs and the strength of evidence for association between a risk factor (an exposure) and a health outcome in relation to different study designs. Descriptive studies cannot be used to establish causal relationships, whereas an analytical approach, which includes observational and experimental/intervention studies, looks for associations between potential causes (exposures) and disease occurrence (outcomes). Experimental or intervention design provides the strongest evidence for association and is considered to be the top level on the hierarchy of all epidemiological study designs, while observational designs, including cross-sectional, case-control and cohort studies, remain important in providing a significant amount of evidence regarding causal inferences in epidemiology.

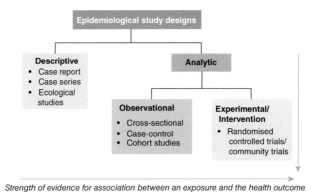

Strength of evidence for association between an exposure and the health outcome

Figure 13.7   Epidemiological study designs and the strength of evidence for association between a risk factor (an exposure) and a health outcome

Descriptive studies

Epidemiological data can be obtained from a broad range of sources and routinely collected data, including death registrations, disease surveillance, vital statistics, census data, hospital records and population surveys. The data can be used to describe the burden of disease in a community and to inform disease patterns and the changes in disease trends by investigating the 'what, who, when and where' (variations in time, place and person) of the health-related events in descriptive studies. They can also be used to generate hypotheses for exploring possible causes of a specified health event or outcome. The hypotheses will be further tested in analytic studies. For example, migrant studies compare the differences in disease rates in migrant populations over generations and between countries to find out whether the differences are due to genetic or environmental reasons (e.g. changes in lifestyles). The other common forms of descriptive studies include case reports and case series of unusual medical occurrences or adverse events. Case series are collections of individual case reports. Data is collected by clinical practitioners and documented if the disease has not been seen before or has been observed in an unusual form among the reported cases. It is crucial to identifying a new disease or a potential epidemic.

Countries and international organisations collect routinely available health statistics to assess the health status of a population or country and to monitor the progress toward specific health indicators and overall goals. For instance, to address the SDGs, the WHO develops health-related indicators to work with the member states toward measurable targets. On the WHO's Global Health Observatory website, such mortality data and global health estimates can be found to compare health levels of different countries or regions and address burdens of disease. These health statistics or population data can be used to address changes in disease patterns in relation to time, place and personal characteristics. For example, in ecological studies, researchers make use of routinely collected data such as disease incidence, prevalence and mortality data to investigate the relationship between the disease rate and the prevalence of a specific factor over time or in different geographic areas. A shortcoming of these studies is that they do not relate exposure and outcome in individuals. There are likely to be many factors other than the exposure being studied, and these also contribute to the occurrence of the disease. Instead, ecological studies compare disease rate and the prevalence of a specific exposure (e.g. unemployment rate) at the population level. This is known as the 'ecological fallacy' (Büttner & Muller, 2015).

Analytic studies

The analytic approach in epidemiology attempts to answer the 'why' and 'how' of the variations in health outcomes observed in different groups, communities and populations. The different outcomes can be attributed to varying demographic characteristics, socio-economic status, genetic factors, immunological status, environmental exposures and other behavioural risk factors that are potentially underlying causes of a disease. Data for analytic studies can be collected in various ways, as detailed in the section on descriptive studies. The general term 'exposure' is used to represent 'potential causes' of a health outcome. The exposure may be a risk factor, a protective factor, or a treatment or intervention, depending on the nature of the exposure factor and the study design. Analytic studies – including observational and experimental or intervention studies – are concerned with the **association** between exposure status and a health event. In observational studies, including *cross-sectional, case-control* and *cohort* studies, researchers observe the study subjects and measure the exposure and outcome variables without providing treatments or interventions to the subjects. On the other hand, experimental or intervention studies enable researchers to control the exposure factor and replace it with a 'treatment' or an 'intervention' to see its effect on the outcome variable (see Figure 13.7).

Association – the statistical dependence between the occurrence of a health-related event and a specific variable or a personal characteristic.

Cross-sectional studies

Cross-sectional studies are also known as 'simple surveys'. The study is conducted at a single point in time (cross-sectionally) without follow-ups. Ideally, the study subjects are randomly selected so that the sample is representative of the source population and the prevalence of a health outcome can be determined. Figure 13.8 presents a model of cross-sectional study. The initial sample selection of a cross-sectional study involves only one group, with no compari-son group. However, the study subjects can be split into two, or more than two, groups based on the status of the main outcome variable or the exposure of interest. The prevalence of the outcome can be studied. Associations between outcome and exposure can be measured.

Many countries conduct large population surveys such as census surveys and health and nutrition surveys on a regular basis to collect information about socio-demographic characteristics of population, health and nutrition status, the use of health services and lifestyle risk factors. Cross-sectional studies are less expensive and time-consuming when compared to other forms of analytic studies. As the outcome and the exposures are measured at the same point in time – the temporal sequence of exposure and outcome events is uncertain – a common problem with cross-sectional studies is the inability to draw causal inferences.

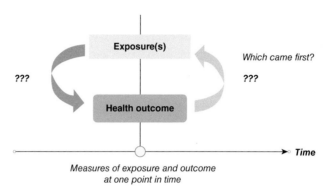

Figure 13.8   A cross-sectional study design

Case-control studies

Case-control studies recruit study participants based on their outcome status. If the health outcome is presence of lung cancer, a group of lung cancer cases and another group of non-cancer individuals (controls) are selected independently. The study works backward in time (retrospectively) to collect and measure the participants' past experience of exposure (e.g. smoking history). The prevalence of exposures are compared between the case and control groups, and the association between the outcome and the exposure can then be assessed. Figure 13.9 displays the design of a case-control study, indicating the direction and timing of data collection.

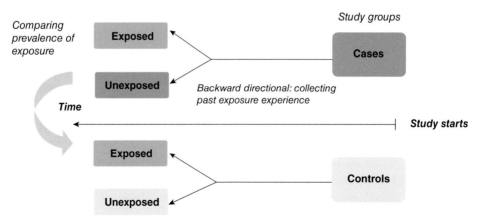

Figure 13.9   A case-control study and direction of data collection

Ideally, the control group in a case-control study should represent the population from which the study subjects have come, and the prevalence of exposure in the control group should be similar to the general population. Any members who have developed the disease in the control group at the beginning of the study should be excluded from the control group or recruited into the case group. In order to minimise potential **confounding** effects from common demographic characteristics, investigators select control subjects by 'matching' the distributions of key confounding variables (e.g. gender and age) in the cases. Some demographic variables such as age, gender and socio-economic status are common confounding factors. They are usually associated with the exposure or the outcome factors. For example, a study may investigate the effect of coffee drinking during pregnancy on low birth weight (LBW) of newborns, and the result shows coffee drinking is associated with LBW. However, after adjusting for the differences in mother's age, socio-economic status and smoking during pregnancy between the study groups, the association no longer exists. In this example, the coffee drinking and LBW relationship is possibly confounded by age, socio-economic status and smoking.

In comparison with cohort and intervention studies, case-control studies are more cost-efficient and less time-consuming as no follow-up is required. All cases can be recruited at the same point in time regardless of the duration of disease latency and the variation in diseased period among the cases. Case-control studies can also assess the effects of multiple exposures or risk factors. However, some limitations have been identified. First, it is difficult to select a representative control group. Second, a **recall bias** may occur if cases tend to recall their experience of exposure differently because of their disease, and results in an underestimation or overestimation of the true effect. In addition, frequency of disease (e.g. incidence) cannot be determined.

A case-control study in the United Kingdom (Chilver et al., 2003) investigated whether post-menopausal hormone replacement therapy (HRT) could reduce the risk of acute myocardial infarction (AMI). The researchers selected 864 women aged 35–65 years diagnosed with AMI and two age-matched controls free of AMI from the same geographic area. The duration of HRT use was calculated, based on the sum of total prescriptions shown in each participant's general practitioner (GP) record. The results of this study demonstrated that HRT use for over 60 months significantly reduced the risk of AMI. As the length and duration of HRT use occurred in the past, it was very likely that the collection of exposure data had involved some levels of recall bias.

Cohort studies

A cohort study, or prospective cohort design, involves a group of people who share the same experience with a particular exposure, such as an occupational hazard, an environmental exposure or a behavioural risk factor. As shown in Figure 13.10, a representative sample from the target population is selected and grouped based on their exposure status. Data collection at baseline (the beginning of the study) includes basic socio-demographic variables, the measures of exposure (duration, frequency and received dose of exposure), and the information of other potential risk or confounding factors. Most importantly, none of the participants should have the disease or health outcome at the initial recruitment stage. Both exposed and unexposed groups are followed up for a specified period of time or until a sufficient number of cases is achieved. The rates, such as incidence or mortality rates, of the outcome are measured and compared between the groups to determine the association between the exposure and the outcome.

Confounding – 'the distortion of a measure of the effect of an exposure on an outcome due to the association of the exposure with other factors that influence the occurrence of the outcome' (Porta, 2008, p. 38). Adjustment of confounding is using appropriate statistical techniques to remove the effects of differences in the distribution of certain confounding factors between the study groups.

Recall bias – in case-control or cross-sectional studies, when a particular group of study subjects is more likely to overestimate or underestimate their past experience of exposure than the other group.

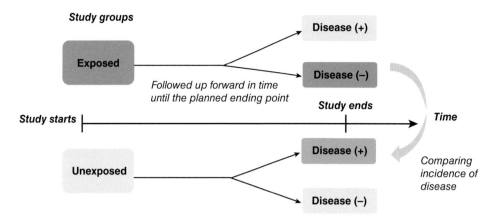

Figure 13.10   A prospective cohort study design and direction of data collection

Of all the observational study designs, cohort studies provide the strongest evidence concerning the most direct measurement of the risk of developing a disease as the temporal sequence of exposure and outcome is certain; that is, exposure precedes the development of the outcome. The most challenging issue with cohort studies is to ensure good follow-ups of all participants. The more people who are 'lost to follow-up', the more likely selection bias will occur in the study. Selection bias arises when there is a systematic difference between the people who are included in a study and those who are not. This systematic difference may result in a distortion in the measure of association. For example, selection bias may be introduced if different sampling methods are used to select samples from exposed and unexposed groups in a cohort study.

Prospective cohort studies are potentially costly and time-consuming when the outcome of interest is a chronic disease. Alternatively, another form of cohort study can be designed – namely, a retrospective cohort study – in which measurement of exposures, follow-up of participants and measurement of outcomes could have occurred in the past. However, it must be certain that the exposure event preceded the outcomes for a retrospective cohort design. Like a prospective cohort design, the study participants are grouped on the basis of their exposure status in a retrospective cohort study.

One of the main strengths of cohort studies is that temporal relationships for determining causality can be established because the exposure factor was present prior to the occurrence of the outcome. A prospective cohort design will also help to understand the natural history of the disease. The incidence of the outcome can be directly measured. It can study withdrawals (using incidence density) and rare exposures. There are some disadvantages associated with cohort studies. They can be very expensive and time-consuming if the disease has a long latency and the study involves a large study sample. Moreover, loss to follow-up would be another potential issue when the duration of the study is long.

Intervention or experimental studies

As shown in Figure 13.11, the design of an intervention or experimental study is fundamentally a prospective cohort study. It enables the investigator to change the exposure to an 'intervention' and control over the factors other than the 'intervention' factor through randomisation. The intervention can be designed to test a new treatment, vaccine, healthcare practice, or health education or promotion program. One group (the study group) is offered the intervention, while the other group (the control group) is offered an alternative treatment – for example, conventional treatment or intervention – or placebo. Participants are randomly allocated into different groups so that all potential confounding factors, such as demographic characteristics like gender and age, are evenly distributed across the groups. Both groups are followed up over a period and are compared with the changes in disease rate at the end of the study.

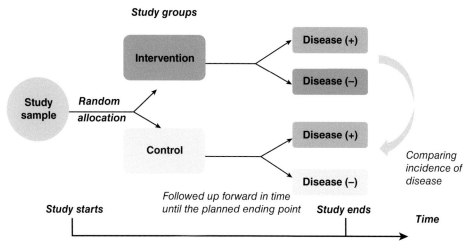

Figure 13.11   An intervention study design and key components of the study

Experimental studies are also known as randomised control trials. There are two main types: clinical and community trials, depending on the randomisation of intervention on individual or community basis. A community-based cluster randomised trial is often used to assign the intervention and compare two or more groups of people from communities. A quasi-experimental design is employed when randomisation is absent. The major advantage of experimental intervention studies over the other forms of analytic study design is that they deal with known potential and unknown confounding factors through randomisation. However, they can be unethical and impractical when applied in human beings. Ethical issues need to be taken into account when an intervention is introduced. The intervention is expected to protect participants against disease, and no harm should be associated with the intervention.

SPOTLIGHT 13.4

Ethical issues arising in experimental studies

Drawing on the results of many observational HRT studies (the example in the case-control studies section is one of them) which reported some benefits of HRT use in menopausal women, such as reducing menopausal symptoms and lowering the risk of heart attack, coronary death, stroke and osteoporosis, a randomised controlled trial was developed by the Women's Health Initiative (WHI, Chlebowski et al., 2003) to provide more substantial evidence on the actual health effects of HRT. A total of 16 608 post-menopausal women aged 50–79 years was recruited and randomised into HRT and placebo groups. Baseline data was collected in 1993 and a total of 8.5 years of follow-up was planned. Although the study found that HRT use reduced the risks of osteoporosis, bone fractures and colorectal cancer, it also showed that HRT was associated with increased risks of heart attacks, stroke, breast cancer and blood clots. As the overall health risks were shown to outweigh the benefits of HRT use, the research study was discontinued three years earlier than planned. This study did not suggest that menopausal women should consider using HRT or alternatives. Based on the results of this trial, the American Heart Association recommended against initiating HRT for the secondary prevention of cardiovascular disease. This issue remains controversial in clinical medicine.

QUESTION

Why was the WHI clinical trial stopped earlier than planned?

Use of surveillance data in epidemiological studies

Surveillance has been defined as 'the ongoing systematic collection, analysis and interpretation of health data, essential to the planning, implementation, and evaluation of public health practice, closely integrated with the timely dissemination of these data to those who need to know' (Thacker & Berkelman, 1998, p. 164). Traditionally, surveillance involves the continuous monitoring of the occurrence and distribution of infectious disease. It has become increasingly important in monitoring changes in non-infectious diseases and other types of health conditions such as injuries, cancer, the coverage of vaccination, the use of prescription drugs, environmental hazards and even risk factors of diseases. Surveillance data can be used to monitor changes in disease frequency in terms of time, place and personal characteristics, as detailed in descriptive studies. Various sources of surveillance data can also be used in analytic studies to identify risk factors of diseases. In epidemiological practice, surveillance data from different sources can be linked to examine associations. For example, some cohort studies collect exposure data at baseline and use surveillance data to follow up the outcomes through linkage to mortality data or cancer register systems, also known as linkage studies. Data linkage is also popularly used in studying vector-borne diseases. For instance, dengue fever surveillance data can be linked with mosquito surveillance data, or even with long-term monitoring of climatic data. Surveillance data can also be used to evaluate the effects of public health programs or interventions. Due to resource constraints, surveillance data in low and middle-income countries are less complete and accurate. The mortality data in those countries are largely based on modelling estimates. This remains one of the major public health challenges. Further readings regarding surveillance and its applications are recommended at the end of this chapter.

Measures of association

According to the evidence shown in descriptive analyses, an analytic study can be developed to determine whether an association between exposure and disease exists. Measures of association are calculated and used to assess a possible causal relationship between an exposure and a health outcome by comparing disease occurrence in groups with and without the exposure. These measures quantify the strength and direction of an effect of exposure on a health outcome and are fundamental to assessing causality. The choice of measure of association is dependent on the study design (such as risk ratio in follow-up studies and odds ratio in case-control studies) and the information available for measure of disease occurrence.

In follow-up studies (cohort and experimental studies), relative risk (RR) is calculated to quantify the risk (incidence) of developing a disease in the exposed group, compared to the unexposed group. The RR measures differ in relation to the choice of measure of disease frequency. A two-by-two table (Table 13.1a) describes exposure status and outcomes between the comparison groups (exposed and unexposed groups) before RR is calculated. For instance, a cohort study investigated the relationship between employment status and mortality among HIV-positive individuals in Vancouver, Canada (Richardson et al., 2013) and the results are presented in Table 13.1b.

Table 13.1a   Relationship between employment status and mortality 1996–2010

| Exposure | Outcome (death) | | Total |
	Yes (+)	No (-)	
Unemployed	178	389	567
Employed	16	83	99
Total	194	472	666

Table 13.1b   Relationship between employment status and mortality 1996–2010 (calculating RR)

| Exposure | Outcome (death) | | CI | RR |
	Yes (+)	No (-)		
Unemployed	178	389	$CI_e = 178/567 = 0.314$	–
Employed	16	83	$CI_0 = 16/99 = 0.162$	$RR = CI_e \div CI_0 = 1.94$

Applying CI formula (as shown in the section on 'Frequency of disease occurrence'), the incidence among unemployed individuals (exposed group) can be expressed and calculated as:

$CIe = 178 \div 567 = 0.314 = 314$ deaths per 1000 over 15 years

Meanwhile, the incidence for employed individuals (unexposed group) is:

$CI_0 = 16 \div 99 = 0.162 = 162$ deaths per 1000 over 15 years

The relative risk is:

$(RR) = CI_e \div CI_0 = 314 \div 162 = 1.94$

The RR result indicates that the exposed group (unemployed) had a higher risk of mortality than the unexposed group. That is, the risk of 15-year mortality in the unemployed group was 1.94 times higher compared with the employed group. This measures the effect in the exposed group relative to the unexposed group.

In case-control or cross-sectional studies, CI or IR cannot be calculated, so an alternative measure, the odds ratio (OR), is used to estimate the association between exposure and outcome. Using the data from a case-control study on vitamin D status and coronary heart disease (Aljefree et al., 2016) shown in Table 13.2 (the numbers of subjects are denoted as **a**, **b**, **c**, **d**), OR is calculated by dividing the odds of exposure in the cases (**a/c**) by the odds of exposure in the controls (**b/d**).

Table 13.2   Vitamin D status and risk of coronary heart disease

Smoking status	Outcome		OR
	Cases	Controls	
Vitamin D deficiency	99 **(a)**	76 **(b)**	5.0
Adequate vitamin D	31 **(c)**	119 **(d)**	1
Total	120	195	

Source: Based on Aljefree et al., (2016).

The OR for vitamin D-deficient subjects compared with those with adequate vitamin D can be expressed as $(\mathbf{a/c}) \div (\mathbf{b/d}) = (\mathbf{a} \times \mathbf{d})/(\mathbf{b} \times \mathbf{c})$.

The odds ratio for individual with vitamin D deficiency compared to those with adequate vitamin D status is:

$$\mathbf{OR} = (\mathbf{a} \times \mathbf{d})/(\mathbf{b} \times \mathbf{c}) = 99 \times 119/76 \times 31 = 5.0$$

$$OR = \frac{(\mathbf{a} \times \mathbf{d})}{(\mathbf{b} \times \mathbf{c})} = \frac{99 \times 119}{76 \times 31} \times 197 = 5.0$$

The result shows that vitamin D deficiency increases the risk of death due to coronary heart disease. The risk is estimated relative to the unexposed group (subjects with sufficient vitamin D).

Measures of association are used to investigate aetiology and prevention of disease. As discussed previously, most diseases are multifactorial and represent the effects of a combination of multiple factors. Although an established association provides important evidence for determining causation, the finding of an association between exposure and disease should not be immediately assumed as causal. More evidence needs to be collected to evaluate causal relationships. Bradford Hill's (1965) criteria for causation are commonly used in epidemiology to establish evidence of a possible causal relationship. The issues of validity, bias and confounding regarding the quality of evidence to assess the true relationship between exposure and disease are beyond the scope of this chapter. Further readings in relation to these issues are recommended at the end of this chapter.

SUMMARY

In this chapter, you have learnt about epidemiology in public health. It is the way that we assess the health of populations. As you have seen throughout the chapter, there are many important issues relating to this. Below is the summary of salient issues relating to epidemiology in public health.

Learning objective 1: Understand the essence of epidemiology and outline the scope and purposes of epidemiology in public health.

In the context of constantly changing environments, the focus of epidemiology has extended from communicable diseases to a broader range of health issues, including chronic diseases, injuries, various health risks and even lifestyle factors. Epidemiology plays an important role in identifying the aetiology of health-related problems and developing disease prevention and control measures in public health and clinical practice. Its scientific methods and critical thinking approach form the basis of evidence-based practice in all health fields and are essential to effective health prevention and promotion in populations. This chapter has explained the purposes, basic principles and applications of epidemiology in public health by breaking down the definition of epidemiology into several key concepts.

Learning objective 2: Calculate measures of frequency of disease or health-related events and be able to compare the patterns of a health event with regard to time, place and personal characteristics in order to identify health issues or problems in the compared populations.

This chapter has also introduced the measures of disease frequency and presented the use of these measures in descriptive epidemiology to compare the patterns of health issues with regard to time, place and personal characteristics in different populations, supplemented with Australian and global examples to reinforce students' understanding of the topics. The comparisons may lead to further analytic studies to identify possible causes of a disease or a health condition.

Learning objective 3: Be familiar with the major features of the commonly used epidemiological study designs and the use of epidemiological studies in relation to determining association between exposure and disease.

This chapter has discussed several study designs and their key features, and has provided real-world examples to strengthen your understanding of different designs. The study design is determined on the basis of whether the study participants are selected by exposure or outcome status, the time dimensions of the study and the information or resources available for the study. The study design directs the approach to data collection in order to establish causal implications in evidence-based practice.

Learning objective 4: Apply appropriate quantitative measures of association to different study designs, in order to identify possible causes of a health outcome.

The quantitative measures of association demonstrated in this chapter are used to identify the possible causes of ill health. The choice of measure of association is dependent on the study design and the data available for measure of disease occurrence. These measures have public health implications in managing the risk factors of a disease or health issue, and to further plan and evaluate public policy and strategies to prevent ill health.

TUTORIAL EXERCISES

According to the AIHW (2014a), at the end of 2009 there were 861 057 people (429 083 males and 431 974 females) diagnosed with cancer at some point in the previous 28 years. In 2010, 65 983 new cancer cases in men and 50 598 in women were identified.

The Australian population at the end of 2009 comprised 10 967 831 males and 11 063 919 females (Australian Bureau of Statistics, 2014).

1 What was the cancer prevalence in the total Australian population at the end of 2009?

2 Calculate and compare the gender-specific cancer prevalence at the end of 2009.

3 Calculate and compare the gender-specific cancer incidence (incidence rates in different genders) in 2010. Is this a measure of CI or IR? Why?

4 Combining the results in questions 2 and 3, what were the public health implications in relation to the gender differences in prevalence and incidence? (Optional)

Note: The denominator for CI is *population at risk of developing cancer at the beginning of 2010* (1 January). The total population at the beginning of 2010 is considered the same as the population at the end of 2009. Those people who already had cancer before the end of 2009 were excluded as they were no longer at risk of developing cancer.

FURTHER READING

Büttner, P., & Muller, R. (2015). *Epidemiology* (2nd ed.). South Melbourne Press.

Gordis, L. (2009). Ethical and professional issues in epidemiology. *Epidemiology* (4th ed.). Saunders Elsevier.

Hill, A. B. (1965). The environment and disease: Association or causation?. *Proceedings of the Royal Society of Medicine*, *58*(5), 295–300.

Webb, P., Bain, C., & Page, A. (2019). *Essential epidemiology: An introduction for students and health professionals* (4th ed.). Cambridge University Press.

Yarnell, J. (2013). Epidemiology in public-health practice. In J. Yarnell, & D. O'Reilly (Eds.), *Epidemiology and disease prevention: A global approach* (2nd ed.). Oxford University Press.

REFERENCES

Aljefree, N. M., Lee, P., Al Saqqaf, J. M., & Ahmed, F. (2016). Association between vitamin D status and cardio-metabolic risk factors among adults with and without coronary heart disease in Saudi Arabia. *Journal of Diabetes & Metabolism*, *7*(10).

Australian Bureau of Statistics (ABS). (2014). *Death rates, summary, states and territories – 2003 to 2013*. Retrieved http://www.abs.gov.au/AUSSTATS/abs@.nsf/mf/3302.0

Australian Government, Department of Health. (2021). Coronavirus case numbers and statistics. Retrieved https://www.health.gov.au/news/health-alerts/novel-coronavirus-2019-ncov-health-alert/coronavirus-covid-19-case-numbers-and-statistics#covid19-summary-statistics

Australian Institute of Health and Welfare (AIHW). (2014a). *Cancer in Australia: An overview 2014.* (Cancer Series #90). AIHW.

——(2014b). *Mortality and life expectancy of Indigenous Australians 2008 to 2012*. AIHW.

Büttner, P., & Muller, R. (2015). *Epidemiology* (2nd ed.). Oxford University Press.

Chilver, C. E. D., Knibb, R. C., Armstrong, S. J., Woods, K. L., & Logan, R. F. A. (2003). Post menopausal hormone replacement therapy and risk of acute myocardial infarction – a case control study of women in the East Midland, UK. *European Heart Journal*, *24*, 2197–2205.

Chlebowski, R. T., Hendrix, S. L., Langer, R. D., Stefanick, M. L., Gass, M., Lane, D., . . . WHI Investigators. (2003). Influence of estrogen plus progestin on breast cancer and mammography in healthy postmenopausal women. *Journal of the American Medical Association*, *289*(24), 3243–53.

Gerstman, B. B. (2013). *Epidemiology kept simple: An introduction to traditional and modern epidemiology* (3rd ed.). John Wiley & Sons.

Hill, A. B. (1965). The environment and disease: Association or causation? *Proceedings of the Royal Society of Medicine, 58*(5), 295–300.

Lambert, H. Gupte, J., Fletcher, H., Hammond, L., Lowe, N., & Pelling, M. (2000). COVID-19 as a global challenge: towards and inclusive future. *Lancet Planetary Health, 4*(8): E312–14.

Lashley, F. R. (2006). Emerging infectious diseases at the beginning of the 21st Century. *Online Journal of Issues in Nursing, 11*(1), 29.

Last J., Spasoff, R., & Harris, S. (2000). *A dictionary of epidemiology*. Oxford University Press.

Pfefferbaum, B., & North, C. S. (2020). Mental health and the Covid-19 pandemic. *New English Journal of Medicine, 383*, 510–12.

Porta, M. S. (Ed.) (2008). *A dictionary of epidemiology* (5th ed.). Oxford University Press.

Richardson, L. A., Milloy, M-J. S., Kerr, T. H., Parashar, S., Montaner, J. S. G., & Wood, E. (2013). Employment predicts decreased mortality among HIV-seropositive illicit drug users in a setting of universal HIV care. *Journal of Epidemiology and Community Health, 68*(1), 93–6.

Thacker, S., & Berkelman, R. L. (1998). Public health surveillance in the United States. *Epidemiologic Review, 10*, 164–90.

Webb, P., Bain, C. & Page, A. (2019). *Essential epidemiology: An introduction for students and health professionals* (4th ed.). Cambridge University Press.

World Health Organization (WHO). (2007). *New health threats in the 21st century. World health report 2007: Global public health ecurity in the 21st century*. WHO.

——(2011). *Implementation of the International Health Regulations (2005): Report of the Review Committee on the Functioning of the International Health Regulations (2005) in relation to pandemic (H1N1) 2009*. WHO.

——(2021a). Timeline: WHO's COVID-19 response. Retrieved http://www.who.int/emergencies/diseases/novel-coronavirus-2019/interactive-timeline#!

——(2021b). Noncommunicable diseases: fact sheets. Retrieved http://www.who.int/news-room/fact-sheets/detail/noncommunicable-diseases

Wouters O. J., Shadlen, K. C., Salcher-Konrad, M., Pollard, A. J., Larson, H. J., Teerawattananon, Y., et al. (2021). Challenges in ensuring global access to COVID-19 vaccines: production, affordability, allocation, and deployment. *Lancet, 397*(10278), 1023–34.

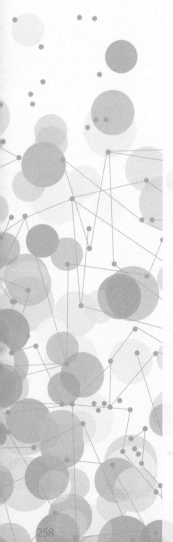

14

Planning and evaluation of public health interventions

Stuart Wark

LEARNING OBJECTIVES

After studying this chapter, you should be able to:

1   describe the roles of planning and evaluation as part of any public health intervention
2   explain the three key concepts that underpin planning and evaluation
3   understand the six-stage model for planning and evaluation
4   determine the most appropriate evaluation approach for different interventions
5   develop a simple plan for a proposed intervention, including an evaluation.

VIGNETTE

The public health implications of blue-green algae

Blue-green algae, or cyanobacteria, can produce toxins that are dangerous to humans, aquatic animals and livestock. It can build up to unsafe levels within freshwater and marine water sources whenever prevailing conditions support this growth (Vu et al., 2020). If there is reduced water flow in combination with increased water temperatures and the right mix of light and nutrient levels, a 'bloom' of blue-green surface scum will result (Kaur et al., 2021). If this occurs within a water supply or a recreational area, it can result in serious public health consequences.

The World Health Organization (WHO) has developed guidelines for safe levels of cyanobacteria to address concerns about the potential poisoning of humans and animals. Health issues in the human population can arise from the ingestion of contaminated water, through dermal (skin) exposure or by consuming animals previously affected. The health effects of exposure to cyanobacteria have been reported to include a wide variety of issues including gastrointestinal problems, such as diarrhoea and vomiting, 'flu-like symptoms, skin rashes, and eye or ear irritations. Ingestion can result in increased severity of these symptoms, and has been reported as resulting in death (WHO, 2015).

As a consequence of the health problems associated with exposure to cyanobacteria, public health interventions are required to support communities that may be affected. These programs could include a variety of disparate options, from distributing general education material to local residents, through to specialist training of paramedics and health practitioners in how to deal with a widespread outbreak. As an example of a current and continuing public health intervention in Australia, rivers and other water sources are regularly checked for blue-green algae levels and, if a bloom is identified, the relevant local or state government department will issue a health warning to the public (e.g. WaterNSW, 2021). But how do we know whether public health interventions such as these are effective in minimising the effects of a bloom on a community? This is where careful planning and evaluation of public health interventions becomes vital.

Introduction

The principles of public health promotion have been outlined in previous chapters within this textbook (see Chapter 3). The importance of planning prior to the development and subsequent implementation of any such public health interventions has been recognised for many decades (e.g. Kok, 1993) and continues to be considered critical to the effectiveness of a program (Thompson, Kent & Lyons, 2014). However, while appropriate evaluation of the intervention is as important as the initial planning, historically it has been an often overlooked aspect of program development (Green & Kreuter, 2005). Planning, implementation and evaluation should be viewed as three equally necessary and complementary components of any **public health program**.

This chapter introduces planning and evaluation with respect to public health promotions and interventions. Entire textbooks have been written on healthcare planning and evaluation (e.g. Issel, Wells & Williams, 2021), so this chapter focuses primarily on overarching

Public health program – a planned and structured project, or series of projects, that includes specific intervention/s designed to address one or more identified public health needs of a community.

Project team – usually a group of people who work together to design, implement and evaluate a public health program; for smaller projects, the 'team' may just be one individual.

concepts. It identifies a simple, six-stage public health planning model that assists **project teams** to move from the initial identification of a need through implementation to assessment of the outcomes, with the evaluation also identifying any needs that remain partially or completely unmet. The concepts of planning and evaluation should be viewed as being part of a continuing process; the planning of public health interventions should be informed through review of outcomes from relevant projects while the evaluation phase should provide observations and recommendations for future programs. If evaluations are not carefully planned and undertaken, it may not be possible to establish whether the program achieved the desired public health outcomes. Subsequent projects may then not be aligned with the needs of the community as valuable knowledge for any follow-up interventions was missed.

Why plan? Development of a public health intervention

The United States Institute for Healthcare Improvement identified three key drivers for any public health intervention, which they named the 'triple aim':

1 'Improving the patient experience of care (including quality and satisfaction);
2 Improving the health of populations; and
3 Reducing the per capita cost of health care' (Institute for Healthcare Improvement, 2021).

If it is possible to achieve these three aims through an intervention, it is likely that a program can be delivered that is effective and efficient, and be perceived by the desired target group as generally beneficial. However, unless appropriate planning and development is undertaken before any intervention commences, there is a high likelihood that the program will not meet all three drivers; or worse, there is the risk of a 'triple fail' in which none of the factors are achieved. It is acknowledged that the 'triple aim' approach was conceptualised for healthcare settings, and that all three drivers may not necessarily be applicable to all public health programs. For example, improving the patient experience of care may not be relevant for programs implemented outside of a health system, like the example of monitoring blue-green algae blooms. Nonetheless, the triple aim is a useful lens through which to begin development of potential programs.

Planning – the process by which a public health intervention is conceptualised, developed, implemented and then evaluated.

Planning is a systematic approach whereby a public health program is conceptualised and developed to allow for future implementation (Glanz & Bishop, 2010). It is often perceived as being just the initial phase; however, it is important to acknowledge that planning must involve careful consideration of the evaluation of the entire program, both during implementation and at its conclusion. A key aspect of the planning phase involves the clear identification of need for the community in question and, by ascertaining these needs, the overall program goals and objectives can be defined. This, in turn, enables an effective **evaluation** of the intervention in achieving the desired health outcomes for the target population and in sustaining any positive changes into the future (Schell et al., 2013).

Evaluation – a systematic approach to assessing the implementation and outcomes of a public health intervention to identify problems and/or determine whether the program has met its nominated goals.

Planning for public health programs is based on three principles:

1 Defining the main and, if appropriate, any secondary outcome/s that the program is trying to achieve

2 Specifying the intervention that is going to be implemented as a mechanism to achieving these outcomes

3 Determining the objective measures that provide evidence to confirm if the program has achieved the nominated outcomes (National Public Health Partnership, 2000).

The first principle, *defining the outcomes*, requires the project team to consider the specific needs of the population, normally by identifying priority health areas (Sansoni, 2016). The team must determine the needs of the population through either gathering new information or reviewing existing information. Desirably, this information is sourced through a variety of methodologies, such as examination of epidemiological or socio-economic data collected through questionnaires, focus groups and/or interviews with stakeholders, including health practitioners, members of the public, police, social workers, teachers and so forth. This data can then be used to identify and prioritise the needs of the stakeholders and, from that point, the desired outcomes that will address the need can be defined.

The second principle, *specifying the intervention*, is where the team matches the project's goals with an intervention designed to achieve the nominated outcomes (MacDonald et al., 2016). This stage requires the team to evaluate a variety of approaches to the problem at hand and nominate the project's methodology. Once the optimal approach has been identified, it is then possible to nominate the resources that are required for the project, develop a working budget and set out a clearly defined list of responsibilities within an action plan. Inherent to the action plan is a timeline for the project, from planning to implementation, evaluation and final reporting.

The third principle, *validating the outcomes*, requires the team determine the objective measures that will enable the evaluation phase, so that the key question: 'Has this intervention been successful?' can be answered. It is vital to ensure that the project's outcomes are directly aligned with mechanisms that enable accurate evaluation. While evaluation is a distinct phase of the project and separate to planning, how the project will be evaluated must be considered in advance and should not be included as an afterthought or following commencement of the project (Rychetnik et al., 2002).

REFLECTION QUESTIONS

1 Governments around the world have struggled to address the public health effects of drug use. Do you think that government decisions relating to the legality of specific substances is derived from carefully developed, planned and evaluated research?

2 Why are some drugs, such as alcohol, caffeine and tobacco, deemed legal, while others such as marijuana are prohibited? What about naturally occurring hormones such as testosterone?

3 What factors, other than public health concerns, could potentially play a role in government decision-making?

4 How could these additional issues affect your implementation of a public health intervention aimed at assisting people with drug addiction?

The six-stage model of public health planning

The three principles, as discussed earlier in this chapter, lead to a six-stage model for planning small public health interventions, and these stages are outlined in Figure 14.1. This simple model has been developed specifically for this chapter, using the concepts and principles outlined in planning documents and reports including: *A Framework for Environmental Health Risk Management* (United States Environment Protection Agency, 1997); *Framework for Program Evaluation in Public Health* (United States Department of Health & Human Services, 1999); *A Planning Framework for Public Health Practice* (National Public Health Partnership, 2000); *Health 2020* (WHO, 2013) and *A Framework for Program Evaluation* (Centers for Disease Control and Prevention, 2017). This model is aimed primarily at local interventions, and may not necessarily be appropriate for large-scale, multifaceted public health programs. For national and international-level interventions, there is often a need for additional and extensive legislative and policy changes, and a more comprehensive planning model may be required to address these aspects.

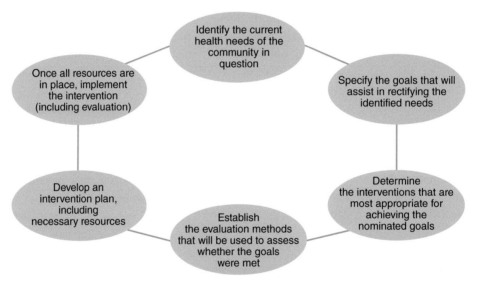

Figure 14.1   The six-stage model of public health planning

While the model commences at the top and progresses clockwise, it is important to recognise that it does not proceed solely in a linear fashion. In fact, it is ideal for previous stages to be reconsidered before implementation commences. As the plan is developed, questions often arise that require previous decisions to be re-evaluated. However, if the project team does return to a previous stage, it is important that the subsequent stages are completed again, taking into account the changing information or knowledge.

This process of review is not an indication that the intervention is fundamentally flawed, but instead enables continuous quality improvement to increase the likelihood of achieving the nominated project goals. The circular model provides for the evaluation to identify unaddressed issues, which in turn can then be recommended for examination in future interventions. Each of the six stages are discussed in detail in the following section.

SPOTLIGHT 14.1

Gun control

In 1996, the small Tasmanian town of Port Arthur was the site of Australia's worst mass shooting, with 35 people killed and another 18 seriously injured. This massacre led the Australian government to introduce the *National Firearms Program Implementation Act 1996* (Commonwealth of Australia, 1996). This legislation and associated public campaigns resulted in the almost-complete elimination of mass shootings in Australia over the following 10 years (Chapman et al., 2006). In contrast, in the United States there have been many incidents of lone and multiple shooters in recent times; in the decade 2011–20 alone, there were 72 different mass shootings (Statista, 2021).

QUESTIONS

1 Do you think that the interventions implemented in Australia to minimise gun-related deaths would be successful in the United States?
2 The number of mass shootings in the United States was 11 in 2017, 12 in 2018 and 10 in 2019. It then dropped to just two in 2020 (Statista, 2021). Was this dramatic reduction the result of an effective public health intervention, or could other factors be responsible?

Stage 1 – Identify the health needs of the community in question

A public health intervention requires an explicit understanding of the community issues the project is aiming to address. Without this knowledge, it is not possible for any program to reliably achieve outcomes that improve the health of the target population. As such, the first stage in a public health intervention is to clearly identify the needs of the community and to prioritise which needs are to be the focus of the intervention.

Determining the health needs of a population is complex. There are many approaches that can be used to gather information, and which may each result in different but equally correct answers (Liamputtong, 2017, 2019). In other chapters within this book, there are examples of methodologies designed to measure the frequency of diseases and patterns of illness (see Chapter 13), while also recognising the contribution that individual perspectives can play in determining health priorities (see Chapter 12). Different approaches can be used to obtain information that will facilitate the assessment of the health needs in a community; however, the variation in data may result in very different priorities being identified.

It is also worth considering different types of 'need' when determining health priorities. Need can be conceptualised on the basis of an identified discrepancy between two or more comparison groups (e.g. residents of a town in central Australia reliant on water supplied through a pipeline, compared to people in another remote location who are able to gain access through a consistent local water source). However, need can also be seen in the light of a failure to conform to nominated standards, such as when either of these water sources are affected by levels of blue-green algae that exceed government guidelines. Individuals can also identify their own needs, and these will vary according to the perspective of either the person or their wider cohort. In considering the vignette example of a blue-green algae outbreak, it may be that local council workers desire updated training in the use of water treatments, to alleviate both the current crisis and to prevent future occurrences, while health practitioners may instead prioritise additional knowledge of how to best assist individuals who have experienced poisoning. Both are equally valid needs but providing the council workers with training in how to provide specialist medical support would not necessarily result in any improvements in health outcomes.

Reviewing the evaluations of previous similar public health interventions is also vital in Stage 1. A well-conducted evaluation should identify what was achieved, but equally it should acknowledge any issues that remain either partially or completely unresolved. It is possible for a new project to therefore build on the achievements of a previous program, but also to address needs of the community that may have emerged during the implementation of a previous intervention and were therefore not addressed at that time.

Stage 2 – Specify the goals that will assist in meeting the identified needs

Once the needs of the community have been identified and priorities determined, the second stage is to define which goals, if achieved, will assist in improving the current situation. The goal of a project may not be to eradicate a problem, but instead may be aimed at alleviating or reducing the effects of a health issue that cannot be completely eliminated.

The setting of clear goals serves several purposes. They assist in understanding the fundamental question of why the project is occurring, and not merely what is going to happen. In Stage 1, the needs of the community are identified and the goals of the project now have to be developed to directly address these needs (the 'why'). At the same time, the goals should also reflect the intervention that is to be attempted (the 'what'), as this facilitates appropriate evaluation of whether the project achieved the desired outcomes for the community. However, goals should not be designed to be easily met, purely to argue for the success of the project. Goals should be aspirational and attainable; they should be sufficiently challenging to ensure that progress occurs and the target population sees an improvement in their health outcomes.

In setting goals, there may be one or more overarching goals, and then sub-goals. An overarching goal is a general statement of what the project is aiming to achieve. The sub-goals are specific statements of outcomes that are proposed to be achieved within the timeframe of the project. Using the case example of blue-green algae, a public health intervention goal could be to 'reduce the number of people hospitalised after exposure', with sub-goals then nominating a very specific outcome, such as 'to provide specialist first-responder training to 10 paramedics in the local area'.

It is worth noting that numerous different terms may be used synonymously with the word 'goal'. Depending upon the model, goals may be referred to as aims, objectives, targets and so forth. In principle though, the purpose is the same: to nominate clearly what is hoped to be achieved and to allow for future evaluation of whether the project has been successful.

Stage 3 – Determine the interventions that are most appropriate for achieving the nominated goals

Intervention approaches can be extremely varied. They may include such disparate methods as national media campaigns, local school education sessions, household pamphlet drops, individual or group onsite training sessions, online courses, physical treatments (such as chemical applications or prophylactic medications), and so on. It is important to recognise that while differing approaches may each nominally meet the project goals, the level of success may vary. Therefore, failure to consider all possible approaches may result in less-than-optimal outcomes. Many public health projects are conceptualised initially with a desired intervention already in mind. This may reflect what the project team is comfortable in organising, is familiar with from previous projects, or even simply because the interventions have been successful in the past. Stage 3 is where the team needs to carefully consider the options that may be available, and should remain open to alternative approaches.

Overall cost is naturally an important factor to take into account, and is often thought to be the first point of consideration. However, the intervention methods should not be determined primarily by what is the cheapest option. It is important to start any consideration of proposed intervention methods by identifying and viewing all possible approaches and then rating them according to their effectiveness in addressing the identified needs (Stage 1) and goals (Stage 2). It is a better outcome for the project team to consider scaling back the overall project goals than to implement a less-expensive intervention that is likely to be ineffective. If two approaches are viewed as being equal in effectiveness, appropriate consideration of the overall project cost may then assist in ranking one method above another.

Time is also a critical component; both in terms of how long it will take to develop the intervention and with respect to when and for how long the program will run. An intervention that is likely to be effective in terms of both cost and outcomes may not be feasible if it does not occur within a desired timeframe. For example, it may be possible to provide a cheap and effective public health advertisement on public TV regarding the dangers of swimming in blue-green algae-affected water. However, if the only time this program ran was during winter, any potential effect may be largely dissipated by the time it is actually needed in summer. Further, it is vital to have clearly nominated the target audience to ensure the approach can be tailored to any known demographic preferences. For example, there is a clear demographic shift occurring in TV viewing habits, with people under the age of 45 years increasingly watching less commercial TV and instead choosing to watch streamed content (Poggi, 2017). Any public health intervention based on TV advertising may therefore be less effective if people in this age bracket represent the key audience.

The final component of Stage 3 is documentation of all resources that will be required. This includes identifying both the existing and any additional resources that are needed. This review process should consider the following factors:

- *Human resources.* This should include the project team itself, members of the local community, subject-matter experts and local, national or international advisors. People can assist in the development, implementation and evaluation of the program by contributing their knowledge, skills, experiences and labour. Influential individuals, such as family members, local community leaders and even popular social media figures may be able to assist in guiding public opinion on important public health issues.
- *Knowledge resources.* There is often a variety of useful existing information sources that can assist in the development of a program. These might include government or an industry body's guidelines and recommendations, such as the *Australian Drinking Water Guidelines* (Water Quality Australia, 2018) for the blue-green algae example. Both state and local governments may also have policies and procedures for dealing with situations unique to their location. The internet is also a source of information, but caution must be exercised whenever reviewing content that is potentially unreliable and

based on opinion rather than the available scientific evidence. This is not to say that individual viewpoints should not be considered, as expert opinion and personal experiences can be important in understanding potential barriers that limit a program's effectiveness, but such information should be carefully evaluated with respect to the wider knowledge base.

- *Physical resources.* This can include existing assets, information and communication technologies (ICT), training rooms and other spaces, and resources to be purposively developed for the intervention. Examples of resources that may need to be designed include information brochures, websites or training materials, and even chemicals or physical barriers such as fencing, netting or cages. A thorough investigation of the physical resources that are available locally may assist in reducing the costs of the project, as there may be no need to replicate items that are already either under-utilised or able to be hired rather than purchased outright.

Establishing the necessary resources prior to commencement is vital so that potential pitfalls, such as unavailable personnel or expensive items, can be recognised. If it is clear that there may be problems with resource allocation in this planning stage, the intervention approach must be re-considered. The best-intentioned project will fail if the necessary resources are not available at the right time.

Stage 4 – Establish the evaluation methods that will be used to assess whether the goals were met

As noted earlier, evaluation is one of the most important but overlooked aspects of any public health intervention. An effective evaluation enables the project team to accurately identify what worked, what did not work and what knowledge may be useful for any future interventions. The proposed evaluation methods should always be mapped in advance against each of the goals and sub-goals, to ensure that accurate assessment of the outcomes, both desired and undesired, can occur without limitation. The importance of ensuring that the evaluation methods are established in advance of commencing the intervention cannot be too strongly emphasised. Attempting to retrospectively 'fit' an evaluation into a project that has already begun can potentially discredit any of the achievements made.

Evaluation methods must be objective and free from actual or perceived bias. While it is naturally desirable for an intervention to be considered 'successful', it is crucial that the evaluation methods are robust and independent of undue influence from the project team. This does not mean that the evaluation must always be undertaken by a third party, but there is the need for the evaluation to clearly demonstrate that the project team has not attempted to skew the findings to make outcomes appear overly beneficial.

The general principles and methods used in evaluation are covered in greater detail later in this chapter. Using the blue-green algae scenario, exemplar evaluations could include pre-testing and post-testing of the knowledge of workers, a review of the number of blooms across a defined location over a set period of time, or an appraisal of any changes in the severity and/ or duration of symptoms in exposed individuals.

Stage 5 – Develop an intervention plan, including necessary resources

Continuous review of the proposed project enables emerging issues to be identified as early as possible. As such, prior to finalising the intervention plan, the project team should review the previous stages to ensure that no new problems are evident. This is part of the circular nature of the model; it may be that the project team will recognise a major flaw in the planning process at this point, and will therefore need to return to Stage 1 to ensure that the entire intervention is not compromised.

Once the team is satisfied that no additional actions are necessary, the intervention plan can be developed. By this time, the team should be clear on the public health need the intervention is going to address, the best way to address this need, the evaluation methods that will determine whether the need has been addressed and the resources required to achieve all of these steps.

The intervention plan must outline exactly:

* Who is going to do each action
* What resources are required to support the nominated person/s to implement the action, and
* The timeframe for each of the actions.

A matrix that specifies each action, the person who is responsible for the action, any necessary resources and the proposed timeframe for completion is a common structure for intervention plans. An example of a very simple plan to provide an information brochure on blue-green algae to local residents in a small town is included in Table 14.1.

Table 14.1   Matrix of a sample intervention plan

Intervention Plan – Blue-green Algae Brochure Mail-out			
Action	**Person/s responsible**	**Resources required**	**Timeframe**
Develop brochure content with focus on effects of blue-green algae through exposure while swimming	• **Team leader** • Content developer • Public health doctor	• Information from health guidelines (Water Quality Australia, 2018) • Advice from doctor • Computer program for brochure design	3 months: commencing 1 July
Print brochure for distribution	• Team Leader	• Final approved version of electronic brochure • $500 for printing costs (to be paid from government grant)	2 weeks: commencing 1 September
Distribute brochure to all households in town	• Team leader • Manager, Disability Employment Service	• 500 brochures • $2500 to pay for household distribution by local disability employment program	1 week: commencing 15 September

Team leader – a project team will normally have a designated team leader who is responsible for overseeing the implementation of the entire project and delegating tasks to team members.

This matrix is simplistic, but more detailed plans could use the same structure with additional detail. Each of the actions (e.g. develop brochure) can be divided up into specific sub-activities with more nuanced allocations of responsibilities, delegations and approvals.

Several specialist software solutions are available, both commercially and free, to assist teams with planning for public health interventions. If the project is complex and requires substantial resources, occurs over a long or multiple time periods, or includes many locations,

a dedicated software package may be beneficial to the planning and implementation processes. However, the time involved for key personnel to learn how to use new software may
ultimately delay the project. If there is not a computer program mandated by either the
employer or funding body, it is feasible to map out simple intervention plans in any
mainstream spreadsheet or free web-based program. If an individual can foresee that they
are going to be planning a few interventions over the following months or years, it is
recommended that they trial some different packages to see which ones best meet their need.
In contrast, if a person is involved in planning a simple, one-off intervention, it is suggested
that specialist software may not be necessary. It is possible to move a project to a more
complex package if necessary, but the money and time spent in purchasing and learning a
program that is not actually required cannot be regained.

Stage 6 – Once all resources are in place, implement the intervention (including evaluation)

The final stage in the model is where the actual implementation of the intervention occurs. If
the planning stages have been rigorous and comprehensive, the intervention will have an
increased chance of achieving the nominated outcomes. However, it is worth remembering
that there is never a guarantee that the goals will be met; it is impossible to accurately predict
in advance exactly how an individual or community may react to an intervention, and there
may be adverse circumstances that cannot be predicted.

Once the program has commenced, it is important to continually review the progress of the
intervention plan. It is likely that unforeseen issues will arise through the duration of this
implementation stage, and if appropriate surveillance of the program is occurring, these issues
can be predicted and rectified before they affect the project. When a problem is identified, it is
important to return to Stage 5 and update the intervention plan to incorporate any new actions,
responsibilities and timeframes. Similarly, a review of the nominated evaluation methods (Stage
4) may be required to ensure that any issues are not inadvertently overlooked or missed.

Finally, once the actual intervention has been completed, it is easy to avoid focusing on
ensuring the evaluation phase. Comprehensive evaluation enables the project team to understand whether the intervention was effective in addressing the initial needs of the community,
and also can help to identify where there are remaining areas for improvement or continuing
gaps that require follow-up. Any evaluation of a project should include observations of what
did and did not work as planned, and should provide specific recommendations for future
interventions to consider. While evaluation is conceptualised and incorporated into the
planning of a project, it requires a specific focus, and any project must have a comprehensive
understanding of what constitutes an appropriate evaluation.

SPOTLIGHT 14.2

Public health interventions: Smoking versus obesity

Smoking remains a major public health issue around the world. It has been reported to cause the
death of approximately 21 000 Australians annually and costs the health system billions of dollars. On
a positive note, the past few decades have seen significant decreases in the number of smokers

(AIHW, 2019). However, it is not clear how much of the reduction in smoking is due to government regulations, such as bans on smoking in public areas and the increased taxes on cigarettes, as opposed to the widespread health behavioural change programs (Sammut, 2008). Like smoking, obesity has emerged as a major public health issue and there is similar need to address this problem (WHO, 2021).

QUESTIONS

1   With regard to the obesity epidemic, do you think that there are any lessons to be learnt from previous public health interventions aimed at reducing smoking?
2   Is government regulation of nutrition likely to be more successful than providing information about healthy eating and exercise to the general community through TV advertising?
3   Should the recommendations from other interventions be considered when developing a new program, even if it is in a different area of health?

The role of evaluation

Evaluation is the systematic and structured review of a public health program, with a focus on the use of objective measures that provide for the identification of strengths and areas for improvement (Dawson, 2019). Without appropriate evaluations being conducted during and following the conclusion of a public health program, any future interventions will not be in a position to build upon the strengths of the previous program, and may struggle to avoid making similar mistakes.

Evaluations are based on a combination of assessing the processes, effects and key outcome indicators. Without this knowledge, it may be impossible to determine whether the goals of the project have been achieved. The evidence gained from evaluations can then assist with the identification of what has been successful, what has not worked as predicted and what improvements for future programs may be appropriate. When future projects undergo evaluation, this iterative approach will enable constant refinement and better targeting of programs.

The purpose of evaluation within a public health context is to examine how effective the project in question has been in achieving the desired outcomes identified within the planning phase (Dawson, 2019). Evaluations should be measured against these nominated goals, and should highlight how well the intervention managed to improve health outcomes for the individuals or populations in question. It considers the overall success of a program, with specific consideration of factors including cost-effectiveness and efficiency of delivery vital for determining the outcome. However, evaluations are not limited just to consideration of how well the goals and objectives are met, but also should examine whether the implementation of the intervention was effective (United States Environment Protection Agency, 1997; WHO, 2001). If the project did not meet its goals and objectives, the failure may have been due to the way in which the intervention was implemented, rather than because there was a problem with the structure of the proposed intervention.

REFLECTION QUESTIONS

The 'Grim Reaper' public health campaign was shown on mainstream TV in Australia for only three weeks in 1987, before being followed up with print advertisements in newspapers. Commissioned by the National Advisory Committee on AIDS, the purpose of the intervention was to raise awareness of the potential spread of HIV/AIDS. The campaign was considered at the time to have been effective in achieving this goal (Morlet et al., 1988).

1 Would this approach be effective for all public health issues?

2 Do you think a 'scare' campaign would be as effective now?

3 Have there been changes within society that mean this style of intervention may now be obsolete?

Evaluation methods

In general, planning and evaluation can be seen as two interrelated elements that both inform and assist in the development of each other. The planning phase involves the development of specific goals and sub-goals, while the evaluation phase attempts to assess how well these nominated goals were met (WHO, 2001; Dawson, 2019). As noted earlier in the six-stage planning model (see Stage 4), how the evaluation of a public health project will occur should be determined during the planning phase and well prior to commencement of any intervention. Evaluations of public health interventions should, whenever appropriate and feasible, measure short, medium- and long-term effects, both in terms of health outcomes for individuals and for determinants of health within a population (National Public Health Partnership, 2000; Green & Kreuter, 2005).

The evaluation plan should specifically consider and nominate responses to each of the following questions:

- What is the purpose of the evaluations (e.g. what are the goals and objectives being measured)?
- What evaluations are to be conducted, and when are these evaluations proposed to occur?
- What indicators must be defined to enable changes to be accurately measured?
- What questions are required to be answered in each evaluation, to enable the correct data to be collected?
- Which key stakeholders are responsible for each of the steps of the proposed evaluations?
- What methodology is going to be used for the evaluations?

While a variety of evaluation types exists, this section focuses on four key types. Two occur generally during the planning and implementation stages of the intervention, while the other two normally take place during or after the intervention has been completed. These four types of evaluation are:

- **Formative evaluation**, which enables the project team to examine whether the intervention is likely to achieve the desired results and to identify any barriers that can be overcome before the intervention is finalised (Stetler et al., 2006).
- **Process evaluation**, which measures how well the intervention itself is being implemented (Moore et al., 2015).
- **Outcome (or summative) evaluation**, which determines whether the overall goals of the project, as defined in the planning phase, have been met (WHO, 2000).

- **Impact evaluation**, which considers how effective the project was in achieving the nominated goals, and whether the outcomes were sustained (Department of Foreign Affairs and Trade, 2012).

Examples of each of these four types of evaluation are included in Table 14.2, along with some reasons for when and why they could be used in a public health intervention, and example questions for each type of evaluation.

Table 14.2 Evaluation types

Evaluation type	Stage of intervention	Reason for using this type of evaluation	Example questions for this type of evaluation
Formative	During the development of an intervention	Formative evaluations enable the project team to identify changes that may be required before the intervention commences, to ensure the greatest chances of success.	• Are the key stakeholders happy with the proposed plan? • Are there any obvious impediments to implementation that have not been considered? • Is there a mismatch between the overall budget for the project and the proposed resources?
Process	During the implementation of the intervention	Process evaluation is, in effect, a monitoring process and occurs during the implementation. It enables the project team to assess whether the intervention is progressing as planned, and to identify any problems that may be able to be overcome without fundamentally changing the project at this late point.	• Are the methods and resources appropriate? • Is the budget on track, or is it costing more than expected? • Are the nominated timeframes being met? • Does the target group already appear to be benefitting from the intervention? • Are the proposed number of participants receiving the intervention? • Is there capacity for additional intervention?
Outcome	During the implementation of the intervention and/or at the conclusion of the intervention and subsequent months	Outcome evaluations are used to objectively assess whether the intervention is having an effect on the community in question. It enables the project team to determine whether the nominated goals have been achieved.	• Has there been measurable change in the target's knowledge, attitudes and/or behaviours? • Has there been measurable change in physical characteristics (individual, community or environment)? • Did the entire project come in on budget?
Impact	At the conclusion of the intervention and in subsequent months/years	Impact evaluation is also used to see whether the nominated goals of the intervention were achieved, but may take place over a longer time period to more accurately measure the extent of the intervention's impact, and whether any identified outcomes were sustained over a period of time.	• What changes arose from the intervention? • Were any observed changes sustained over time? • Were there any secondary changes that may not have been expected? • Does the cost of the project reflect good value for money when considering any short and longer-term changes?

It is worth noting that economic evaluation is sometimes considered to be a completely separate category to the above four evaluation types (see e.g. Drummond et al., 2015). However, it is often possible to incorporate economic considerations (e.g. a cost–benefit evaluation) into another evaluation. If it is identified that there is a need for a strong focus on the financial effects or cost benefits of an intervention, it may be worthwhile to consider including a specific sub-category on economic analysis into the outcome or impact evaluation. This may be particularly applicable for larger projects that are reliant on government funding and where clear evidence of value for money is required.

SPOTLIGHT 14.3

The vaccination debate

In 1998, a study was published in *The Lancet*, a highly reputable medical journal, titled 'Ileal-lymphoid-nodular hyperplasia, non-specific colitis, and pervasive developmental disorder in children' (Wakefield et al., 1998). Although this paper did not report a causal relationship between the measles, mumps and rubella (MMR) vaccination and autism, it was a catalyst for a widespread drop in vaccination rates in many countries, due to concerns about MMR causing autism in children. Widespread misconceptions about vaccinations and autism continue to persist (Zerbo et al., 2018), and the emergence of the COVID-19 pandemic was associated with a further rise in 'vaccination hesitancy' (Razai et al., 2021).

QUESTION

If you were asked to lead a team to design a public health campaign on social media to combat community misunderstandings about vaccinations, what factor do you think would be most important to consider when developing a plan for this intervention?

SUMMARY

Planning and evaluation are key components underpinning the success of any public health program. Appropriate planning prior to implementation is vital if the target community is to achieve any short, medium or long-term health benefits, while rigorous evaluation will also provide valuable insights for future interventions. This chapter introduced the concepts of planning and evaluation, and provided a six-stage model to guide the development, implementation and review of a public health program.

Learning objective 1: Describe the roles of planning and evaluation as part of any public health intervention.
Planning and evaluation are integral components of any program that is aiming to improve a public health issue. The ideas underpinning both planning and evaluation are examined across the chapter, with a particular focus in the first section on the generic concepts.

Learning objective 2: Explain the three key concepts that underpin planning and evaluation.
Three principles of *defining the outcomes, specifying the intervention* and *validating the outcomes* underpin the development of successful public health programs. If these three concepts are not carefully considered prior to commencement, the chances of a program achieving optimal results are greatly diminished.

Learning objective 3: Understand the six-stage model for planning and evaluation.
There are several different models for planning a health intervention. A simple six-stage model was proposed that outlines a circular approach, moving from identification of community need through to evaluation of the intervention and recommendations for future programs.

Learning objective 4: Determine the most appropriate evaluation approach for different interventions.
The final section of the chapter examined the concept of evaluating an intervention. It discussed four different evaluation types (formative, process, outcome and impact) and outlined when these evaluation types should be undertaken and what information they could provide.

Learning objective 5: Develop a simple plan for a proposed intervention, including an evaluation.
The chapter introduced to the concepts of planning and evaluation. The six-stage model provides a framework for developing a public health intervention, and a possible template for planning is provided.

TUTORIAL EXERCISES

1   Imagine that you are employed at a local council and are responsible for ensuring the health of the community in relation to local water quality. What public health issues would you need to consider, and what types of skills, knowledge and attitudes might you need to focus on improving to avoid issues with blue-green algae blooms?
2   Critically analyse your own capacity to implement a public health intervention to address concerns relating to a blue-green algae bloom in the local water source. What strengths would you bring and, equally, in what areas would you require advice and input from other experts?
3   Using the six-stage model and the intervention plan template, develop a simple intervention to address one concern relating to blue-green algae blooms.
4   Find an existing evaluation of a public health intervention. Read your chosen report and consider whether the planning processes undertaken by the project team were appropriate. Nominate why the report did or did not effectively evaluate the program, and identify what possible intervention could now build on knowledge gained through the completed project.

FURTHER READING

Centers for Disease Control and Prevention. (2017). *A framework for program evaluation*. Retrieved https://www.cdc.gov/eval/framework/index.htm

Dooris, M. (2006). Healthy settings: challenges to generating evidence of effectiveness. *Health Promotion International, 21*(1), 55–65.

Drummond, M., Sculpher, M., Claxton, K., Stoddart, G., & Torrance, G. (2015). *Methods for the economic evaluation of health care programmes*. Oxford University Press.

Issel, L. M., Wells, R., & Williams, M. (2021). *Health program planning and evaluation: A practical, systematic approach for community health* (5th ed.). Jones and Bartlett Publishing.

REFERENCES

Australian Institute of Health & Welfare (AIHW). (2019). Burden of tobacco use in Australia. Retrieved https://www.aihw.gov.au/reports/burden-of-disease/burden-of-tobacco-use-in-australia/summary

Centers for Disease Control and Prevention. (2017). A framework for program evaluation. Retrieved https://www.cdc.gov/eval/framework/index.htm

Chapman, S., Alpers, P., Agho, K., & Jones, M. (2006). Australia's 1996 gun law reforms: Faster falls in firearm deaths, firearm suicides, and a decade without mass shootings. *Injury Prevention, 12*(6), 365–72.

Commonwealth of Australia. (1996). *National Firearms Program Implementation Act 1996*. Retrieved https://www.legislation.gov.au/Details/C2004A05054

Dawson, A. (2019). Evaluation research in public health. In P. Liamputtong (Ed.), *Handbook of research methods in health social sciences*. Springer.

Department of Foreign Affairs and Trade. (2012). Impact evaluation. Retrieved https://dfat.gov.au/aid/how-we-measure-performance/ode/Documents/impact-evaluation-discussion-paper.pdf

Drummond, M., Sculpher, M., Claxton, K., Stoddart, G., & Torrance, G. (2015). *Methods for the economic evaluation of health care programmes*. Oxford University Press.

Glanz, K., & Bishop, D. B. (2010). The role of behavioral science theory in development and implementation of public health interventions. *Annual Review of Public Health, 31*(1), 399–418.

Green, L., & Kreuter, M. (2005). *Health program planning: An educational and ecological approach* (4th ed.). McGraw Hill.

Institute for Healthcare Improvement. (2021). The triple aim for populations. Retrieved http://www.ihi.org/Topics/TripleAim/Pages/Overview.aspx

Issel, L. M., Wells, R., & Williams, M. (2021). *Health program planning and evaluation: A practical, systematic approach for community health* (5th ed.). Jones and Bartlett Publishing.

Kaur S., Srivastava A., Ahluwalia A.S., & Mishra Y. (2021) Cyanobacterial blooms and cyanotoxins: Occurrence and detection. In S. K. Mandotra, A. K. Upadhyay, & A. S. Ahluwalia (Eds.), *Algae*. Springer.

Kok, G. (1993). Why are so many health promotion programs ineffective? *Health Promotion Journal of Australia, 3*(2), 12–17.

Liamputtong, P. (2017) The science of words and the science of numbers. In P. Liamputtong (Ed.), *Research methods in health: Foundations for evidence-based practice* (3rd ed.) (pp. 3–28). Oxford University Press.

——(2019). Qualitative inquiry. In P. Liamputtong (Ed.), *Handbook of research methods in health social sciences*. Springer Nature.

MacDonald, M., Pauly, B., Wong, G., Schick-Makaroff, K., van Roode, T., Strosher, H. W. . . . Ward, M. (2016). Supporting successful implementation of public health interventions: protocol for a realist synthesis. *Systematic Reviews*, *5*, 54.

Moore, G. F., Audrey, S., Barker, M., Bond, L., Bonell, C., Hardeman, W. . . . Baird, J. (2015). Process evaluation of complex interventions: Medical Research Council guidance. *Medical Journal*, *350*.

Morlet, A., Guinan, J., Diefenthaler, I. & Gold J. (1988). The impact of the 'grim reaper' national AIDS educational campaign on the Albion Street (AIDS) Centre and the AIDS Hotline. *Medical Journal of Australia*, *148*(6), 282–7.

National Public Health Partnership. (2000). *A planning framework for public health practice*. Retrieved www.health.nsw.gov.au/research/Documents/planning-framework.pdf

Poggi, J. (2017). Nearly half of millennials and gen xers don't watch any traditional TV. *AdAge*. Retrieved http://adage.com/article/media/half-young-consumers-watching-content-traditional-tv-study/310564/

Razai, M. S., Chaudhry, U. A. R., Doeholt, K., Bauld, L., & Majeed, A. (2021). Practice Pointer: Covid-19 vaccination hesitancy. *British Medical Journal*, *373*(n1138).

Rychetnik, L., Frommer, M., Hawe, P., & Shiell, A. (2002). Criteria for evaluating evidence on public health interventions. *Journal of Epidemiology and Community Health*, *56*(2), 119–27.

Sammut, J. (2008). *The false promise of GP super Clinics. Part 1: Preventive care*. The Centre for Independent Studies.

Sansoni, J. (2016). *Health outcomes: An overview from an Australian perspective*. Australian Health Outcomes Collaboration, Australian Health Services Research Institute.

Schell, S. F., Luke, D. A., Schooley, M. W., Elliott, M. B., Herbers, S. H., Mueller, N. B., & Bunger, A. C. (2013). Public health program capacity for sustainability: a new framework. *Implementation Science*, *8*(1), 15.

Statista. (2021). Number of mass shootings in the United States between 1982 and May 2021 (Webpage). Retrieved https://www.statista.com/statistics/81148//number-of-mass-shootings-in-the-us/

Stetler, C. B., Legro, M. W., Wallace, C. M., Bowman, C., Guihan, M., Hagedorn, H. . . . Smith, J. L. (2006). The role of formative evaluation in implementation research and the QUERI experience. *Journal of General Internal Medicine*, *21*(Suppl 2), S1–8.

Thompson, S., Kent, J., & Lyons, C. (2014). Building partnerships for healthy environments: research, leadership and education. *Health Promotion Journal of Australia*, *25*(3), 202–8.

United States Department of Health & Human Services. (1999). Framework for program evaluation in public health. *Morbidity and Mortality Weekly Report (MMWR)*, *48*(RR-11), 1–35.

United States Environment Protection Agency. (1997). *A framework for environmental health risk management. The US Presidential Congressional Commission on Risk Management 1997*. Retrieved https://cfpub.epa.gov/ncea/risk/recordisplay.cfm?deid=55006

Vu, H. P., Nguyen, L. N., Zdarta, J., Nga, T. T. V., & Nghiem, L. D. (2020). Blue-green algae in surface water: Problems and opportunities. *Current Pollution Reports*, *6*(2), 105–22.

Wakefield, A. J., Murch, S. H., Anthony, A., Linnell, J., Casson, D. M., Malik, M., . . . Walker-Smith, J. A. (1998). RETRACTED: Ileal-lymphoid-nodular hyperplasia, non-specific colitis, and pervasive developmental disorder in children. *The Lancet*, *351*(9103), 637–41.

Water Quality Australia. (2018). Australian drinking water guidelines (2011) – updated November 2018 (Webpage). Retrieved https://www.waterquality.gov.au/guidelines/drinking-water

WaterNSW. (2021). Water quality: Algae (Webpage). Retrieved https://www.waternsw.com.au/water-quality/algae#:~:text=Blue%2Dgreen%20algae%20may%20be,from%20Red%20Alert%20warning%20areas

World Health Organization (WHO). (2000). Outcome evaluations. Retrieved www.emcdda.europa.eu/attachements.cfm/att_5869_EN_7_outcome_evaluations.pdf

——(2001). *Evaluation in health promotion: Principles and perspectives*. WHO.

——(2013). Health 2020. A European policy framework and strategy for the 21st century. Retrieved http://www.thehealthwell.info/node/583943

——(2015). Guidelines for safe recreational water environments. Retrieved https://www.who.int/publications/i/item/WHO-FWC-WSH-15.03

——(2021). Obesity and overweight. Retrieved https://www.who.int/news-room/fact-sheets/detail/obesity-and-overweight

Zerbo, O., Modaressi, S., Goddard, K., Lewis, E., Fireman, B., Daley, M., . . . Klein, N. (2018). Vaccination patterns in children after autism spectrum disorder diagnosis and in their younger siblings. *JAMA Pediatrics*, *172*(5), 469–75.

PART 4

Public health issues and special populations

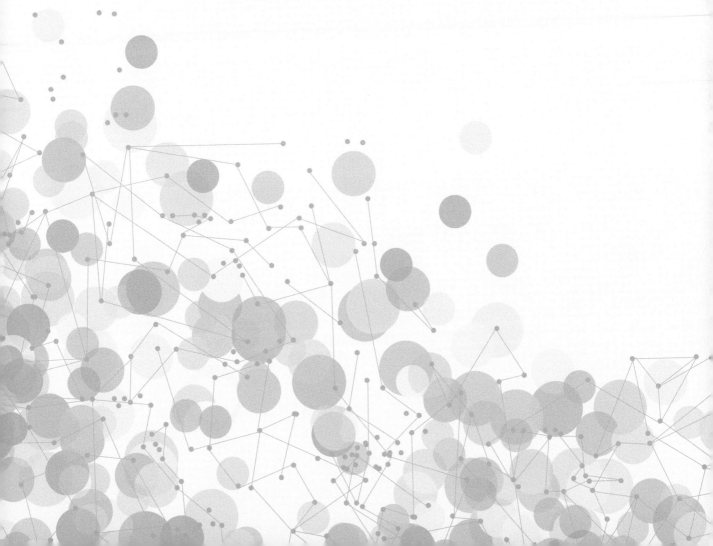

The health of children: The right to thrive

15

Lisa Gibbs, Elise Davis, Simon Crouch and Lauren Carpenter

LEARNING OBJECTIVES

After studying this chapter, you should be able to:

1   describe how social changes have led to increased child overweight and obesity
2   apply a socio-ecological model to identify multi-level factors influencing children's oral health and wellbeing
3   explain how the health and wellbeing of children living in same-sex parented families is directly influenced by broader social attitudes and can benefit from resilience-building strategies
4   describe the importance of prevention, early intervention and post-trauma support for children's mental health, including settings-based approaches to support children's social and emotional wellbeing.

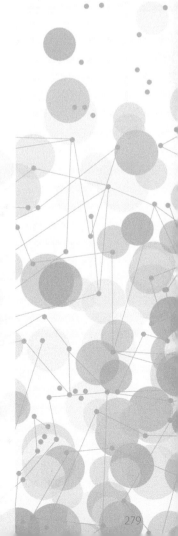

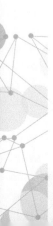

VIGNETTE

Children and young people's capacity in times of adversity

In January 2020, teenagers Lachie* and Jack* helped their mother to pack the car of clothes and valuables, and then cleared flammable things away from the house. The worst part was clearing the dried leaves and litter from the roof gutters. It was so hot and windy! They all moved quickly and were finally able to drive to the nearest bushfire evacuation centre in the next town. They could not relax once they got there because the threat of the fires was everywhere, in the orange sky and the dust-filled air. They waited with all of the other families, simultaneously anxious and bored. Everybody needed a distraction, so Lachie and Jack decided to do what they do best. They had experience in performing at festivals and, of course, their performing gear was the first thing they had packed into the car, so they put on a show for their fellow evacuees: stilt-walking and juggling in spectacular costumes. They also held free workshops in circus arts, which were especially popular with the kids.

This example demonstrates the capacity of children and young people to contribute to their own wellbeing and the wellbeing of others in times of stress. During COVID-19 lockdowns, children created chalk drawings on the footpaths outside their homes, and placed stuffed toys and pictures of rainbows in their windows to signal support for their own and community wellbeing. These examples provide an important reminder that keeping children and young people safe from physical and mental harm during times of adversity includes keeping them informed about what is happening and giving them age-appropriate opportunities to contribute to safety strategies and to demonstrate their competence.

* names have been changed

Introduction

Children and young people have the right to be healthy and to maximise their opportunities for a fulfilling life. This is enshrined in the 1989 United Nations (UN) *Convention on the Rights of the Child,* which articulates children's rights to health, safety, wellbeing and citizenship (UN, 1989). This convention defines childhood as being under the age of 18 years but acknowledges that in some countries the age of adulthood is considered to begin before 18 years. Age ranges for youth services extend up to 25 years in some countries. This highlights that childhood is a social construct that has shifted throughout history and across nations and cultures, influencing theoretical frameworks for childhood and hence opportunities for children. For example, the notion of the 'child at risk' represents children as vulnerable and in need of protection; the 'developing child' represents children as in the process of becoming adult and therefore in need of support and representation until their maturity and competencies have fully developed; and the 'citizen child' conceptualises children as capable of contributing to decisions affecting their lives (Morrow, 2003; Gill, 2007; Leonard, 2007; MacDougall, 2009). These theoretical frameworks are not necessarily mutually exclusive and can have a combined influence. For example, in a post-disaster setting, children can be provided with opportunities to participate in post-disaster research (citizen child), using child-friendly methods that are positive and relevant to the age and stage of the child (developing child), and ensuring a sensitive and ethical approach is employed so as not to exacerbate the experience of trauma (child at risk) (Gibbs et al., 2013).

Children's smaller size and developing but not fully matured physical, intellectual and social competencies mean they are often more vulnerable than adults to threats to their physical and mental health and wellbeing. Children's life circumstances and the health behaviours they develop also influence their health over their life course (Halfon & Hochstein, 2002). The various elements of their life circumstances, such as parenting, family income, parental level of education, housing, neighbourhood and education, are known as the social determinants of health and they are reliable indicators of inequalities in health and social outcomes (Marmot & Wilkinson, 2005; see also Chapter 7). Therefore, child public health considerations do not just need to address the current health status of the child; they also need to address the health concerns that may emerge from children's circumstances and lifestyle.

A socio-ecological framework is helpful in recognising the multi-level influences on health and wellbeing. Socio-ecological frameworks acknowledge the biological elements of health and the importance of individual behaviours (Bronfenbrenner, 1979; Dahlgren & Whitehead, 1991; Lynch, 2000). At the same time, they recognise many other social and environmental influences that essentially align with the social determinants of health. They include the family and sociocultural contexts; school and community settings; and the macrophysical, political and economic environments that alter living conditions and opportunities for health-promoting behaviours. Children's direct interaction with these different levels of influence increases progressively over time as they mature, and is mediated throughout by adult guardians, including parents and teachers. The role of these mediators needs to be included in any efforts to implement change in the spheres of influence on child health and wellbeing, such as in the home, school and community settings.

This chapter explores socio-ecological influences on child health and wellbeing by examining overweight or obesity prevention, oral health, the experiences of children in same-sex parent families and mental health. In doing so, opportunities to reduce child health inequalities and to increase resilience and quality of life are discussed.

Social determinants of health – the social and economic conditions in which people are born, grow, live, work, play and age, and which influence their health, such as poverty, unemployment, civic participation and social relationships (WHO, 2008).

Socio-ecological framework – a model taking into account the range of influences on individuals arising from interacting genetic and biological factors, individual behaviours, and social, cultural, physical, political and economic environments.

Prevention of overweight and obesity in childhood

Overweight and obesity is an international public health issue affecting children at unprecedented levels (World Health Organization [WHO], 2017). It is estimated that 38.2 million children worldwide under the age of five years and 340 million children and adolescents aged 5–19 years were overweight or obese in 2016, with rates having increased fourfold between 1975 and 2016 (WHO, 2021a). The health implications of overweight and obesity in childhood and adolescence are severe, and include increased risk of cardiovascular conditions, diabetes, joint problems, sleep apnoea and poor self-esteem. They are also associated with increased risk of adult obesity and higher adult morbidity and mortality. The establishment of healthy dietary and physical activity behaviours in young children may help to prevent the onset of overweight or obesity in adolescence and adulthood. However, the population-level epidemic reflects the fact that individual behaviours are being driven by broader social and environmental changes.

Obesogenic environments

The term 'obesogenic environments' describes conditions that make it harder to be healthy by reducing opportunities for physical activity and healthy eating in everyday life (Swinburn, Egger & Raza, 1999). For example, neighbourhoods with limited public transportation, unsafe cycling conditions and lack of direct walking routes force a reliance on vehicular transport rather than active transport. Similarly, public spaces such as sporting facilities that offer only high-sugar and high-fat food and drinks for purchase, and sporting clubs that hand out fast-food vouchers to children as rewards, make it difficult for healthy eating choices to be made.

REFLECTION QUESTION

The world has seen major changes in lifestyles over the past 20 years. In what ways might this influence children's and adolescents' risk of overweight and obesity?

Obesity prevention initiatives

Childhood obesity prevention initiatives ideally involve a multi-level approach to effecting sustainable change in target communities (Waters et al., 2011). This includes a combination of policy, program and environmental strategies in recognition of the different levels of influence on children's health and behaviours. Interventions are commonly situated in settings such as schools, early child care and communities, to allow for multi-level strategies. It is important in these settings to account for the local social, cultural and historical contexts.

Systems approaches – examining and understanding how the different components of systems interact and thus, how they can be strengthened or new systems created to help promote health.

More recently, **systems approaches**, or systems thinking, have been proposed as a way to address challenges of sustainability and scalability when implementing community-based childhood obesity interventions (Swinburn et al., 2019). A recent trial, the Whole of Systems Trial of Prevention Strategies for Obesity (WHO STOPS Childhood Obesity) worked with community members to identify and map characteristics of their community that were contributing to childhood obesity, and how they fit together. For example, junk-food con-sumption was linked to a several factors, including the influence of parents on children's eating behaviours, food marketing and the culture of using food as a reward (Allender, 2015).

Public health effects

There is some evidence that increased awareness and changing environments arising from multi-level public health initiatives have contributed to differences at the population level (Olds et al., 2010), with recent measures of child overweight and obesity in Australia indicating that prevalence rates are settling at around 25 per cent (Australian Institute of Health and Welfare [AIHW], 2021). However, persistent prevalence of one in four children being overweight or obese is not acceptable for optimal long-term population health.

An additional concern is that rates may continue to be increasing for disadvantaged population groups.

SPOTLIGHT 15.1

Changing trends

Multi-generational changes in lifestyles have contributed to the escalating rates of child overweight and obesity internationally. The car is now the primary form of transport, reflecting a significant shift from children previously walking or riding to school. This is partly due to parents' concerns about children's safety as pedestrians and cyclists. It has also shifted because of the increasing trend of both parents being in paid work and an increase in single-parent households, and consequently many children are now being dropped at school on the way to work. Families tend to be smaller, so children have fewer siblings to play with outside after school. Parents are less likely to allow their children to go to a park by themselves because of concerns about 'stranger danger'. Busy parents are relying on the increased availability of high-density packaged foods for their children's lunchboxes. Families are regularly eating unhealthy foods that used to be occasional parts of the family diet. The increasing popularity of screen activities means that children are also less engaged in active play during and after school, and on weekends. Children are being given mobile phones at younger ages as a means of maintaining contact with their parents. Computers and tablet devices are also being used by schools as part of children's education. There has been a major shift during the COVID-19 pandemic, with many students experiencing extended periods of learning from home.

QUESTION
How can these social shifts towards unhealthy lifestyles be influenced to promote healthy eating and physical activity for children?

Child oral health

Oral health includes the health of teeth, gums and other tissues of the mouth. Pain, disease or disorders affecting oral health can also affect many other aspects of people's lives, including speech, eating, smiling and general wellbeing. The importance of oral health as a major public health concern internationally was demonstrated when a resolution on oral health, calling for the development of a global oral health strategy by 2022 and action plan by 2023, was adopted at the WHO's 2021 World Health Assembly (WHO, 2021b).

The main oral health concern affecting children is dental caries (dental decay), and a particularly severe form of this occurring in very young children is early childhood caries (ECC). ECC is defined as the presence of any decayed, missing or filled tooth surfaces in the primary teeth of children under the age of six years and is one of the most common and preventable diseases of early childhood (Phantumvanit et al., 2018). It is an international public health problem but rates of prevalence vary considerably from less than 5 per cent to 98 per cent, with higher rates more evident in developing countries (Phantumvanit et al., 2018).

Gingivitis is another common condition affecting child oral health. It is characterised by swelling, redness and bleeding of the gums. If left untreated, gingivitis can progress to periodontitis, an advanced inflammatory form of gum disease affecting the structures that surround and support the teeth. However, this can be prevented and treated through regular tooth brushing, flossing and professional dental care.

Inequalities in child oral health appear as early as two years of age, with those from socially disadvantaged circumstances, particular geographic locations, Indigenous families, and immigrant and refugee families showing poorer oral health than the wider population (Verlinden et al., 2019; Kilpatrick et al., 2012; Riggs et al., 2014). ECC is often dismissed as unimportant because children's first teeth (primary dentition) are eventually replaced by their adult teeth (permanent dentition). However, ECC can cause illness, pain, abscesses, disturbed sleep, difficulty eating and speaking, and can lead to poor oral health in adolescence and adulthood (United States Department of Health and Human Services, 2000; Cunnion et al., 2010). It can also affect self-esteem and social interactions, as well as school attendance and academic outcomes (Sheiham, 2006; Jackson et al., 2011). Severe cases can result in hospitalisation and the need for surgery and anaesthesia, with associated health risks (Tennant et al., 2000; Nalliah et al., 2010).

Dental service use

The key oral health promotion messages for prevention of ECC are to eat well, drink well, clean well and stay well. 'Eat well' and 'drink well' refer to the importance of reducing the consumption of high-sugar foods and sweetened drinks. 'Clean well' refers to the importance of brushing teeth twice daily with toothpaste (Mejàre et al., 2015). The message of 'stay well' is to visit dental health practitioners to check on children's oral health and to receive treatment if required. The first stages of ECC are not always visible to non-professionals, and research has shown that parents of children with early stage ECC have not taken their children to see a dentist because they think they do not need it and because of a lack of understanding of the need to take care of the primary dentition (Christian et al., 2015). Other barriers to service use can include cost, time and cultural and linguistic barriers (Riggs et al., 2014). In Australia, public dental services and the Child Dental Benefits Schedule have been implemented in addition to private dental services to mitigate cost as a barrier to accessing dental services. Some Aboriginal Community Controlled Health Services (ACCHS) also provide dental care for their patients. In some states and territories of Australia there are additional initiatives to increase access to public services, such as mobile dental clinics that visit schools and remote areas, and dental voucher schemes that enable public patients to access care in private clinics.

Water fluoridation

Oral public health efforts have been introduced in Australia to reduce rates of ECC, including the addition of fluoride to drinking water for most Australian towns and cities (Australian Government, Department of Health, 2017). Despite this approach to oral health promotion, there are many rural and remote areas where 'town water' is not used and therefore many children miss out on the benefits of fluoridation (Gussy et al., 2006; Lucas et al., 2011). The published evidence on fluoridation strongly supports its use in reducing dental caries (National Health and Medical Research Council [NHMRC], 2007; Lucas et al., 2011).

When water fluoridation is extended to new areas it tends to generate considerable public debate over its merit because of concerns that it is 'artificial and imposed, and any risks were not personally controllable' (Armfield & Akers, 2010). Opponents to water fluoridation cite health risks; however, there is insufficient evidence to support these concerns (NHMRC, 2017).

Childhood oral-health interventions

The National Oral Health Plan 2015–2024 was released by the Australian government to guide strategies for improving oral health across the Australian population, including population groups at particular risk of inequity in oral health. Australia's performance against the plan is monitored and reported by the AIHW (Oral Health Monitoring Group, 2015; AIHW 2020).

Oral health promotion and educational interventions can be targeted at the level of individual, family and/or community to address disadvantage and health inequality. They can be delivered in various ways and contexts to promote oral health behaviours and reduce dental caries. Child dental screenings conducted in community settings can contribute to parents' understanding of their children's oral health needs. Survey instruments have been developed to support oral health-risk assessments, including measures specifically for children and young people (Sischo & Broder, 2011; Gao et al., 2010).

The core health promotion principles outlined in the *Ottawa Charter for Health Promotion* (see also Chapter 3) can guide child oral health promotion interventions (WHO, 1986). In the example in Spotlight 15.2, the relevant health promotion principle is noted in italics alongside each corresponding intervention strategy.

SPOTLIGHT 15.2

Cultural influences on child oral health

The Teeth Tales study identified a range of sociocultural risk and protective factors affecting child oral health in families with a refugee or immigrant background living in Melbourne, Victoria. As part of the study, immigrant families from Iraq, Lebanon and Pakistan were invited to participate in a trial of a community program co-developed and implemented by The University of Melbourne in partnership with community, health, cultural and government representatives *(strengthening community action; building healthy public policy; re-orienting health services)*. Dental screenings were conducted on 667 children aged one to four years, and 151 families attended community oral health-education sessions led by someone from their own language and cultural background *(develop personal skills)*. The sessions included information and discussions about the key oral healthcare messages with the peer educator, a visit to the local community dental service, provision of a family oral health pack with information, toothbrushes and toothpaste, and follow-up reminder messages to eat well, drink well, clean well and stay well. At the same time, the participating community health and local government organisations underwent a cultural competence review and re-orientation of services to increase their accessibility *(create supportive environments)*.

The trial evaluation showed improved oral hygiene in children from intervention families, compared to the comparison group, as well as increased parental knowledge on tooth-brushing technique and the role of fluoride in water (Gibbs et al., 2015). The participating organisations also demonstrated changed policies and programs to improve cultural competence. The study informed the refugee access policy for Dental Health Services Victoria *(building healthy public policy)*. Continuing outcomes from the Teeth Tales study include publication of the Cultural Competence Organisational Review resources (Centre for Culture, Ethnicity and Health, 2018). The lead agency, Merri Community Health Services, also re-oriented its dental services to include a new oral health program called Little Smiles, in which dental screenings and oral health education are provided to children in preschool settings, with treatment referrals provided as required *(re-orienting health services)*.

QUESTION
What strategies may be helpful to target child oral health interventions for families from diverse cultural and linguistic backgrounds?

Children in same-sex parent families

An increasing number of children in Australia are growing up with at least one parent who identifies as being same-sex attracted. Commonly referred to as 'same-sex parent families', these families have been formed in a variety of ways, with a range of intra-familial relationships. **Same-sex parent families** include families with gay male parents, lesbian parents, bisexual parents and transgender parents. Children may come into these families from previous heterosexual relationships, through the use of assisted reproductive technologies and surrogacy, or through fostering and adoption. Regardless of how same-sex parent families are formed, child health and wellbeing in this context garners much social and political interest and is an example of how family structure more broadly can affect child health.

Same-sex parent family – any family in which at least one parent identifies as being same-sex attracted.

Biological or social parenting?

Same-sex families have evolved over recent decades. They have moved from 'stories of impossibilities' through to 'stories of opportunities' and 'stories of choice' (Weeks et al., 2001). Having a family used to be thought an impossible concept for non-heterosexual people, as 'coming out' ruled out marriage, then the only realistic option for having children. Instead, LGTBIQ+ people would form families among their peers and friendship groups. The 'opportunity' to have children evolved as social and cultural shifts changed public perceptions of what constituted a 'real family'. Stacey (1996) puts this in the context of the 'sexual revolution and feminist assertions of autonomy' (p. 110). These changes enabled lesbian women to join the growing group of women having children outside the context of marriage. Research, media attention and the increased visibility of same-sex families enabled a growing confidence in non-heterosexual people who wanted to be parents (Weeks et al., 2001). With the recent options presented by new and emerging reproductive technologies, same-sex families are now able to make 'choices' about how they achieve parenthood. Where Weeks and colleagues (2001) talk about 'doing *parenting*', others describe 'doing *family*' – meaning that family is constructed in everyday practice and experience rather than by biological definition alone (Oswald et al., 2005; Perlesz et al., 2006). In both contexts, same-sex families have gradually found a position in society in which social parenting is given equal prominence with biological parenting. Despite a lack of community role models, negotiated social parenting plays an important role in many same-sex families.

Health and wellbeing

It is increasingly understood that, in terms of their overall health and wellbeing, children with same-sex attracted parents are developing well (Dempsey, 2013). Early research focused on the psychosocial aspects of health, but more recently an holistic understanding of child health in this context has been described. Evidence is emerging that suggests the health of children with same-sex attracted parents shows benefits in some areas, particularly in relation to family cohesion. Australian research has identified that child health related to family processes benefits from the ways in which same-sex parent families 'do family', particularly in terms of shared parental responsibilities and non-gendered parenting (Crouch et al., 2014).

Stigma

Despite these positive outcomes overall, there is clear evidence that experiences of stigma in same-sex parent families can have a negative effect on child health (Crouch et al., 2014). **Stigma** essentially refers to an 'undesired differentness' (Goffman, 1963). It is an outcome of negative social attitudes. In the 1960s, Goffman categorised homosexuality as a 'blemish of individual character', or unnatural passion, which is unfortunately a perspective that persists for many people today. LeBel (2008) highlights a more recent definition of stigma that brings into play the importance of social identity and notes a general understanding that members of stigmatised groups are both devalued and discriminated against, thus leading to social exclusion and loss of status. Major and O'Brien (2005) build on Goffman's categorisations, suggesting that stigmatisation can result from three key attributes: behaviour, appearance and group membership. They also propose that members of stigmatised groups are at greater risk of mental and physical health problems, as is the case for many same-sex attracted people and their families, than their heterosexual counterparts. While laws that recognise same-sex marriage go some way to combatting the stigma that same-sex parent families are subjected to, there is still a long way to go before there is complete acceptance. Likewise, other families also are stigmatised, including single-parent families and families from culturally and linguistically diverse backgrounds. Public health practice should aim to minimise stigma and any potential harms.

Stigma – negative social attitudes in relation to a behaviour seen as different from the norm, leading to discrimination and social exclusion.

Resilience

Resilience in same-sex parent families has often been considered in relation to stigma (van Gelderen et al., 2009). The American Psychological Association (APA) defines resilience as 'the ability to adapt well to adversity, trauma, tragedy, threats or even significant sources of stress' (APA, 2018), although there is little consistency across the literature on a single definition. For children, personal characteristics as well as family and community influences combine to determine an overall ability to cope (Ungar, 2011). Masten and Powell (2003) suggest that emotional regulation and well-developed coping strategies are key to resilience at the individual level (Masten & Powell, 2003). These characteristics can be the result of a secure family environment, which is itself often influenced by quality parenting (Frosch &

Resilience – the capacity to adapt to major disruption or stress.

Mangelsdorg, 2001). One possible factor in developing resilience is the warmth of a child's relationships with their parents, particularly as this can provide a sense of safety and security. By being involved with neighbourhood networks and schools, children can benefit from social participation and shared responsibilities, building resilience at the community level (van Gelderen et al., 2009). Same-sex attracted parents employ a range of resilience-building strategies to combat stigma and to maximise health outcomes for their children. This includes seeking safe environments, developing parental supports, identifying role models, strengthening family communication and educating institutions (Crouch et al., 2017).

SPOTLIGHT 15.3

Stigma and child health in same-sex parent families

Experiences of stigma can have a significant effect on the lives of young children growing up with same-sex attracted parents. Jane worked as a nurse in a remote Australian community, where she lived with her female partner and daughter, Tina. Concerns in the local community about her same-sex relationship surfaced when she entered negotiations to extend her short-term work contract to a continuing position. A significant change to her employment conditions for the new contract made an ongoing position in the community untenable, and Jane was informed by a friend, who was privy to the decision-making process, that her same-sex relationship had played a role in the new offer. This experience led Jane to moving her family, including Tina, who had been settled in the remote community, back to the state capital to seek a more inclusive work environment.

As Jane settled into her new urban community she sought out supports from her friends and extended family to provide numerous role-models for her daughter. She selected a school that did not have strong religious affiliations, as she perceived some of the local Catholic schools as not being welcoming to same-sex parent families, and made a special effort to meet with the teachers from Tina's new school to explain her family context and emphasise the need for inclusive teaching practices.

QUESTIONS

1   How might Tina's health and wellbeing have been affected by experiences of stigma?

2   What resilience-building strategies does Jane employ to support Tina's health?

Children and mental health

Mental health is 'a state of wellbeing in which an individual realises their own abilities, can cope with the normal stresses of life, can work productively and make a contribution to their community' (WHO, 2004). A recent systematic review of 21 studies reported that mental health problems were identified in 17 per cent of preschool-aged children within primary healthcare settings (Charach et al., 2020). Similarly, a separate meta-analysis of 41 studies showed mental health problems were highly prevalent internationally, with almost 1 in 7 children and adolescents aged 4–18 years (13.4 per cent) meeting clinical diagnostic criteria (Polanczyk et al., 2015). This shows that mental health problems can start early in life. They can also be persistent, sometimes continuing into later childhood, adolescence and adulthood.

Mental health risk and protective factors

Childhood mental health problems are the result of multidimensional interactions between biological vulnerabilities, sociocultural interactions, and lifelong and situational environmental stressors. Key risk factors include insecure child-caregiver attachment, harsh parenting styles, adverse childhood experiences (such as abuse and neglect, exposure to family violence, parental mental illness), bullying and harassment from peers, exposure to disasters, racism and discrimination, and low socio-economic status (Carbone, 2020; Bonanno et al., 2010). Key protective factors include social support and connections, positive home and learning environments (child care/school) and higher socio-economic status (Carbone, 2020). The presence of risk factors does not necessarily mean that a child will develop a mental health problem; however, when a child is exposed to several risk factors, their combined effects can lead to difficulties (Masten, 2014). There is emerging evidence that interventions that address risk factors and promote protective factors can improve health and wellbeing, and potentially can prevent mental health problems or avoid extension of problems into adulthood (Carbone, 2020).

Childhood mental health – psychological, social and emotional wellbeing, involving children's thoughts, feelings and behaviours.

REFLECTION QUESTION

During the COVID-19 pandemic, many countries around the world required families to isolate at home for extended periods and for children to engage in home-schooling through videoconferencing platforms. How might this have improved and/or worsened the mental health of children? What key protective factors are likely to reduce the risk of harms?

Support strategies for child mental health

Childhood mental health problems can be successfully treated but tend to be under-treated (Radez et al., 2021). There are four main barriers that prevent children and families from getting mental health support, including limited mental health knowledge, social stigma, fears around confidentiality and cost (Radez et al., 2021). In recognition of these barriers, there is an important role for public health interventions that focus on systems and settings in which children are engaged. Support strategies should follow a stepped-care approach that provides: step 1– universal care to build resilience; step 2– targeted psychosocial support programs for those showing signs of distress or sub-clinical signs of a mental health disorder; and step 3– psychological treatment by trained mental health professionals for those with mental health concerns (Phoenix Australia, 2020). For example, evidence shows that school-based psychosocial programs can support child and adolescent recovery from disasters and other forms of mass trauma (Brown et al., 2017).

SPOTLIGHT 15.4

Protecting children's mental health

Gaby is 12 months old. She has just started walking and is making babbling sounds. She is being raised by her single mother, Brenda, who separated from Gaby's father when she was pregnant. Brenda found the first three months of Gaby's life particularly hard, and struggled to get out of bed sometimes to meet Gaby's needs. She was diagnosed with postnatal depression and was prescribed anti-depressants. Brenda's mother was able to help take care of Gaby, emotionally and financially. When Gaby was six months old, Brenda needed to return to work. Gaby started attending a long daycare centre. All of the educators are qualified, and they have regular training on child development. The room leader in the babies' room has developed a strong relationship with Gaby. The childcare centre regularly holds social events, and Brenda and Gaby enjoy attending and have met other families with children the same age as Gaby.

QUESTION
Using a socio-ecological understanding of children's mental health, to which risk and protective factors has Gaby been exposed?

SUMMARY

In this chapter, child public health in general, and health issues and life circumstances that have potential to affect children's wellbeing and capacity to thrive, have been discussed. Socio-ecological models have been described as a useful means of identifying multi-level influences on children's health and wellbeing. Health promotion principles, as outlined in the Ottawa Charter, have also been noted as a useful guide to development of intervention strategies. Specifically, this chapter provides insights into the following.

Learning objective 1: Describe how social changes have led to increased child overweight and obesity.

Social and environmental changes have resulted in generational shifts in family lifestyles that are associated with high rates of child overweight and obesity. There are opportunities to promote increased healthy eating and physical activity through public health campaigns, community initiatives and school-based changes addressing environment, knowledge and behaviours.

Learning objective 2: Apply a socio-ecological model to identify multi-level factors influencing children's oral health and wellbeing.

The development of decay in children's first teeth can have a severe effect on their health and wellbeing, and can compromise their future oral health. Families living in poverty, those with a refugee-like background and children living in areas with non-fluoridated water are at risk of poor childhood oral health. Community based interventions can improve oral health behaviours and reduce early childhood caries, particularly if they engage parents, involve community service providers and are communicated through shared culture and language.

Learning objective 3: Explain how the health and wellbeing of children living in same-sex parented families is directly influenced by broader social attitudes and can benefit from resilience-building strategies.

Same-sex parent families include any families where at least one of the parents identifies as same-sex attracted. As social and cultural shifts have broadened perceptions of families, there has been an increase in, and recognition of, same-sex parent families. Stigma remains a concern for these families and has been shown to have an influence on the mental health and wellbeing of the children in those families. However, in other respects children in same-sex parent families have been shown to have good health and, in some cases, experience additional benefits, particularly in relation to shared parental responsibilities and non-gendered parenting.

Learning objective 4: Describe the importance of prevention, early intervention and post-trauma support for children's mental health, including settings-based approaches to support children's social and emotional wellbeing.

Childhood mental health problems are highly prevalent and result from interactions between biological vulnerabilities, sociocultural interactions and environmental stress. Risk and protective factors have been identified at the individual, family, school, childcare and community levels. Treatment is feasible but can be lengthy and expensive, and some people may be reluctant to seek help due to stigma. In order to support the mental health of children at the population level, prevention, early intervention and post-trauma support are important, including services and systems that support children's social and emotional wellbeing.

TUTORIAL EXERCISES

1 Socio-ecological frameworks outline different levels of influence on individual health behaviours and outcomes. How could the core health promotion principles outlined in the Ottawa Charter be used to plan a child oral health promotion intervention in your local area?

2 Development and implementation of child health promotion interventions involves working with adults in children's settings. How might parents be involved in planning mental health interventions in primary school settings?

3 How would child obesity-prevention interventions need to be different for this generation of children when compared to their parents or grandparents?

FURTHER READING

Brown, R. C., Witt, A., Fegert, J. M., Keller, F., Rassenhofer, M., & Plener, P. L. (2017). Psychosocial interventions for children and adolescents after man-made and natural disasters: A meta-analysis and systematic review. *Psychological Medicine*, *47*(11), 1893–905.

Gibbs, L., Waters, E., Christian, B., Gold, L., Young, D., de Silva, A., Calche, H., Gussy, M., . . . Moore, L. (2015). Teeth Tales – A community based child oral health promotion trial with migrant families in Australia. *BMJ Open*, 5(6), e007321.

Odgers, C., & Jensen, M. R. (2020). Annual research review: Adolescent mental health in the digital age: Facts, fears, and future directions. *Journal of Child Psychology and Psychiatry, and Allied Disciplines*, *61*(3), 336–48.

Swinburn, B. A., Kraak, V. I., Allender, S., Atkins, V. J., Baker, P.I., Bogard, J. R., Brinsden, H., Calvillo, A., . . . Dietz, W. H. (2019). The global syndemic of obesity, undernutrition, and climate change: *The Lancet* Commission report. *The Lancet*, *393*(10173), 791–846.

Weeks, J., Heaphy, B., & Donovan, C. (2001). *Same sex intimacies: Families of choice and other life experiments*. Routledge.

REFERENCES

Allender, S., Owen, S., Kuhlberg, J., Lowe, J., Nagorcka-Smith, P., Whelan, J., & Bell, C. (2015). A community based systems diagram of obesity causes. *PLoS ONE*, *10*(7), e0129683.

American Psychological Association (APA). (2018). Introduction: Resilience guide for parents & teachers (Webpage). Retrieved http://www.apa.org/helpcenter/resilience.aspx#

Armfield, J. M., & Akers, H. F. (2010). Risk perception and water fluoridation support and opposition in Australia. *Journal of Public Health Dentistry*, *70*, 58–66.

Australian Government Department of Health. (2017). Fluoridation of drinking water (Webpage). Retrieved http://www.health.gov.au/internet/main/publishing.nsf/Content/dentalfluoridation

Australian Institute of Health and Welfare (AIHW). (2020). *Australia's National Oral Health Plan 2015–2024: Performance monitoring report in brief*. Cat. No. DEN 234. AIHW.

——(2021). *Childhood overweight and obesity – the impact of the home environment*. Cat. No. PHE 283. AIHW Retrieved https://www.aihw.gov.au/getmedia/eb8c3fe2-09bb-4f9e-8905-47b6baad06bd/aihw-phe-283.pdf.aspx?inline=true

Bonanno, G. A., Brewin, C. R., Kaniasty, K., & La Greca, A. M. (2010). Weighing the costs of disaster: Consequences, risks, and resilience in individuals, families, and communities. *Psychological Science in the Public Interest*, *11*(1), 1–49.

Bronfenbrenner, U. (1979). *The ecology of human development: Experiments by nature and design.* Harvard University Press.

Brown, R. C., Witt, A., Fegert, J. M., Keller, F., Rassenhofer, M., & Plener, P. L. (2017). Psychosocial interventions for children and adolescents after man-made and natural disasters: a meta-analysis and systematic review. *Psychological Medicine, 47*, 1893–1905.

Carbone, S. (2020) *Evidence review: The primary prevention of mental health conditions.* Victorian Health Promotion Foundation. Retrieved https://www.vichealth.vic.gov.au/-/media/ResourceCentre/Evidence-review-prevention-of-mental-health-conditions-August-2020.pdf?la=en&hash=6CDC96F267CBED73CC3EFB8803C2E6EBCD169C43

Centre for Culture, Ethnicity and Health. (2018). Cultural competence organisational review resources. Retrieved http://www.ceh.org.au/cultural-competence-organisational-review-tool/

Charach, A., Mohammadzadeh, F., Belanger, S.A., Easson, A., Lipman, E.L., McLennan, J.D., Parkin, P., & Szatmari, P. (2020). Identification of preschool children with mental health problems in primary care: Systematic review and meta-analysis. *Journal of the Canadian Academy of Child and Adolescent Psychiatry, 29*(2).

Christian, B., Young, D., Gibbs, L., de Silva, A., Gold, L., Riggs, E., Calache, H., Tadic, M., Hall, M., Moore, L., & Waters, E. (2015). Exploring child dental service use among migrant families in metropolitan Melbourne. *Australian Dental Journal, 60*, 200–4.

Crouch, S. R., McNair, R., & Waters, E. (2017). Parent perspectives on child health and wellbeing in same-sex families: Heteronormative conflict and resilience building. *Journal of Child and Family Studies, 26*(8), 2202–14.

Crouch, S. R., Waters, E., McNair, R., Power, J., & Davis, E. (2014). Parent-reported measures of child health and wellbeing in same-sex parent families: A cross-sectional survey. *BMC Public Health, 14*, 635.

Cunnion, D. T., Spiro, A., Jones, J. A., Rich, S. E., Papageorgiou, C. P., Tate, A., Casamassimo, P., Hayes, C., & Garcia, R. I. (2010). Pediatric oral health-related quality of life improvement after treatment of early childhood caries: A prospective multisite study. *Journal of Dentistry for Children, 77*(1), 4–11.

Dahlgren, G., & Whitehead, M. (1991). *Policies and strategies to promote equity in health.* Institute for Future Studies.

Dempsey, D. (2013). *Same-sex parented families in Australia.* CFCA Paper No. 18, Australian Institute of Family Studies.

Frosch, C. A., & Mangelsdorg, S. C. (2001). Marital behavior, parenting behavior, and multiple reports of preschoolers' behavior problems: Mediation or moderation? *Developmental Psychology, 37*, 502–19.

Gao, X. L., Hsu, C. Y., Xu, Y., Hwarng, H. B., Loh, T., & Koh, D. (2010). Building caries risk assessment models for children. *Journal of Dental Research, 89*, 637–43.

Gibbs, L., Mutch, C., O'Connor, P., & MacDougall, C. (2013). Research with, by, for, and about children: Lessons from disaster contexts. *Global Studies of Childhood, 3*(2), 129–41.

Gibbs, L., Waters, E., Christian, B., Gold, L., Young, D., de Silva, A., Calche, H., Gussy, M., ... Moore, L. (2015). Teeth Tales – A community based child oral health promotion trial with migrant families in Australia. *BMJ Open, 5*(6), e007321.

Gill, T. (2007). *No fear: Growing up in a risk averse society.* Calouste Gulbenkian Foundation.

Goffman, E. (1963). *Stigma: Notes on the management of spoiled identity.* Prentice-Hill.

Gussy, M. G., Waters, E. G., Walsh, O., & Kilpatrick, N. M. (2006). Early childhood caries: Current evidence for aetiology and prevention. *Journal of Paediatrics and Child Health, 41*(1–2), 37–43.

Halfon, N., & Hochstein, M. (2002). Life course health development: An integrated framework for developing health, policy, and research. *Milbank Quarterly, 80*(3), 433–79.

Jackson, S. L., Vann Jr, W. F., Kotch, J. B., Pahel, B. T., & Lee, J. Y. (2011). Impact of poor oral health on children's school attendance and performance. *American Journal of Public Health, 101*(10), 1900–6.

Kilpatrick, N., Neumann, A., Lucas, N., Chapman, J., & Nicholson, J. M. (2012). Oral health inequalities in a national sample of Australian children aged 2–3 and 6–7 years. *Australian Dental Journal, 57,* 38–44.

LeBel, T. P. (2008). Perception of and responses to stigma. *Sociology Compass, 2*(2), 409.

Leonard, M. (2007). Trapped in space? Children's accounts of risky environments. *Children & Society, 21*(6), 432–45.

Lucas, N., Neumann, A., Kilpatrick, N., & Nicholson, J. (2011). State-level differences in the oral health of Australian preschool age children. *Australian Dental Journal, 56,* 56–62.

Lynch, J. (2000). Social epidemiology: Some observations about the past, present and future. *Australasian Epidemiologist, 7*(3), 3.

MacDougall, C. (Ed.) (2009). *Understanding twenty-first century childhood.* Oxford University Press.

Major, B., & O'Brien, L. T. (2005). The social psychology of stigma. *Annual Review of Psychology, 56,* 393–421.

Marmot, M., & Wilkinson, R. (Eds.). (2005). *Social determinants of health.* Oxford University Press.

Masten, A. S. (2014). *Global perspectives on resilience in children and youth. Child Development, 85*(1), 6–20.

Masten, A. S., & Powell, J. L. (2003). A resilience framework for research, policy, and practice. In S. S. Luthar (Ed.), *Resilience and vulnerability: Adaptation in the context of childhood adversities* (pp. 1–25). Cambridge University Press.

Mejàre, I. A., Klingberg, G., Mowafi, F. K., Stecksén-Blicks, C., Twetman, S. H., & Tranæus, S. H. (2015). A systematic map of systematic reviews in pediatric dentistry – what do we really know? *PLoS One, 10*(2), e0117537.

Morrow, V. (2003). Perspectives on children's agency within families: A view from the sociology of childhood. In L. Kuczynski (Ed.), *Handbook of dynamics in parent-child relations* (pp. 109–29). Sage.

Nalliah, R. P., Allareddy, V., Elangovan, S., Karimbux, N., & Allareddy, V. (2010). Hospital based emergency department visits attributed to dental caries in the United States in 2006. *Journal of Evidence Based Dental Practice, 10*(4), 212–22.

National Health and Medical Research Council (NHMRC). (2007). *A systematic review of the efficacy and safety of fluoridation.* Australian Government.

——(2017). *Public statement, Water fluoridation and human health in Australia.* Australian Government. Retrieved https://nhmrc.gov.au/about-us/publications/2017-public-statement-water-fluoridation-and-human-health

Olds, T. S., Tomkinson, G. R., Ferrar, K. E., & Maher, C. A. (2010). Trends in the prevalence of childhood overweight and obesity in Australia between 1985 and 2008. *International Journal of Obesity, 34*(1), 57–66.

Oral Health Monitoring Group. (2015). Healthy mouths healthy lives: Australia's National Oral Health Plan 2015–2024. COAG Health Council. Retrieved http://www.coaghealthcouncil.gov.au/Portals/0/Australia%27s%20National%20Oral%20Health%20Plan%202015-2024_uploaded%20170216.pdf

Oswald, R. F., Blume, L. B. & Marks, S. R. (2005). Decentering heteronormativity: A model for family studies. In V. L. Bengston, A. C. Acock, K. R. Allen, P. Dilworth-Anderson & D. M. Klein (Eds.), *Sourcebook of family theory and research.* Plenum.

Perlesz, A., Brown, R., Lindsay, J., McNair, R., De Vaus, D., & Pitts, M. (2006). Family in transition: Parents, children and grandparents in lesbian families give meaning to 'doing family'. *Journal of Family Therapy, 28,* 175–99.

Phantumvanit P., Makino, Y., Ogawa, H., Rugg-Gunn, A., Moynihan, P., Petersen, P. E., Evans, W., Feldens, C.A., … Ungchusak, C. (2018). WHO Global Consultation on Public Health Intervention against Early Childhood Caries. *Community Dentistry and Oral Epidemiology, 46,* 208–87.

Phoenix Australia, Centre for Posttraumatic Mental Health. (2020). Australian guidelines for the prevention and treatment of acute stress disorder, posttraumatic stress disorder and complex posttraumatic stress disorder. Retrieved https://www.phoenixaustralia.org/australian-guidelines-for-ptsd/

Polanczyk, G.V., Salum, G.A., Sugaya, L.S., Caye, A., & Rohde, L.A. (2015). Annual research review: A meta-analysis of the worldwide prevalence of mental disorders in children and adolescents. *Journal of Child Psychology & Psychiatry, 56*(3), 345–65.

Radez, J., Reardon, T., Creswell C., Lawrence, P.J., Evdoka-Burton, G., & Waite, P. (2021). Why do children and adolescents (not) seek and access professional help for their mental health problems? A systematic review of quantitative and qualitative studies. *European Child and Adolescent Psychiatry, 30*, 183–211.

Riggs, E., Gussy, M., Gibbs, L., van Gemert, C., Waters, E., & Kilpatrick, N. (2014). Hard to reach communities or hard to access services? Migrant mothers' experiences of dental services. *Australian Dental Journal, 59*, 201–7.

Riggs, E., Gussy, M., Gibbs, L., van Gemert, C., Waters, E., Priest, N., . . . Kilpatrick, N. (2014). Assessing the cultural competence of oral health research conducted with migrant children. *Community Dent Oral Epidemiology 42*(1), 43–52.

Sheiham, A. (2006). Dental caries affects body weight, growth and quality of life in pre-school children. *British Dental Journal, 201*(10), 625–6.

Sischo, L., & Broder, H. L. (2011). Oral health-related quality of life: What, why, how, and future implications. *Journal of Dental Research, 90*(11), 1264–70.

Stacey, J. (1996). *In the name of the family: Rethinking family values in the postmodern age.* Beacon Press.

Swinburn, B., Egger, G. J., & Raza, F. (1999). Dissecting obesogenic environments: The development and application of a framework for identifying and prioritising environmental interventions for obesity. *Preventative Medicine, 29*, 563–70.

Swinburn, B. A., Kraak, V. I., Allender, S., Atkins, V. J., Baker, P. I., Bogart, J. R., . . . Dietz, W. H. (2019) The global syndemic of obesity, undernutrition, and climate change: *The Lancet* Commission report. *The Lancet, 393*, 791–846.

Tennant, M., Namjoshi, D., Silva, D., & Codde, J. (2000). Oral health and hospitalization in Western Australian children. *Australian Dental Journal, 45*, 204–7.

Ungar, M. (2011). The social ecology of resilience: Addressing contextual and cultural ambiguity of a nascent construct. *American Journal of Orthopsychiatry, 81*, 1–17.

United Nations (1989). *Convention on the Rights of the Child.* G.A. res. 44/25, annex, 44 U.N. GAOR Supp. (No. 49) at 167, U.N. Doc. A/44/49 (1989), entered into force 2 September 1990. /C/93/Add.5 of 16 July 2003.

United States Department of Health and Human Services. (2000). *Oral health in America: A report of the Surgeon General.* US Department of Health and Human Services, National Institute of Dental and Craniofacial Research, National Institutes of Health.

van Gelderen, L., Gartrell, N., Bos, H., & Hermanns, J. (2009). Stigmatization and resilience in adolescent children of lesbian mothers. *Journal of GLBT Family Studies, 5*(3), 268–79.

Waters, E., de Silva-Sanigorski, A., Hall, B. J., Brown, T., Campbell, K. J., Gao, G., Armstrong, R., Prosser, L., & Summerbell, C. D. (2011). Interventions for preventing obesity in children. *The Cochrane Library,* December (12) Art. No. CD001871.

Weeks, J., Heaphy, B., & Donovan, C. (2001). *Same sex intimacies: Families of choice and other life experiments.* Routledge.

World Health Organization (WHO). (1986). *Ottawa Charter for Health Promotion.* WHO.

——(2004) *Promoting mental health: concepts, emerging evidence, practice (Summary Report).* WHO

——(2008). *Closing the gap in a generation: Health equity through action on the social determinants of health. Final report of the Commission on the Social Determinants of Health.* WHO. Retrieved http://apps.who .int/iris/bitstream/10665/43943/1/9789241563703_eng.pdf

——(2017). *Report of the Commission on Ending Childhood Obesity.* Retrieved https://apps.who.int/iris/ bitstream/handle/10665/259349/WHO-NMH-PND-ECHO-17.1-eng.pdf?sequence=1&isAllowed=y

——(2021a). Obesity and overweight fact sheet. Retrieved https://www.who.int/news-room/fact-sheets/ detail/obesity-and-overweight

——(2021b). Oral health. Executive Board Resolution WHA74/A74.R5. 31 May.

Verlinden, D. A., Reijneveld, S. A., Lanting, C. I., van Wouwe, J. P., & Schuller, A. A. (2019). Socio-economic inequality in oral health in childhood to young adulthood, despite full dental coverage. *European Journal of Oral Sciences, 127,* 248–53

Adolescence, health, social problems and public health

16

Jessica Heerde and Sheryl Hemphill

LEARNING OBJECTIVES

After studying this chapter, you should be able to:

1   explain what internalising and externalising problems are, risk factors for these problems, and how they can be addressed through public health approaches
2   understand adolescent homelessness and its contributing factors and effects on health, and discuss public health approaches to addressing homelessness
3   identify key risk factors for adolescent alcohol, tobacco and other drug use and their effects on health, and discuss multifaceted public health approaches for addressing the use of these substances
4   understand the features of, and risk factors for, bullying perpetration and victimisation, and use your understanding of relationships along with health and public health approaches to respond to bullying.

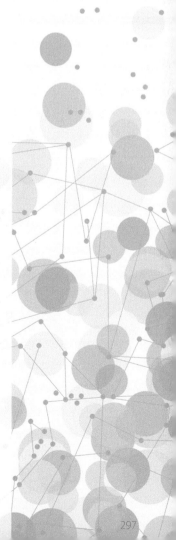

VIGNETTE

Adolescents, health and wellbeing

Kate left home at 15 years of age, after being physically assaulted by her mother and told to leave and not return. Kate lived with foster carers for a year, but after her 18th birthday she was required to move into independent living. Consequently, Kate moved into transitional housing with four other people of similar ages to her. From this point, Kate had to live her life as an independent adult. She secured a part-time job, but the income she received from this job was not enough to cover her costs of living (e.g. food, clothing, household bills). Kate was unable to obtain full-time work and, after missing several rental payments, was forced to leave the share house and transitioned into homelessness. She had just turned 20 years old. During the time Kate experienced homelessness, she frequently moved between sleeping rough (i.e. on the streets) and couch-surfing (staying temporarily in other people's homes). When she was sleeping rough, Kate was very afraid for her personal safety. For this reason she regularly stayed awake overnight, only taking short naps in the daytime. She also regularly went for multiple days at a time with very little to eat.

While she was homeless, Kate regularly became angry, often threatening or hitting other people. Sometimes, she engaged in behaviours that were not socially acceptable, to obtain money or a place to stay for a night. She experimented with alcohol and drugs to try to make herself feel better about who she was and the behaviour she was engaging in while homeless.

Kate is now 21 years old. With assistance from a homelessness support service, she recently moved into short-term crisis housing. Kate's caseworker has just advised her that this accommodation will only be available for a 'few' days, and then she will need to find somewhere else to live. Living in crisis housing provides Kate with a temporary safe place to stay, a bed to sleep in, and bathroom and communal laundry facilities.

Introduction

Adolescence – a distinct phase of human development spanning the period from childhood to adulthood.

Adolescent health, development and behaviour lay the foundation for future population health (Patton et al., 2018; Sawyer et al., 2012). **Adolescence** now occupies a greater portion of the life-course. It is commonly framed as the period of 10–24 years of age, moving beyond former definitions of adolescence being aged 10–19 years (Sawyer et al., 2018). Globally, there are approximately 1.8 billion young people aged 10–24 years (Sawyer et al., 2018). Adolescence precipitates changes in the ways in which young people interact with their families, peers and wider society. Disadvantage, social inequality and a range of harmful health and social problems often become prominent during adolescence. Some of these, as discussed in this chapter, include mental health problems (e.g. psychological distress, depression and anxiety symptoms, deliberate self-harm and suicidal behaviour), engagement in anti-social behaviours, homelessness, substance use (alcohol, tobacco, other drugs) and bullying (perpetration and victimisation). Although not all adolescents experience these types of health and social problems, when they do occur, they are likely to affect health and wellbeing over the long term. Understanding the drivers of these problems and the benefits of public health interventions designed to address them, are central to improving the health and wellbeing of all adolescents.

While public health approaches have previously been embedded within biomedical paradigms focusing predominantly on education as a means of improving health, more recent public health approaches acknowledge the influence of lifestyle and lifestyle choices on health and the social determinants of health (see also chapters 1 and 2). Many approaches aiming to reduce harmful health and social problems in adolescence are underpinned by a determinants approach that seeks to understand the social, economic, environmental and political factors influencing health and social behaviour, and related health problems and outcomes (see chapters 7, 8 and 10). In developing public health approaches that aim to reduce harmful health and social problems, it is important to understand the factors that contribute to these, the social context in which they occur, and whether there are related factors associated with health problems for specific groups of adolescents (e.g. those experiencing homelessness).

This chapter explores some of the common health and social problems experienced by adolescents, including internalising and externalising problems, homelessness, substance use, and traditional and cyberbullying perpetration and victimisation. We also discuss some of the contextual factors (herein referred to as risk and protective factors) that may increase or decrease the likelihood of these health and social problems (Hawkins & Weis, 2017). Risk and protective factors can be categorised by the social context in which adolescents interact, including the family, peer group, school and community, as well as the personal characteristics of the adolescent. We conclude by discussing some of the public health approaches used by practitioners and researchers to target these health and social problems.

Internalising and externalising problems

Internalising and **externalising problems** among adolescents affect not only their immediate health and wellbeing, but also many of the social determinants that influence health. These include, but are not limited to, adolescents' engagement at school, completing high school and pursuing further education or higher education, entering the workforce, and their attainment of adult roles within health, social and economic contexts (e.g. employment and job security, housing, social inclusion). The Australian Institute of Health and Welfare's (AIHW, 2021) *Australia's Youth* report suggests that 20 per cent of young people aged 11–17 years describe psychological distress at either high or very high levels, and 26 per cent of young people aged 15–24 years describe long-term mental ill health. Deliberate self-harm (DSH) among adolescents is of high concern, with approximately 1 in 10 young people reporting having deliberately injured themselves (AIHW, 2021). Suicide also remains a leading cause of death for young Australians, with the rate of suicide among young men double that for young women (AIHW, 2021). Adolescence frequently sees a peak in externalising problems, with the prevalence of anti-social behaviours estimated to be approximately 17 per cent (Hemphill & Heerde, 2019). Both internalising and externalising problems are of concern due to their association with increased risk for reduced life chances, as well as their association with other health and social problems (e.g. other forms of mental ill health, substance use, victimisation and homelessness).

Internalising problem – occurs when an adolescent directs their emotional symptoms within (e.g. psychological distress, anxiety and depressive symptoms, deliberate self-harm).

Externalising problem – occurs when an adolescent directs their difficulties into the surrounding environment (e.g. aggression, anti-social behaviour, delinquency).

Factors contributing to internalising and externalising problems

Internalising problems, including depression, anxiety, DSH and suicide, are influenced by a range of risk and protective factors within individual, family, school and community contexts. Consistently reported risk factors for internalising problems include family factors such as violence and conflict, poor communication and low levels of parent–adolescent problem-solving (Kelly et al., 2016). Low levels of school connectedness are associated with depressive symptoms (Rowland et al., 2022) while school-based programs aimed at reducing behavioural problems have positive effects on student–teacher relationships, school connectedness and academic achievement (Freiberg & Lapointe, 2006). Community based factors, including violence, victimisation and high levels of poverty, increase risk for depressive symptoms, while high numbers of transitions across schools and community-based crimes are linked to internalising problems (Shortt & Spence, 2006).

Risk and protective factors for externalising problems span individual, peer group, family, school and community risk factors. At the individual level, adjustment problems, low impulse control and interpersonal difficulties are risk factors (Loeber & Farrington, 2000). At the family level, coercive and inconsistent disciplinary strategies are associated with child and adolescent-onset externalising problems (Loeber & Farrington, 2000). Poor parental supervision and monitoring, low levels of interaction within the family, family violence and conflict, and parental attitudes favourable to violence also are risk factors for externalising problems (Loeber & Farrington, 2000). Interaction with delinquent peers is an established risk factor for externalising problems (Hawkins et al., 2014). At the community level, risk factors include neighbourhood disadvantage and crime, low perceived risks of punishment, unemployment and high levels of social disorganisation (Wikstrom & Sampson, 2013). Protective factors for both internalising and externalising problems are less frequently examined; however, factors such as opportunities and recognition for prosocial involvement in the family, closeness to parents, interactions with prosocial peers and higher levels of school achievement and connection have been cited as reducing risk for internalising and externalising problems (Hawkins et al., 2014; Kelly et al., 2016).

The relationship between internalising and externalising problems and health

Adolescent internalising problems can lead to the disruption of developmental pathways and achievement of adult milestones, and a wide range of health and social problems linked to later health inequities including adult internalising problems, suicidality – including DSH, suicidal ideation and suicide attempt (Borschmann et al., 2017) – externalising problems, substance use (Moran et al., 2012), academic underachievement, and unemployment and job insecurity (Stice, Ragan & Randall, 2004).

Negative developmental, health and social outcomes are reported for externalising problems, and include substance use, continued engagement in externalising problems, relationship problems, academic underachievement and involvement with the criminal justice system (Hemphill & Heerde, 2019). Researchers have argued that the developmental consequences associated with externalising problems are more severe, leading to contact with the criminal justice system, when the onset of these behaviours occurs in childhood than in adolescence (Hemphill & Heerde, 2019).

Public health approaches to addressing internalising and externalising problems

The **prevention science** paradigm, targeting risk and protective factors and the social context in which they occur across the life course, has commonly been adopted in devising approaches to address and reduce rates of adolescent health and social problems, including internalising and externalising problems. Public health approaches designed to address these problems often use multiple components, relying on multi-sectoral partnerships between community-based organisations. For instance, prior initiatives such as MindMatters (Wyn et al., 2000) and more recently Be You (BeyondBlue, 2021), are examples of national adolescent mental health promotion programs. More broadly, the National Suicide Prevention Strategy is a policy-driven example of a suicide and self-harm prevention approach designed to focus on mental health across all stages of the life course. Other approaches include mental health campaigns distributed through mass media and designed to modify societal and cultural norms and perceptions, while increasing awareness of common mental health problems, and where help can be sought (e.g. R U OK?). The need for multifaceted approaches targeting multiple risk and protective factors have been addressed through universal and secondary prevention approaches for externalising problems. These programs aim to increase adolescents' social and problem-solving skills, as well as to address family-related risk factors such as increasing parental supervision, monitoring and positive family interactions, while decreasing family violence, conflict and parental attitudes favourable to these behaviours.

Prevention science – a research approach characterised by examining risk and protective factors across individual, family, peer group and community contexts over time, and how these can be modified to influence behaviour.

SPOTLIGHT 16.1

Developing a family resources workshop

Jennifer is a social worker specialising in reconnecting homeless young people with their families (frequently referred to as 'family reunification'). Services provided by the organisation Jennifer works with are delivered using a developmental framework, which is a framework that classifies risk and protective factors and their influence on growth and behaviour according to defined developmental periods. The emphasis is on improving both adolescent health and family relationships. Using this framework permits the organisation to build its public health strategies in a way that matches the developmental needs of their clients, and to implement these strategies at key periods in development, when they are likely to have the most benefit.

Jennifer has been asked to present a whole-day workshop to colleagues and clinicians from community-based organisations in her local government area, focusing on the development and prevention of adolescent internalising and externalising problems, and provision of family-based treatment. Also to be explored through the workshop, and to further develop the organisation's services, are the delivery of mental health services to adolescents, their families, local schools and community groups.

QUESTIONS

1   Identify and explain the various risk and protective factors that could be discussed in Jennifer's workshop.

2   What strategies might be devised for service provision to ensure organisational approaches respond to the diverse and changing health needs of adolescents, families and schools within the local community?

Homelessness

Young people who are homeless face major adversity during their adolescent years, with consequences that extend across their later lives. The daily experience of what it is like to be homeless, and the damage it does to adolescents' health, welfare and life chances are often hidden from view. Homeless adolescents are an unseen group, commonly moving between rough sleeping, staying in crowded dwellings or supported accommodation, couch-surfing, or staying temporarily with others. This group faces many health and social inequalities that have devastating effects on their health and wellbeing. In Australia, rates of **homelessness** continue to rise. The 2019–20 specialist homelessness services annual report of the AIHW (2020) shows that, of the 290 500 Australians who sought specialist homelessness services (SHS) over this period, over 40 per cent were aged under 25 years. Homelessness has disruptive effects on adolescents' educational pathways and achievement, their transition into higher education and employment, capacity to establish a stable and nurturing social network, and the attainment of young adult milestones that set a foundation for adult health and social wellbeing (Heerde & Patton, 2020). These disruptive effects are frequently compounded by histories of child and adolescent abuse and often are further complicated by violence experienced while homeless (Heerde & Patton, 2020). To reduce the number of homeless adolescents, and the health and social effects of homelessness, public health approaches must intervene when adolescents are at serious risk of falling into homelessness or are already homeless, and they must also address the underlying drivers of homelessness in young people before its consequences arise for health across the later life course.

Homelessness – the situation of having either no occupancy at a residence or occupancy at a residence that is limited and non-renewable, and where there is no control of, or space for, social interactions (AIHW, 2020).

Factors contributing to homelessness

Understanding the modifiable drivers of adolescent homelessness is critical to identifying points of intervention for reducing the transition into homelessness. A broad range of risk factors have been identified as influencing homelessness, across the range of social settings in which adolescents interact. Prior experiences of child or adolescent homelessness (including family homelessness), substance use, mental ill health and contact with youth justice settings are commonly cited, individual-level risk factors (Heerde, Bailey, Kelly et al., 2021). Characteristics of the family environment, including child abuse and family violence, parental financial and employment insecurities, low-quality parent–adolescent relationships, less positive family management practices, high levels of family conflict and the transition from out-of-home care, are associated with adolescent homelessness (Heerde, Bailey, Kelly et al., 2021; Heerde, Bailey, Toumbourou et al., 2020, 2021). With regard to peer-level risk factors, low-quality peer relationships, interacting with peers engaged in problem behaviour and engaging with substance-using peers have been associated with later homelessness (Heerde, Bailey, Kelly et al., 2021; Heerde, Bailey, Toumbourou et al., 2021). Risk for homelessness is also increased when adolescents report having been suspended from school, academic underachievement, low commitment to school and having few opportunities for, and engagement in, school-based activities (Heerde, Bailey, Kelly et al., 2021; Heerde, Bailey, Toumbourou et al., 2020, 2021). At the community level, high levels of community poverty and victimisation and low attachment to ones' neighbourhood are thought to increase risk for homelessness (Heerde, Bailey, Toumbourou et al., 2020).

The relationship between homelessness and health

Homelessness is as much a health issue as it is a social issue, and the health burden it places on adolescents is cause for concern. Homeless adolescents experience a range of morbidities including mental ill health, injury, violence, communicable and non-communicable diseases, and substance abuse (Heerde & Patton, 2020). Risk for sexually transmitted infections and unplanned pregnancies are increased by sexual exploitation. Sexual (and physical) victimisation is often accepted as normal when it occurs, leading adolescents to experience significant shame and internalised stigma. Homeless adolescents typically lack regular and consistent health care, despite often experiencing a recognised need for treatment or care (Heerde & Pallotta-Chiarolli, 2020). This includes a lack of access to required medications and vaccinations, opportunity for rest and recuperation from illness and/or injury, as well as basic hygiene and sanitation. The shame and stigma adolescents often associate with being homeless is an additional barrier to their seeking health or medical care. They frequently report unequal provider–client relationships in healthcare settings, a distrust of service providers, and feeling that their dignity and identity have been de-valued (Heerde & Patton, 2020). Thus, the health consequences of homelessness for later life, including premature death, are likely to be profound among adolescents, and necessitate targeted, public health responses.

Public health approaches to addressing homelessness

Few public health approaches have specifically focused on increasing health-service access and utilisation among young homeless people. Social housing has been, and remains, a key pillar for reducing homelessness and its health burden; yet this system remains underfunded and overwhelmed. There remains a lack of robust evidence on the health of homeless young Australians, and the roles that health care may play in preventing it. The health burden of homelessness can be seen as a failure of multiple sectors to work together effectively for the homeless. Multi-sectoral approaches are required to prevent, address and reduce the health burden associated with homelessness. These approaches should be designed to address the complex needs of homeless young people. Approaches that address the shame, stigma and disempowerment frequently expressed by young homeless people, that are collaborative and respectful, and that seek to address young people's vulnerabilities are also desperately needed as part of a person-centred approach to addressing their health (Heerde, Bailey, Toumbourou & Patton, 2020). Engaging homeless people in appropriate health care, using a person-centered, multi-sectoral response, is part of an intersectoral strategy to reduce homelessness and its health burden.

SPOTLIGHT 16.2

Responding to homelessness and violence

Jack is 18 years old and currently living in a supported accommodation residential setting. He was born in Australia and was 13 years old when he first experienced homelessness (i.e. when he first ran away from home). At this time, Jack could not return home and as such he was placed into residential care by Child Protective Services. He had been physically and psychologically abused by both his mother and father. Jack left residential care and lived on the streets, in parks and in abandoned buildings up to a year ago, when he was referred to his current supported accommodation housing. While homeless, Jack would not eat for days at a time, and regularly used alcohol, tobacco and marijuana. Jack currently uses alcohol and tobacco. While homeless, Jack regularly experienced (and engaged in) violence and other threatening behaviours. On one of these occasions, weapons were used and Jack was physically assaulted and stabbed.

QUESTIONS
1   Describe three key factors that may have contributed to Jack transitioning into homelessness.
2   Describe three factors encountered by Jack while he was homeless that may have influenced his state of health and wellbeing.
3   Considering the knowledge you have gained through the previous sections in this chapter, what types of healthcare approaches would you, as a health worker, implement with Jack if you were his case manager?

REFLECTION QUESTION

Public health approaches have traditionally relied on intervening only when young people are at serious risk of falling into homelessness or are already homeless. These approaches are unlikely to treat the underlying causes of homelessness among young people. Nor do they address the health burden associated with homelessness. Using what you have read in this chapter, what can be done to reduce the number of young people experiencing homelessness and to address their health concerns?

Alcohol, tobacco and other drug use

Adolescence is a period of heightened risk for alcohol, tobacco and other drug use (e.g. marijuana and other illicit drugs). The use of these substances is associated with disruption to the development of peer relationships, the acquisition of social skills and the achievement of adult milestones (e.g. adult social relationships and employment). The use of these substances interferes with, and may impair, adolescent physical, psychological, and emotional health and functioning (Hill et al., 2000; Hemphill, Heerde et al., 2011). Rates of alcohol and tobacco use have decreased among Australian adolescents in recent times, with risky drinking (binge drinking at least once a month) decreasing from 47 to 30 per cent, and daily smoking decreasing from 19 to 6 per cent, among 14–24-year-olds in 2019 (AIHW, 2021). Despite these decreases, adolescents remain a priority target group in national drug strategies (Department of Health, 2017), particularly in preventing uptake and delaying first use, due to the major consequences use of these substances has for adolescents, their families and the broader community. Complex combinations of risk factors play a role in the development of adolescent substance use, with alcohol, tobacco and marijuana use in early adolescence associated with frequent use of these substances in mid to late adolescence, and posing increased risks for abuse and dependence in adulthood (Chan et al., 2013; Lubman et al., 2007).

Factors contributing to alcohol, tobacco and other drug use

Complex relationships exist between those risk factors that influence adolescents' use of alcohol, tobacco and other drugs. These risk factors may not necessarily be direct causes of substance use but rather may be associated with engagement in this behaviour. Individual factors include the deterioration of family relationships (e.g. child abuse), childhood display of aggressive behaviour and other personality-based characteristics (e.g. sensation-seeking behaviour, attitudes favourable to drug use) (Lubman et al., 2007; Hemphill, Heerde et al., 2011). Family characteristics, including social disadvantage and family breakdown (Lubman et al., 2007), increase the likelihood of use of these substances. In addition, young people are more likely to use substances when there are lower levels of parental monitoring, and lenient rules and favourable attitudes towards the use of alcohol, tobacco and other drugs (Mathers et al., 2006; Hemphill, Heerde et al., 2011).

School and peer factors linked with adolescents' use of alcohol, tobacco and other drugs are varied. Early school failure (Lubman et al., 2007) and low levels of school engagement have shown strong associations with substance use (Bond et al., 2005). In relation to peers, substance use has been linked to low levels of social support (Newcomb & Bentler, 1988) and interactions with anti-social (Hemphill, Heerde et al., 2011) and substance-using peers (Lubman et al., 2007). Social interactions with peers often present opportunities for underage alcohol use (Mathers et al., 2006). Community factors associated with adolescent substance use include high levels of drug availability and use within the community (Lubman et al., 2007; Hemphill, Heerde et al., 2011) and low levels of desirability to conform to social rules and norms.

The relationship between alcohol, tobacco, other drug use and health

A range of acute and chronic health and behavioural problems has been shown to result from adolescent substance use, including internalising problems, substance abuse and addiction, injury resulting from victimisation or engagement in externalising behaviours, physical health problems (e.g. gastrointestinal disorders, hepatitis, HIV/AIDS) and relationship difficulties. For example, adolescent alcohol use has been linked to disruptions in the process of developing peer relations, the development of adult relationships (Toumbourou et al., 2014), progression to the use of multiple substances, low school engagement and completion (Bond et al., 2005) and continued engagement in externalising problems (Hill et al., 2000).

Public health approaches to addressing alcohol, tobacco and other drug use

Alcohol use in adolescence is one influential factor in later alcohol use and poor health outcomes (Toumbourou et al., 2014). Public health approaches have sought to target individual, family, peer group, school and community-based risk factors for substance use (including alcohol and tobacco) through multifaceted prevention approaches. Such approaches aim to address adolescents' characteristics, as well as peer group, family, school and community level factors that have been associated with increased use of these substances (Hemphill, Heerde et al., 2011). For instance, multifaceted and comprehensive prevention approaches, including the Seattle Social Development Project (Hawkins et al., 1992) and Communities That Care

(Hawkins & Catalano, 2002) use established, community focused strategies shown to decrease adolescents' engagement in externalising problems and substance use, informing legislation and policy debates

---

SPOTLIGHT 16.3

Developing approaches to adolescent substance use and abuse

Penny is 18 years old and a single mother to an eight-month-old boy, Sam. Penny first left home when she was 15 years old and lived on the streets, but she has been in stable transitional housing for over a year. While she was homeless, Penny used LSD and other illicit drugs, and does not recall much of her homeless experience. She states that she has been experiencing physical pain because of abuse she had experienced in her childhood. Penny has been diagnosed with depression and is currently taking prescribed medication (antidepressants). Sometimes Penny describes her depression as something that people around her do not believe in, so she feels lonely and like there is no one to talk to. Penny smokes cigarettes and approximately three nights a week, after she has put her son to bed, Penny has several alcoholic drinks. She has been increasingly feeling like these drinks help her get to sleep at night but is worried that she might be becoming dependent on alcohol. She is worried that if she talks to her caseworker about her drinking, she will have to place her son in the care of Child Protective Services.

QUESTIONS

1   Identify and explain some of the risk factors that may be influencing Penny's behaviour, particularly in relation to her health and wellbeing.
2   Considering the important dimensions of Penny's background experiences, what would need to be considered in developing strategies to assist her? What range of healthcare approaches and settings would you draw on as a health practitioner assisting Penny?

Bullying and cyberbullying perpetration and victimisation

Traditional bullying perpetration – behaviour by an individual(s) against another person or people that is repeated, intended to cause harm and characterised by an imbalance of power, including physical bullying (e.g. hitting and kicking), verbal bullying (e.g. name-calling and insulting) and psychological or social bullying (e.g. lying and spreading rumours).

Cyberbullying perpetration – repeated behaviour by an individual(s) against another person or people using electronic or digital programs or devices in ways intended to inflict harm or discomfort.

Perpetration of **traditional bullying** has been a serious concern for students, their families and schools for many decades. Its more recent counterpart, **cyberbullying perpetration**, has also generated great concern due to the potential for perpetrators to remain anonymous and for bullying to occur anywhere, at any time. Although there is debate among researchers about whether the defining characteristics of traditional bullying and cyberbullying are the same, in general, similar definitions are used. Even though cyberbullying has received much attention in recent times, the rates of cyberbullying perpetration (3.5 per cent) and victimisation (6.6 per cent) are typically lower than traditional bullying (9 per cent and 27 per cent, respectively) (Cross et al., 2009).

Prevention science approaches have contrasted the factors contributing to, and the health effects of, bullying and cyberbullying. Although there are many similarities between bullying and cyberbullying, there are also important differences. In one comparison of factors predicting bullying and **cyberbullying victimisation** (Casas, Del Rey & Ortega-Ruiz, 2013), lack of empathy and perceived school climate (e.g. teacher support and clarity of school rules and expectations for behaviour) were found to be predictors of both forms of victimisation. Another study reported similarities (e.g. negative self-concept, characteristics of the parent–child relationship) and differences in being bullied in internet chatrooms and at school (e.g. popularity, bullying behaviour) (Katzer, Fetchenhauer & Belschak, 2009). Williams and Guerra (2007) examined predictors of bullying and cyberbullying perpetration and found that shared predictors were normative beliefs accepting of bullying perpetration, a negative school climate and perceived lack of peer support.

Cyberbullying victimisation – the experience of being bullied by others using technology.

The relationship between bullying and cyberbullying perpetration and health

The effects of bullying and cyberbullying perpetration can be pervasive. Cyberbullying is a relatively new phenomenon, and longitudinal studies on its effects in adolescents are still underway. Bullying perpetration has been linked with an increased likelihood of engaging in externalising behaviours (Hemphill, Kotevski et al., 2011). According to Gibb and colleagues (2011), bullying perpetration at age 13–15 years was associated with internalising problems, as well as alcohol and illicit drug use and externalising problems at age 16–30 years. In a meta-analysis of 131 studies, Kowalski and colleagues (2014) reported associations between cyberbullying perpetration and drug and alcohol use, and small associations with anxiety and depression.

The relationship between traditional and cyberbullying victimisation and health

Traditional bullying victimisation affects physical, social and emotional health. Longitudinal studies have demonstrated that bullying victimisation leads to internalising problems including depression and anxiety (Hemphill, Kotevski et al., 2011). In addition, Gibb and colleagues (2011) found links with alcohol dependence, illicit drug dependence and externalising problems. One meta-analysis of 34 studies that included three studies of being cyberbullied showed that associations between being cyberbullied and suicidal ideation were stronger than for traditional bullying (van Geel, Vedder & Tanilon, 2014). In the meta-analysis by Kowalski and colleagues (2014), being cyberbullied was associated with suicidal ideation, anxiety and depression, as well as there being weak associations with conduct and emotional problems, and drug and alcohol use.

Traditional bullying victimisation – the occurrence of being traditionally bullied by others.

Public health approaches addressing bullying and cyberbullying perpetration and victimisation

The literature on prevention and intervention strategies and programs aiming to reduce bullying perpetration and victimisation is extensive. Current recommendations for cyberbullying are to draw on programs that were developed for traditional bullying, until there is good evidence for effective approaches specific to cyberbullying. Anti-bullying interventions have been implemented in the United Kingdom, the United States, Canada, Australia and European countries including Norway (Hazelden Foundation, 2016), Finland, Belgium, Germany, Italy, Spain and Switzerland. For 'traditional' bullying, schools are generally considered the best sites to teach students essential social and interpersonal skills to reduce bullying. Although cyberbullying does occur outside of the school context, schools can play a role in teaching students the skills they need to prevent cyberbullying. In a recent review, Gaffney and colleagues (2021) found that the components linked to greater reductions in bullying perpetration were a whole-school approach, school anti-bullying policies, classroom rules about behaviour, information for parents, informal peer involvement and working with victims. For bullying victimisation, the effects of programs were greater when the components of informal peer involvement and information for parents were included.

SPOTLIGHT 16.4

Responding to bullying victimisation in the school and family contexts

Maddie is in Year 9. She lives with her mother and younger brother. She has not seen her father in a long time (and cannot remember what he looks like). Maddie tries hard at school but does not find learning easy and is not sure if she wants to complete school. She has a couple of friends, but none of them is part of the popular group. Out of the blue, one of the popular girls shoves Maddie into the wall at school. Finances at home are tight, so she wears a second-hand school uniform. The popular girls notice this and make mean comments about how she looks. Recently, these same girls posted negative comments on Facebook about Maddie's 'unattractive' appearance. Maddie feels like there's no escape and is finding it hard to sleep. Her mother has noticed that she seems withdrawn and unhappy but is not sure what is going on.

QUESTIONS

1   Identify and explain the risk factors in Maddie's life and the possible effects of her recent experiences on her health and wellbeing.
2   Consider how this information can be used to develop strategies to assist Maddie to handle her current situation. What can Maddie's mother do to assist her daughter? What role might school staff play in addressing the issues that Maddie is facing?

REFLECTION QUESTION

We know that many students who bully (perpetration) have been bullied themselves (victimised) through traditional bullying or cyberbullying, or both, and represent a so-called 'combined group'. We also know that bullying happens in a range of settings outside of school and the internet, such as in workplaces, sports clubs and community groups. At the broader society level, what can we do to prevent bullying in our communities?

SUMMARY

Together, adolescent health, development and behaviour lay a foundation for future population health and wellbeing. Adolescence is frequently a period within which disadvantage, social inequality and a range of harmful health and social problems become prominent. These health and social problems pose risks for health consequences that extend into later adulthood. In this chapter, we have considered four common health and social problems experienced by adolescents: (1) internalising and externalising problems; (2) homelessness; (3) use of alcohol, tobacco and other drugs; and (4) traditional and cyber-bullying perpetration and victimisation. We have discussed some of the risk factors that are known to influence the likelihood of these problems, and some of the public health approaches used by practitioners to address these problems.

Learning objective 1: Explain what internalising and externalising problems are, risk factors for these problems, and how they can be addressed through public health approaches.

Adolescent internalising and externalising problems affect adolescents' immediate wellbeing, as well as engagement in education, entering the workforce and the attainment of other adult social and economic goals. These problems are influenced by a range of risk and protective factors within individual, family, school and community contexts. Both internalising and externalising problems have negative effects on later health and social wellbeing, including mental ill health, homelessness and substance use. Public health approaches designed to address these problems often use multiple components, relying on multi-sectoral partnerships between community organisations.

Learning objective 2: Understand adolescent homelessness and its contributing factors and effects on health, and discuss public health approaches to addressing homelessness.

Young homeless people represent one group facing major adversity during their adolescent years, with consequences that extend across their later lives. Understanding modifiable drivers of adolescent homelessness is critical to identifying points of intervention for preventing the transition into homelessness. Homelessness is as much a health issue as it is a social issue, and its health burden on adolescents is concerning. Multi-sectoral approaches are required to prevent, address and reduce the health and social costs associated with homelessness.

Learning objective 3: Identify key risk factors for adolescent alcohol, tobacco and other drug use and their effects on health, and discuss multifaceted public health approaches for addressing the use of these substances.

Whether it be alcohol, tobacco or other drug use, or any other of the health concerns discussed in this chapter, it is important to understand that many approaches designed to improve adolescent health do so by attempting to understand and modify risk and protective factors at the individual, family, school and community levels that influence the behaviour. Adolescents' use of substances such as alcohol, tobacco and other drugs is associated with a range of acute and chronic health and behavioural problems, hence multifaceted approaches are important in seeking to prevent these effects on later health and wellbeing.

Learning objective 4: Understand the features of, and risk factors for, bullying perpetration and victimisation, and use your understanding of relationships with health and public health approaches to respond to bullying.

This chapter has explored a range of risk factors that may contribute to adolescent traditional and cyberbullying perpetration and victimisation. Anti-bullying interventions have been implemented internationally; however, in general, whole-school approaches may be effective in reducing bullying behaviours.

TUTORIAL EXERCISES

1 Find out more about one of the adolescent health concerns discussed in this chapter and the public health approaches designed to address this concern. How does knowledge of risk factors (1) inform this public health approach, and (2) help you to better understand the context in which this public health approach has been developed?

2 Choose one of the adolescent health concerns discussed in this chapter. Create a conceptual diagram of risk factors from within individual, family, school, peer, family and community domains that may influence the development of this health concern. Choose one risk factor from each domain and devise a strategy for addressing this health concern.

3 Imagine you are working as a health professional in a community setting to provide services for adolescents. What things would you need to consider, and what types of skills would you need to develop, to devise a public health approach designed to enhance the health of the adolescents attending your community setting? You can choose to focus on one or more of the health concerns discussed in this chapter.

FURTHER READING

Hawkins, J. D., & Catalano, R. F. (2002). *Investing in your community's youth: An introduction to the Communities That Care system*. Channing-Bete Company.

Hawkins, J. D., & Weis, J. G. (2017). The social development model: An integrated approach to delinquency prevention. In *Developmental and life-course criminological theories* (pp. 3–27). Routledge.

Heerde, J. A., & Patton, G. C. (2020). The vulnerability of the young homeless. *The Lancet Public Health*, 5.

Patton, G. C., Olsson, C. A., Skirbekk, V., Saffery, R., Wlodek, M. E., Azzopardi, P. S., . . . Francis, K. (2018). Adolescence and the next generation. *Nature*, *554*, 458.

Sawyer, S. M., Afifi, R. A., Bearinger, L. H., Blakemore, S.-J., Dick, B., Ezeh, A. C., & Patton, G. C. (2012). Adolescence: A foundation for future health. *The Lancet*, *379*, 1630–40.

REFERENCES

Australian Institute of Health & Welfare (AIHW). (2020). *Specialist homelessness services annual report 2019*. Cat. No. HOU 322. AIHW.

——(2021). *Australia's youth*. (Cat. No. CWS 81).

BeyondBlue. (2021). *Be you evidence summary*. BeyondBlue. Retrieved https://beyou.edu.au/about-be-you

Bond, L., Toumbourou, J. W., Thomas, L., Catalano, R. F., & Patton, G. (2005). Individual, family, school, and community risk and protective factors for depressive symptoms in adolescents: A comparison of risk profiles for substance use and depressive symptoms. *Prevention Science*, *6*(2), 73–88.

Borschmann, R., Becker, D., Coffey, C., Spry, E., Moreno-Betancur, M., Moran, P., & Patton, G. C. (2017). 20-year outcomes in adolescents who self-harm: a population-based cohort study. *The Lancet Child & Adolescent Health*, *1*, 195–202.

Casas, J. A., Del Rey, R. & Ortega-Ruiz, R. (2013). Bullying and cyberbullying: Convergent and divergent predictor variables. *Computers in Human Behavior*, *29*(3), 580–7.

Chan, G. C., Kelly, A. B., Toumbourou, J. W., Hemphill, S. A., Young, R. M., Haynes, M. A., & Catalano, R. F. (2013). Predicting steep escalations in alcohol use over the teenage years: age-related variations in key social influences. *Addiction*, *108*, 1924–32.

Cross, D., Shaw, T., Hearn, L., Epstein, M., Monks, H., Lester, L., & Thomas, L. (2009). *Australian covert bullying prevalence study (ACBPS)*. Child Health Promotion Research Centre, Edith Cowan University.

Department of Health. (2017). *National Drug Strategy 2017–2026*. Commonwealth of Australia.

Freiberg, H. J., & Lapointe, J. M. (2006). Research-based programs for preventing and solving discipline problems. In C. M. Evertson, & C. S. Weinstein (Eds.), *Handbook of classroom management* (pp. 735–86). Erlbaum.

Gaffney, H., Ttofi, M. M., & Farrington, D. P. (2021). What works in anti-bullying programs? Analysis of effective intervention components. *Journal of School Psychology, 85*, 37–56.

Gibb, S. J., Horwood, L. J. & Fergusson, D. M. (2011). Bullying victimization/ perpetration in childhood and later adjustment: Findings from a 30 year longitudinal study. *Journal of Aggression, Conflict and Peace Research, 3*(2), 82–8.

Hawkins, J. D., & Catalano, R. F. (2002). *Investing in your community's youth: An introduction to the Communities That Care system*. Channing-Bete Company.

Hawkins, J. D., Catalano, R. F., Morrison, D. M., O'Donnell, J., Abbott, R. D., & Day, L. E. (1992). The Seattle social development project: Effects of the first four years on protective factors and problem behaviors. In J. McCord, & R. Tremblay (Eds.), *The prevention of antisocial behaviour in children* (pp. 139–61). Guilford Press.

Hawkins, J. D., Oesterle, S., Brown, E. C., Abbott, R. D., & Catalano, R. F. (2014). Youth problem behaviors 8 years after implementing the Communities That Care prevention system: A community-randomized trial. *JAMA Pediatrics, 168*, 122–9.

Hawkins, J. D., & Weis, J. G. (2017). The social development model: An integrated approach to delinquency prevention. In *Developmental and life-course criminological theories* (pp. 3–27). Routledge.

Hazelden Foundation. (2016). *Olweus bullying prevention program*. Hazelden Publishing. Retrieved http://www.violencepreventionworks.org/public/olweus_bullying_prevention_program.page

Heerde, J., Bailey, J., Kelly, A., McMorris, B. J., Patton, G. C., & Toumbourou, J. W. (2021). Life-course predictors of homelessness from adolescence into adulthood: A population-based cohort study. *Journal of Adolescence, 91*, 15–24.

Heerde, J., Bailey, J., Toumbourou, J. W., & Patton, G. C. (2020). Homelessness among young people: Advancing prevention approaches. *Parity, 33*, 39–40.

Heerde, J., Bailey, J., Toumbourou, J. W., Rowland, B., & Catalano, R. F. (2020). Longitudinal associations between early-mid adolescent risk and protective factors and young adult homelessness in Australia and the United States. *Prevention Science, 21*, 557–67.

——(2021). Adolescent antecedents of young adult homelessness: A cross-national path analysis. *Prevention Science, 23*(1), 85–95.

Heerde, J. A., & Pallotta-Chiarolli, M. (2020). 'I'd rather injure somebody else than get injured': An introduction to the study of exposure to physical violence among young people experiencing homelessness. *Journal of Youth Studies, 23*, 406–29.

Heerde, J. A., & Patton, G. C. (2020). The vulnerability of the young homeless. *The Lancet Public Health, 5*(6), e302–3.

Hemphill, S., & Heerde, J. (2019). Delinquency and health in Australian youth. In C. Salas-Wright, M. Vaughan, & D. Jackson (Eds.), *The Routledge international handbook of delinquency and health*. Routledge.

Hemphill, S. A., Heerde, J. A., Herrenkohl, T. I., Patton, G. C., Toumbourou, J. W., & Catalano, R. F. (2011). Risk and protective factors for adolescent substance use in Washington State, the United States and Victoria, Australia: A longitudinal study. *Journal of Adolescent Health, 49*(3), 312–20.

Hemphill, S. A., Kotevski, A., Herrenkohl, T. I., Bond, L., Kim, M. J., Toumbourou, J. W., & Catalano, R. F. (2011). Longitudinal consequences of adolescent bullying perpetration and victimisation: A study of students in Victoria, Australia. *Criminal Behaviour and Mental Health*, *21*(2), 107–16.

Hill, K. G., White, H. R., Chung, I. J., Hawkins, J. D. & Catalano, R. F. (2000). Early adult outcomes of adolescent binge drinking: Person- and variable-centered analyses of binge drinking trajectories. *Alcoholism: Clinical and Experimental Research*, *24*(6), 892–901.

Katzer, C., Fetchenhauer, D., & Belschak, F. (2009). Cyberbullying: Who are the victims? A comparison of victimization in internet chatrooms and victimization in school. *Journal of Media Psychology*, *21*(1), 25–36.

Kelly, A. B., Mason, W. A., Chmelka, M. B., Herrenkohl, T. I., Kim, M. J., Patton, G. C., . . . Catalano, R. F. (2016). Depressed mood during early to middle adolescence: A bi-national longitudinal study of the unique impact of family conflict. *Journal of Youth and Adolescence*, *45*, 1604–13.

Kowalski, R. M., Giumetti, G. W., Schroeder, A. N., & Lattanner, M. R. (2014). Bullying in the digital age: A critical review and meta-analysis of cyberbullying research among youth. *Psychological Bulletin*, *140*(4), 1073–137.

Loeber, R., & Farrington, D. P. (2000). Young children who commit crime: Epidemiology, developmental origins, risk factors, early interventions, and policy implications. *Development and Psychopathology*, *12*, 737–62.

Lubman, D. I., Hides, L., Yücel, M. & Toumbourou, J. W. (2007). Intervening early to reduce developmentally harmful substance use among youth populations. *Medical Journal of Australia*, *187*(7), S22–4.

Mathers, M., Toumbourou, J., Catalano, R., Williams, J., & Patton, G. (2006). Consequences of youth tobacco use: A review of prospective behavioural studies. *Addiction*, *101*(7), 948–58.

Moran, P., Coffey, C., Romaniuk, H., Olsson, C., Borschmann, R., Carlin, J. B., & Patton, G. C. (2012). The natural history of self-harm from adolescence to young adulthood: a population-based cohort study. *The Lancet*, *379*, 236–43.

Newcomb, M. D., & Bentler, P. M. (1988). Impact of adolescent drug use and social support on problems of young adults: A longitudinal study. *Journal of Abnormal Psychology*, *97*(1), 64–75.

Patton, G. C., Olsson, C. A., Skirbekk, V., Saffery, R., Wlodek, M. E., Azzopardi, P. S., . . . Francis, K. (2018). Adolescence and the next generation. *Nature*, *554*, 458.

Rowland, B., Kelly, A. B., Benstead, M., Heerde, J. A., Clancy, E., Bailey, J., . . . Horner, R. (2022). School influences on adolescent depression: A 6-year longitudinal study amongst Catholic, government and independent schools in Victoria, Australia. *Journal of Religion and Health*, doi.org/10.1007/s10943-022-01515-7.

Sawyer, S. M., Afifi, R. A., Bearinger, L. H., Blakemore, S.-J., Dick, B., Ezeh, A. C., & Patton, G. C. (2012). Adolescence: A foundation for future health. *The Lancet*, *379*, 1630–40.

Sawyer, S. M., Azzopardi, P. S., Wickremarathne, D., & Patton, G. C. (2018). The age of adolescence. *The Lancet Child & Adolescent Health*, *2*, 223–8.

Shortt, A. L., & Spence, S. H. (2006). Risk and protective factors for depression in youth: Towards a developmental-ecological model. *Behavior Change*, *23*(1), 1–30.

Stice, E., Ragan, J., & Randall, P. (2004). Prospective relations between social support and depression: Differential direction of effects for parent and peer support? *Journal of Abnormal Psychology*, *113*(1), 155–9.

Toumbourou, J., Evans-Whipp, T., Smith, R., Hemphill, S., Herrenkohl, T., & Catalano, R. (2014). Adolescent predictors and environmental correlates of young adult alcohol use problems. *Addiction*, *109*, 417–24.

van Geel, M., Vedder, P., & Tanilon, J. (2014). Relationship between peer victimization, cyber-bullying, and suicide in children and adolescents: A meta-analysis. *JAMA Pediatrics*, *168*(5), 435–42.

Wikstrom, P. H., & Sampson, R. J. (2013). Social mechanisms of community influences on crime and pathways in criminality. In B. B. Lahey, T. E. Moffit, & A. Caspi (Eds.), *Causes of conduct disorder and juvenile delinquency* (pp. 118–48). The Guilford Press.

Williams, K. R., & Guerra, N. G. (2007). Prevalence and predictors of Internet bullying. *Journal of Adolescent Health*, *41*(6, Suppl.), S14–21.

Wyn, J., Cahill, H., Holdsworth, R., Rowling, L., & Carson, S. (2000). MindMatters: A whole school approach promoting mental health and wellbeing. *Australian and New Zealand Journal of Psychiatry*, *34*(4), 594–601.

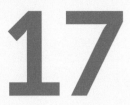

17 Healthy ageing

Elizabeth Cyarto and Frances Batchelor

LEARNING OBJECTIVES

After studying this chapter, you should be able to:

1 describe current models of healthy ageing
2 describe the World Health Organization's public health framework for healthy ageing, including the Decade of Healthy Ageing 2021–2030
3 identify the major health problems experienced by older people
4 identify the barriers and enablers to healthy ageing.

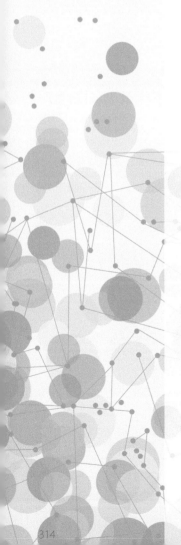

Introduction

Healthy ageing is gaining momentum as an important goal for societies experiencing population ageing. This chapter presents the public health issues relevant to the wellbeing of older people, now and into the future.

The world's population is ageing. The United Nations (UN) (2019) estimates that, globally, the number of people aged 65 years and over will increase from 693 million in 2019 to 1.6 billion in 2050 and 2.5 billion in 2100. In addition, the number of people aged 80 years and over is expected to triple by 2050, increasing from 143 million in 2019 to 426 million in 2050, and 881 million in 2100 (UN, 2019). While the proportion of older people is increasing in developed countries, the growth rate of the older population in developing countries will also rise dramatically and outpace that of developed regions. In four global regions (Africa, Asia, Latin America and the Caribbean), the proportion of the population aged 65 years or over is expected to double between 2019 and 2050 (UN, 2019). In 2019, 55 per cent of the global population aged 65 years or over and 61 per cent of those aged 80 years or over was female.

Population ageing is a result of increased **life expectancy** (reduced mortality) and decreased fertility rates (UN, 2019). For the first time in history, in 2018, people aged 65 years and over outnumbered children under five years of age (UN, 2019).

Australia's population is also ageing. In 2018, about 3.9 million Australians were aged 65 years and over, representing 16 per cent of the total estimated population (Australian Institute of Health and Welfare [AIHW], 2020a). Just over half (53 per cent) was female. Thirteen per cent of Australians (3.2 million) were aged 85 years and over (AIHW, 2020a). By 2066, the number of older Australians is expected to increase to 8.7 million (22 per cent of the population) and by 2096 to 12.8 million (25 per cent) (AIHW, 2020a). The profile of Australia's ageing population is also changing, with the largest proportional increases predicted in those aged 85 years and over. In 2017, 57 per cent (2.1 million) of older Australians were aged 65–74 years, 30 per cent (1.2 million) in the 75–84 years range and 13 per cent (497 000) aged 85 years and over (AIHW, 2018). By 2047, it is predicted that the proportion in the 65–74 years age range will reduce to 45 per cent (3.4 million), whereas in the older age brackets, the relative proportion will increase, with 35 per cent (2.6 million) for the age range 75–84 years and 20 per cent (1.5 million) for people aged 85 years and over (AIHW, 2018).

Life expectancy – the average number of years a person can expect to live, usually from birth. It is based on age and gender-specific death rates.

What is healthy ageing?

Healthy ageing defined

Ageing is the 'process of growing old' (Oxford Advanced Learner's Dictionary, 2015). Although there are commonly used definitions of **old age**, there is no general agreement on the age at which a person becomes old. Calendar age, or the age at which one can receive pension benefits, is often used to mark the beginning of old age (World Health Organization [WHO], 2015). This assumes that chronological age equals biological age, yet it is generally accepted that these two are not necessarily synonymous. There are wide variations in health status, participation and levels of independence among older people of the same age. Gender, culture and social factors also need to be considered. The WHO considers an older person to be aged 60 years or over (WHO, 2002), whereas 65 years is the UN standard to define older people (UN, 2019).

Old age – defined by the WHO as being over the age of 60 years and by the UN as being over the age of 65 years.

The phrase 'healthy ageing' has become commonplace in mainstream and scientific literature because of increasing interest in the wellbeing and independence of the growing proportion of older adults. One of the early conceptualisations of healthy ageing was 'successful ageing' (Rowe & Khan, 1997; Bowling & Dieppe, 2005; Bowling & Iliffe, 2006).

Bowling and Dieppe (2005) propose three models of successful ageing. The first, based on biomedical theories, defines successful ageing as the presence of high levels of physical and cognitive functioning. The second model emphasises psychological resources, life satisfaction and social functioning (Bowling & Dieppe, 2005). The third model is based on older people's perceptions of successful ageing (Bowling & Dieppe, 2005). To the first two models, having a sense of humour, learning new things, financial security, productivity and spirituality were added. Upon further investigation, Bowling and Iliffe (2006) found this multidimensional model to be most predictive of successful ageing (measured using self-reported quality of life). The authors provide a strong argument for an holistic approach and for including older people's views when defining successful ageing.

Healthy ageing is also known as active ageing (WHO, 2002; Bowling, 2008), positive ageing (Kendig & Browning, 1997), productive ageing (Kerschner & Pegues, 1998), and more recently adaptive or constructive ageing (Scharlach, 2017). However, it is accepted that healthy ageing involves more than just physical or functional health. Since 1948, the WHO has defined health 'as a state of complete physical, mental and social wellbeing, and not merely the absence of disease or infirmity' (WHO, 2011, p. 1). Bowling and Iliffe's (2006) multidimensional model of healthy ageing was the foundation for the WHO's healthy ageing frameworks.

REFLECTION QUESTION

How does the concept of healthy ageing relate to the concept of longevity or a long life-expectancy? Should research focus on extending longevity?
   Why or why not?

International policy frameworks on ageing

In 2002, the member states of the UN endorsed the Madrid International Plan of Action on Ageing (the Madrid Plan), with its goal of 'successful adjustment to an ageing world' (UN, 2002, p. 18). That same year, the WHO's Active Ageing framework was developed. Active ageing was defined as 'the process of optimizing opportunities for health, participation and security in order to enhance quality of life as people age' (WHO, 2002, p. 12), allowing people to 'realize their potential for physical, social and mental wellbeing throughout the **life course**' (p. 12).

Another key component of the active ageing framework was consideration of the broad **determinants of health** on ageing. Culture and gender are overarching factors because they shape the way one ages and influence all other determinants. This framework also includes behavioural, social, economic, health and social service systems, physical environment and personal determinants. For more information on the determinants of health, see the chapters in Part 1 of this book.

Life course – all stages of life, from early life to adulthood and old age.

Determinant of health – a factor within and external to the individual that determines health; the specific social, economic and political circumstances into which individuals are born and live.

Redefining healthy ageing

In 2011, the UN undertook a review of the Madrid Plan. The review revealed that, since 2002, only about half the 130 member countries had adopted new policies, strategies and plans with respect to ageing (UN Population Fund & HelpAge International, 2011).

The WHO recognised that to achieve the goals of the Madrid Plan and the Active Ageing framework, systemic change in response to population ageing was required (WHO, 2015). In its *World report on ageing and health*, the WHO (2015) put forth a 'public health framework for action', with a new definition of healthy ageing.

Healthy ageing is defined as 'the process of developing and maintaining the functional ability that enables well-being in older age' (WHO, 2015, p. 28). Within this definition,

Healthy ageing – the process of developing and maintaining the functional ability that enables wellbeing in older age.

functional ability refers to the health-related attributes that enable a person to 'be and do what they have reason to value' (WHO, 2015, p. 28). Functional ability combines two elements: intrinsic capacity and environments, which are interrelated. According to the WHO (2015), **intrinsic capacity** is the 'composite of all the physical and mental capacities that a person can draw on' at any point in time (p. 29). Furthermore, intrinsic capacity is influenced by genetic inheritance, personal characteristics (e.g. gender, ethnicity, education, wealth) and health characteristics (e.g. risk factors, diseases, injuries) (WHO, 2015). **Environments** are not just the built environments of home and community, but also broader society. They include people and their relationships, attitudes, values, and health and social policies, systems or services (WHO, 2015). Environments can compensate for declining intrinsic capacity, enabling a person's functional ability to be greater. For example, if a person with osteoarthritis uses assistive devices and receives home support for heavy household tasks, they may be able to live independently in their own home for longer (commonly referred to as 'ageing in place').

The WHO's public health framework and recommendations describes three broad sub-populations of older adults: those with high and stable intrinsic capacity, those with decreasing capacity and those with substantial loss of capacity (Beard et al., 2016). To maximise functional ability for all, and foster healthy ageing, three key areas for action have been identified. First, health systems and services need to meet the multidimensional needs of the older populations they serve and 'deliver care built around a common goal of functional ability' (Beard et al., 2016, p. 2150). Second, all countries should have systems to provide

Intrinsic capacity – consists of all the physical and mental capacities a person can draw on.

Environments – include the home, community and broader society.

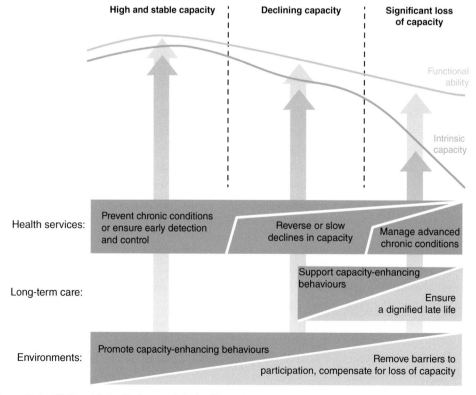

Figure 17.1   WHO's public health framework for healthy ageing
Source: WHO, 2015, p. 33.

comprehensive long-term care, with the goal of maintaining functional ability in those who are dependent on care. Third, 'age-friendly' environments need to be widespread. Age-friendly environments contribute to functional ability by enabling an older person to 'age safely in a place that is right for them, to continue to develop personally and to contribute to their community while retaining autonomy and health' (Beard et al., 2016, p. 2152). Figure 17.1 shows the WHO's healthy ageing framework across the three sub-populations of older adults and how the three key action areas can optimise functional ability.

Decade of Healthy Ageing 2021–2030

In 2016, all 194 WHO member states committed to creating 'a world in which everyone can live a long and healthy life' (WHO, 2017a). From 2016 to 2020, the *Global strategy and action plan on healthy ageing* (WHO, 2017a) focused on five strategic objectives:

- leadership and commitment to action on healthy ageing
- developing age-friendly environments
- aligning health systems to the needs of older populations
- developing an integrated system of long-term care
- improving measurement, monitoring and research.

The final milestone of the global strategy was the plan for the Decade of Healthy Ageing (WHO, 2020a). The Decade promises to be older person-centred and, in each member state, requires a whole-of-government and whole-of-society response (WHO, 2020a). Its overarching goal is to improve the lives of older people by 2030 by optimising their functional ability (WHO, 2020b). The attributes that enable functional ability include people's ability to:

- meet their basic needs to achieve an adequate standard of living (being able to afford the necessities of life)
- learn, grow and make decisions (enhancing autonomy, dignity and independence)
- be mobile (undertaking everyday tasks and participating in activities)
- build and maintain relationships (connecting with family, friends, neighbours and wider community)
- contribute to society (helping people, caregiving, working and volunteering (WHO, 2020b).

Recall that functional ability comprises a person's intrinsic capacity and the environments in which they live (WHO, 2015).

The WHO has further refined intrinsic capacity to include:

- physical movement
- sensory function (hearing, vision)
- cognitive function
- vitality
- psychological function (WHO, 2020b).

The environment, encompassing home, community and wider society, has also been further delineated to comprise:

- products, equipment and technology that facilitate physical, sensory, and cognitive capacity, and daily functioning

- the natural or built environment
- emotional support, assistance and relationships provided by other people and animals
- attitudes (these influence behaviour both negatively and positively)
- services, systems and policies (WHO, 2020b).

The environment can compensate for declining intrinsic capacity. The interaction between a person's intrinsic capacity and their environment influences what they can be and do.

To facilitate multi-sectoral and multi-stakeholder partnering, an online platform has been established (Decade of Healthy Ageing, 2022), where visitors can find and use knowledge in five areas:

- voices (submit stories and listen to stories of older people and their support networks)
- resources (submit and access publications, multimedia, databases and news)
- connect (link with like-minded people)
- innovate (announce research/implementation projects, advocacy campaigns and funding opportunities)
- support (access freely available tools, toolkits and training).

The platform is 'designed to be an inclusive, collaborative space where all knowledge relevant for the Decade can be accessed, shared, and interacted with in one place by everyone around the world' (Decade of Healthy Ageing, 2021). The Decade has become a global collaboration that brings together diverse stakeholders dedicated to creating 'a world in which everyone can live a long and healthy life'.

SPOTLIGHT 17.1

First Nations Peoples of Australia and ageing

by Paulene Mackell and Leona Kosowicz

Perspectives on what constitutes healthy ageing vary between and within cultural groups. In Australia, an emerging body of research has explored the concepts of wellbeing and healthy ageing from the perspectives of First Nations Peoples. Australia's First Nations Peoples are highly diverse in culture, customs, language and laws, and are represented by at least 250 distinct groups. While their individual views on wellbeing and healthy ageing are equally diverse, there remains an overall sense that the healthy ageing frameworks of developed nations are not relevant to older people in First Nations.

In contrast to the individualistic worldview that typically dominates cultures in developed nations, First Nations Peoples more commonly hold holistic and collectivist worldviews that emphasise the wellbeing of the community over the wellbeing of the individual. The National Aboriginal Community Controlled Health Organisation (NACCHO) defines health and wellbeing as:

> Aboriginal health means not just the physical well-being of an individual but refers to the social, emotional and cultural well-being of the whole Community in which each individual is able to achieve their full potential as a human being thereby bringing about the total well-being of their Community. It is a whole of life view and includes the cyclical concept of life-death-life (NACCHO, 2010).

Connection to community is one of several dimensions that sit within the concept of social and emotional wellbeing (SEWB) (Butler et al., 2019; Garvey et al., 2021). SEWB describes the holistic notion of health adopted by many First Nations Peoples, and encompasses social, emotional, physical, cultural and spiritual dimensions of wellbeing. As well as connection to community, SEWB and a recent conceptual model of wellbeing emphasise intrinsic connection to:

- family and kinship
- culture
- land and waters or Country
- spirit, spirituality and ancestors
- mind and emotions
- body.

SEWB is a source of strength and resilience for First Nations Peoples, and may be protective against social, political and historical determinants that have and continue to undermine individual and collective wellbeing. Maintenance of these connections throughout and beyond one's own life course is therefore considered a key component of healthy ageing, with participants in one study highlighting healthy ageing as 'having the physical and mental ability to pass on traditional values, cultural knowledge and cultural spirituality' (Coombes et al., 2018, p. 363). Viewing healthy ageing through an intergenerational and holistic lens means that healthy ageing programs should be led by and co-designed with First Nations Peoples (Wettasinghe et al., 2020). Doing so is methodologically rigorous and aligns with the Uluru Statement from the Heart (First Nations National Constitutional Convention and Central Land Council, 2017). It also highlights an ethical imperative in contemporary colonial Australia, where structural inequity and its effects on healthy ageing remains an everyday reality for First Nations Peoples (Radford & Garvey, 2021).

QUESTION

The Uluru Statement from the Heart invites all Australians to listen to, learn from and walk with First Nations Peoples. How might this invitation influence your approach to support healthy ageing?

SPOTLIGHT 17.2

Experiences of retirement village living

Choice of housing is one of our most basic needs. While most older people prefer to live in their own homes as they age, a proportion considers moving into retirement villages. Approximately 5 per cent of Australians over the age of 65 years live in retirement villages, and this is expected to increase. Reasons cited for considering retirement village living include wanting or needing to 'downsize', the opportunity to participate in activities, and needing a feeling of safety (Malta et al., 2018). Although it has been reported that quality of life and life satisfaction improve when older people move into retirement villages, residents' member organisations have expressed concerns that negative aspects of retirement village living may be under-reported. Researchers at the National Ageing Research Institute, with support from the Residents of Retirement Villages of Victoria, wanted to gain an understanding of the experience of living in retirement villages, positive or negative. The results of a survey of

1876 retirement village residents have been reported in a paper by Malta and colleagues (2018). Residents reported a range of reasons for moving into retirement villages, with the top five reasons being:

- having a safe environment and emergency support
- downsizing
- village facilities on offer
- availability of onsite maintenance.

Residents rated their life satisfaction and emotional health as positive, and 77 per cent rated their physical health as good to excellent. Overall, residents found retirement village life very positive. The negative aspects reported by respondents related to disputes and dispute-resolution processes, particularly around maintenance and contractual issues.

QUESTIONS

1   What processes or systems could enhance residents' experience of retirement village living?
2   What aspects of retirement village living could contribute to healthy ageing, and how does this differ from other settings, such as in one's own home or in residential aged care, for example?

The health of older people

Life expectancy

Globally, there have been gains in life expectancy at birth since the 1950s (UN, 2013). Life expectancy at birth of the global population was 72.6 years, on average, in 2019 and it is projected to increase to 77.1 years in 2050 (UN, 2019). In Australia, life expectancy has also increased. People born in the early 1900s lived to approximately 53 years of age (AIHW, 2020b). A female born in 2017–19 can expect to live to the age of 85 years, and a male may live to 80.9 years (AIHW, 2021a), However, for the Aboriginal and Torres Strait Islander population born in 2015–17, life expectancy is estimated to be 7.8 years lower than that of the non-Indigenous population for females and 8.6 years lower for males (AIHW, 2021a). In 2017–10, in the general population, a female aged 65 years could expect to live an additional 22.7 years and a male of the same age another 20 years (AIHW, 2021a).

Importantly, increases in life expectancy at birth have been matched by improvements in **healthy life expectancy**. This refers to the number of years spent without disease or **disability**, and reflects the time that an individual at a certain age can expect to live in full health (AIHW, 2020b).

The WHO provides global estimates of health-adjusted life expectancy (HALE), with the difference between life expectancy and HALE reflecting years of ill-health or disability (WHO, 2020b). Between 2000 and 2019, life expectancy increased faster than HALE for both males and females, which means people spend more time in ill-health (WHO, 2020b). In 2019, the gap between life expectancy and HALE for males was 8.3 years (69 years versus 61 years) and for females 11 years (76 years versus 65 years). In Australia in 2015, HALE at birth was 71.5 for males and 74.4 for females (AIHW, 2020a). Compared to life expectancy at birth, older males can expect to live 8.9 years in ill health and older females 10.2 years.

Healthy life expectancy – the number of years a person can be expected to live in full health; often used as a synonym for 'disability-free life expectancy'.

Disability – a physical, sensory, intellectual or mental impairment which, combined with social and environmental barriers, may limit a person's activities and participation in society.

Causes of death, health conditions and disability

The increase in life expectancy experienced by older adults has been largely a result of fewer deaths due to vascular disease (AIHW, 2021a). However, in 2017–19, lung cancer was the leading cause of death for older Australians aged 65–74 years while coronary heart disease was the leading causes of death in those aged 75–84 years. Dementia was the leading cause of death for people aged 85 years and over (AIHW, 2021a). In 2019, dementia, coronary heart disease and cerebrovascular disease were the leading underlying causes of death in females, (AIHW, 2021a). For males, coronary heart disease was the leading cause of death, followed by dementia and lung cancer.

Over the past century, the major cause of illness (also known as **morbidity**) in most developed countries has shifted from infectious diseases to chronic conditions. Globally, they caused 42 million deaths in 2019 (Global Burden of Disease Collaborative Network, 2020). Over time, the proportion of deaths worldwide due to chronic conditions increased from 67 per cent in 2010 to 74 per cent in 2019.

According to the AIHW (2020c), chronic diseases are characterised by the following features:

- complex and multi-factorial causation
- exposure to risk factors and gradual onset
- disability and functional limitations leading to reduced quality of life
- prolonged and progressive
- contributing to premature **mortality**.

People with **multimorbidity** are living with two or more diagnosed chronic conditions (AIHW, 2021b).

Age is an important determinant of several chronic diseases. Many conditions (such as cancer) have long latency periods and may not be apparent until middle or old age (AIHW, 2020c). Most chronic illnesses are not immediately life-threatening, and many people manage their conditions well. The most common, self-reported chronic health problems affecting older people in Australia include arthritis, back problems, mental health conditions (depression and anxiety) and cardiovascular disease (AIHW, 2021b). In 2017–18, 80 per cent of Australians aged 65 years and over reported having one or more long-term health problem (AIHW, 2021b). Just over 50 per cent of older Australians are experiencing multimorbidity, including:

- 68.5 per cent of people reporting two chronic conditions
- 46.3 per cent reporting three chronic conditions
- 22.6 per cent reporting four chronic conditions
- 13 per cent reporting five or more chronic conditions (AIHW, 2021b).

A disability is characterised by limitation, restriction or impairment that affects daily living activities lasting (or expected to last) for at least six months (Australian Bureau of Statistics [ABS], 2019). Limitations in activities such as self-care, mobility and communication range from mild to severe or profound. The chronic diseases most associated with activity limitations include dementia, arthritis, hypertension and back problems (ABS, 2019).

Disability rates increase with age. In those aged between 15 and 64 years, 13 per cent were experiencing disability, compared to 49 per cent in those aged 65 years and over (AIHW, 2020d). In 2018, 49.6 per cent of older people had a disability (ABS, 2019). Although the

Morbidity – an indication of ill health in a person; also refers to levels of ill health in a population or group.

Mortality – the rate of death in a particular population.

Multimorbidity – living with two or more chronic conditions.

number of older Australians increased from 2015 to 2018, the prevalence of disability has remained stable among older people living with disability:

- 35.4 per cent had profound or severe limitation
- 15.0 per cent had moderate limitation
- 40.1 per cent had mild limitation.

Burden of disease

Mortality, disability, impairment, illness and injury all contribute to the 'burden of disease', which is a way of measuring the magnitude and effects of diseases on a population's health (AIHW, 2019). A disability-adjusted life year (DALY) is one year of 'healthy life' lost due to a health condition. A DALY takes account of both premature death, and 'healthy' life lost due to disability (AIHW, 2019). In Australia, across all age groups, illness or premature death resulted in a loss of 4.8 million DALYs in 2015 (AIHW, 2019). For adults over the age of 65 years, chronic conditions contributed to 39 per cent of the total disease burden in 2015 (AIHW, 2020a). Coronary heart disease and dementia were the leading causes of total disease burden for people aged 65 years and over in 2015 (AIHW, 2019). Chronic obstructive pulmonary disease (COPD), cerebrovascular disease, dementia, lung cancer and osteoarthritis also contributed to total burden (AIHW, 2019).

Health status

Self-assessed health status is used as a measure of overall population health (AIHW, 2020b). In 2015, 68 per cent of Australians aged 15–24 years self-rated their health as 'excellent' or 'very good', compared to 42 per cent in people aged 65 and over (AIHW, 2018). Despite the associations between ageing, chronic disease and disability, 73 per cent of people aged over 65 years, rated their health as excellent, very good or good (AIHW, 2018). Even though people aged 85 years and over had the highest proportions of fair and poor health (34 per cent compared to 25 per cent in those 65–74 years), 67 per cent rated their health as excellent, very good or good. (AIHW, 2018). More females than males aged 65–84 years reported their health as being excellent or very good. Of those aged 85 years and over, males were slightly more likely to report excellent or very good health.

SPOTLIGHT 17.3

The WHO approach to reducing morbidity and mortality

The WHO has recognised that for individuals aged over 60 years the major burden of disability and death results from age-related losses in intrinsic capacity (WHO, 2015). As a follow-up to the *World report on ageing and health*, the WHO has developed Integrated Care for Older People (ICOPE) guidelines (WHO, 2017b). These guidelines are based on the premise that primary healthcare professionals are well-placed to detect and manage declines in patients' physical and cognitive abilities, if they are trained to do so. The ICOPE guidelines provide practitioners with evidence-based recommendations on community-based approaches to addressing declining intrinsic capacity. In addition to a module on intrinsic capacity (mobility loss, malnutrition, visual and hearing impairment, cognitive impairment and depressive symptoms), ICOPE includes recommendations for addressing geriatric syndromes (urinary incontinence and falls) and for providing interventions to support caregivers (WHO, 2017b). The ICOPE Handbook provides guidance for person-centred assessment and care plan development in primary care (WHO, 2019a). The ICOPE Implementation Framework provides guidance for policymakers and program managers to measure the capacity of health and social care services to deliver integrated care in community settings (WHO, 2019b). These resources exemplify action being taken to align health services with healthy ageing.

QUESTION
According to the ICOPE guidelines (WHO, 2017b), what are the recommendations for managing declines in intrinsic capacity in older people?

Barriers and enablers to healthy ageing

Healthy ageing results from the interaction between an individual's intrinsic capacity and the broader social and physical environment. For individuals and communities to achieve healthy ageing, barriers and enablers at individual, social and physical environmental levels need to be considered. Barriers and enablers can be considered according to the ecological framework proposed by Lak and colleagues (2020), consisting of 'micro (person), meso (process), and macro systems (place and policy making), based on health (prime) environments' (Lak et al., 2020, p. 1), or the 5P approach (Figure 17.2). From their systematic review of the literature, 15 sub-themes across the five major themes emerged, all of which can be considered determinants of healthy or active ageing. In Lak's model, the 'prime' theme is an overarching theme, in which physical, social and mental health influence, and are influenced by, all other determinants.

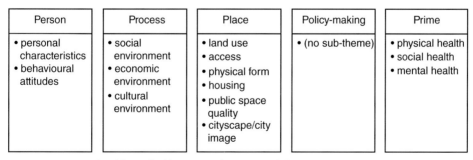

Person	Process	Place	Policy-making	Prime
• personal characteristics • behavioural attitudes	• social environment • economic environment • cultural environment	• land use • access • physical form • housing • public space quality • cityscape/city image	• (no sub-theme)	• physical health • social health • mental health

Figure 17.2   Barriers and enablers to healthy ageing: Themes and subthemes
Source: Adapted from Lak et al. (2020).

Enabling people to age well therefore requires not only actions that address individual factors – for example, primary prevention of disease – but action at many other levels including at the societal level. One example of a barrier to healthy ageing is **ageism**. Ageism 'refers to the stereotypes, prejudice and discrimination towards others and oneself based on age' (WHO, 2021a, p. xix), and can be both individual and structural (Chang et al., 2020).

Ageism – stereotypes, prejudice and discrimination based on age.

The WHO has recognised the widespread existence and effects of ageism (WHO, 2021a). For example, approximately 50 per cent of people across the world are ageist against older people and one-third of Europeans have experienced ageism (WHO, 2021a). The effects of ageism can be seen across the life course, but the health of older people can be affected by age discrimination, negative stereotypes about age and negative self-perceptions about ageing in general (Chang et al., 2020). At the individual level, it has been shown that negative self-perceptions of ageing are associated with, or predict, reduced life expectancy, decreased quality of life, unhealthy lifestyle choices, depression, cognitive impairment and acute and chronic conditions (Chang et al., 2020). Structural ageism; that is, policies, practices and institutional and societal processes that discriminate against older people, can lead to older people being de-valued, having fewer work opportunities, being denied access to health care on the basis of age and being excluded from health research (Chang et al., 2020).

SPOTLIGHT 17.4

Healthy ageing and the COVID-19 pandemic

COVID-19 has had significant effects on all aspects of society globally, but the pandemic and subsequent restrictions have disproportionately affected older people. In addition to the fact that older people are at higher risk of serious illness and death from COVID-19 than younger people, the rapidly imposed restrictions introduced by many countries, including physical distancing, travel and border restrictions, stay-at-home recommendations and avoiding contact with others, have profoundly affected older people's lives. Negative effects on both physical and psychological health have been seen in the short-term, and also are expected to continue over the longer term. These include:

- reduction in physical activity due to lockdown or stay-at-home requirements, potentially accelerating decline in physical and cognitive function
- social isolation and loneliness due to lack of contact with family and friends, and being unable to participate in usual activities such as social groups, church groups, volunteering and work
- mental health effects including anxiety and fear about contracting COVID-19, concern about family members who may be vulnerable (e.g. spouse in residential aged care) and limited opportunities to be with loved ones at end of life, which can compound grief
- possible delays in medical care such elective procedures being postponed, and exacerbation of chronic conditions or delayed treatment.

In order to address the potential negative effects of stay-at-home recommendations on physical function, a coalition of Australian physiotherapists with academic and clinical expertise in exercise for older people undertook rapid development of a website to provide older people and health professionals with information and resources on exercising safely at home. The Safe Exercise At Home Website (www.safeexerciseathome.org.au), provides older people with written instruction and videos demonstrating exercises that can be safely performed at home according to a person's level of fitness and ability. Importantly, the website was codesigned with older people to ensure the information was presented appropriately for the intended audience.

QUESTION

In what ways has the COVID-19 pandemic influenced society's view of older people and the importance of healthy ageing?

SUMMARY

This chapter has discussed issues relevant to the health of older people.

Learning objective 1: Describe current models of healthy ageing.

Healthy ageing is about much more than maintenance of physical health. It is about having opportunities for lifelong participation, adequate food and housing in older age, feeling safe and secure, and having meaningful activities and relationships. There are several models of healthy ageing, including the lay model, in which older people define for themselves what is meant by healthy ageing. This model has been found to be the best predictor of health in older age, reinforcing the importance of including the voices of older people in promoting healthy ageing.

Learning objective 2: Describe the World Health Organization's public health framework for healthy ageing, including the Decade of Healthy Ageing 2021–2030.

In 2002, member states of the UN endorsed the Madrid Plan for action on ageing, with its 'specific goal of successful adjustment to an ageing world' (UN, 2002, p. 18). That same year, the WHO's Active Ageing framework was developed to support people to 'realize their potential for physical, social and mental wellbeing throughout the life course' (WHO, 2002. p. 12). Almost a decade later, widespread global implementation of actions and achievement of objectives had not been achieved. In response, in its *World report on ageing and health* (WHO, 2015), the WHO redefined healthy ageing to be the 'process of developing and maintaining the functional ability that enables well-being in older age' (p. 28). Functional ability comprises the interrelated components of intrinsic capacity and environments. Subsequently, the WHO developed its *Global strategy on ageing and health* (WHO, 2017a), including the 2016–2020 action plan. The current *Decade of Healthy Ageing 2021–2030* is the second action plan to emerge from the WHO's global strategy (WHO, 2020a).

Learning objective 3: Identify the major health problems experienced by older people.

Although older people tend to rate their health as good to excellent, there is a much greater chance of developing chronic illnesses in older age. Until the mid-20th century, the main causes of death worldwide were infectious diseases, such as tuberculosis, measles and malaria. While these continue to account for almost half of all deaths in low-income countries, they account for less than 15 per cent of deaths in high-income countries (WHO, 2021b). Non-communicable diseases such as cancer, heart disease and dementia have taken over as the highest causes of death and disability. The increase in chronic diseases, many of which can be prevented by adopting healthy lifestyle practices, has led to a greater focus on management of health (including self-management) rather than cure, and a focus on educating people of all ages about healthy lifestyle choices.

Learning objective 4: Identify the barriers and enablers to healthy ageing.

Barriers and enablers can be classified using the 5P approach: person, process, place, policymaking and prime (physical, social and mental health). Enabling people to age well requires actions at all levels. A global barrier to healthy ageing, as identified by the WHO, is ageism. Negative self-perceptions of ageing can result in poor health and reduced life expectancy. Ageist policies, practices and processes can unfairly restrict opportunities and disadvantage older people.

TUTORIAL EXERCISES

1   Complete the Healthy Ageing Quiz (see the website of the National Ageing Research Institute, www.nari .net.au) and see if you are on track to age healthily or, if not, what changes you should make.

2 Discuss the following statements:

  a Older adults' perceptions of healthy ageing correspond with current models or frameworks in the literature.

  b Older people are the most frequent users of hospital emergency departments.

  c Ageing well is an individual's responsibility.

  d People should give up work when they turn 65 years of age.

3 What strategies or interventions in the areas of health services, long-term care and environment could be implemented to optimise functional ability for an older person experiencing decreasing intrinsic capacity? (see Figure 17.1)

FURTHER READING

Beard, J. R., Officer, A., Araujo de Carvalho, I., Sadana, R., Pot, A. M., Michel, J-P., . . . Chatterji, S. (2016). The world report on ageing and health: A policy framework for healthy ageing. *Lancet*, *387*, 2145–54.

Bowling, A., & Iliffe, S. (2006). Which model of successful ageing should be used? Baseline findings from a British longitudinal survey of ageing. *Age and Ageing*, *35*, 607–14.

World Health Organization (WHO). (2017). *Integrated care for older people: guidelines on community-level interventions to manage declines in intrinsic capacity*. WHO. Retrieved https://apps.who.int/iris/handle/10665/258981

——(2020). *Decade of healthy ageing: Baseline report*. WHO. Retrieved https://apps.who.int/iris/handle/10665/338677

——(2021). *Global report on ageism*. WHO. Retrieved https://apps.who.int/iris/handle/10665/340208

REFERENCES

Australian Bureau of Statistics (ABS). (2019). *Disability, Ageing and carers, Australia: Summary of findings*. Retrieved https://www.abs.gov.au/statistics/health/disability/disability-ageing-and-carers-australia-summary-findings/latest-release#older-people

Australian Institute of Health and Welfare (AIHW). (2018). *Older Australia at a glance*. Cat. No. AGE 87. AIHW. Retrieved https://www.aihw.gov.au/reports/older-people/older-australia-at-a-glance/report-editions

——(2019). *Australian burden of disease study: Impact and causes of illness and death in Australia 2015 – Summary report. Australian Burden of Disease Study series no. 18*. Cat. No. BOD 21. AIHW. Retrieved https://www.aihw.gov.au/reports/burden-of-disease/burden-disease-study-illness-death-2015-summary/summary

——(2020a). *Health of older people*. Retrieved https://www.aihw.gov.au/reports/australias-health/health-of-older-people

——(2020b). *Australia's health 2020 data insights. Australia's health series no. 17*. Cat. No. AUS 231. AIHW.

——(2020c). *Chronic conditions and multimorbidity. Australia's health 2020*. Retrieved https://www.aihw.gov.au/reports/australias-health/chronic-conditions-and-multimorbidity

——(2020d). *People with disability in Australia*. Retrieved https://www.aihw.gov.au/reports/disability/people-with-disability-in-australia/contents/people-with-disability/prevalence-of-disability#Sex

——(2021a). *Deaths in Australia*. Retrieved https://www.aihw.gov.au/reports/life-expectancy-death/deaths-in-australia/contents/life-expectancy

——(2021b). *Chronic condition multimorbidity. Cat. No. PHE 286*. Retrieved https://www.aihw.gov.au/reports/chronic-disease/chronic-condition-multimorbidity/contents/chronic-conditions-and-multimorbidity

Beard, J. R., Officer, A., Araujo de Carvalho, I., Sadana, R., Pot, A. M., Michel, J-P., . . . Chatterji, S. (2016). The world report on ageing and health: a policy framework for healthy ageing. *Lancet*, *387*, 2145–54.

Bowling, A. (2008). Enhancing later life: How older people perceive active ageing? *Aging and Mental Health*, *12*(3), 293–301.

Bowling, A., & Dieppe, P. (2005). What is successful ageing and who should define it? *British Medical Journal*, *331*, 1548–51.

Bowling, A., & Iliffe, S. (2006). Which model of successful ageing should be used? Baseline findings from a British longitudinal survey of ageing. *Age and Ageing*, *35*, 607–14.

Butler, T. L., Anderson, K., Garvey, G., Cunningham, J., Ratcliffe, J., Tong, A., . . . Howard, K. (2019). Aboriginal and Torres Strait Islander people's domains of wellbeing: A comprehensive literature review. *Social Science & Medicine 233*, 13–157.

Chang, E. S., Kannoth, S., Levy, S., Wang, S. Y., Lee, J. E., & Levy, B. R. (2020). Global reach of ageism on older persons' health: A systematic review. *PloS One*, *15*(1), e0220857.

Coombes, J., Lukaszyk, C., Sherrington, C., Keay, L., Tiedemann, A., Moore, R., & Ivers, R. (2018). First Nation Elders' perspectives on healthy ageing in NSW, Australia. *Australian and New Zealand Journal of Public Health*, *42*(4), 363.

Cyarto, E. V., Meyer, C., Dickins, M., & Lowthian, J. A. Cycling Without Age: meaningful activity for care home residents. *Australasian Journal on Ageing*, in press.

Cycling Without Age (CWA). (2021). *Welcome to the world of Cycling Without Age* (Webpage). Retrieved https://cyclingwithoutage.org/about/

Decade of Healthy Ageing. (2021). *Decade of healthy ageing: The Platform* (Website). Retrieved https://www.decadeofhealthyageing.org/

First Nations National Constitutional Convention and Central Land Council (Australia). (2017). *Uluru Statement from the Heart*. Retrieved http://nla.gov.au/nla.obj-484035616

Garvey, G., Anderson, K., Gall, A., Butler, T. L., Whop, L. J., Arley, B., . . . Tong, A. (2021). The fabric of Aboriginal and Torres Strait Islander wellbeing: a conceptual model. *International Journal of Environmental Research and Public Health*. *18*(15), 7745.

Global Burden of Disease Collaborative Network. (2020. *Global burden of disease study 2019 (GBD 2019) Results*. IHME.

Gow, A. J., Bell, C., & Gray. R. (2020). *Cycling Without Age – research and evaluation report 2019/20*. The Ageing Lab, Heriot-Watt University. Retrieved https://www2.hw.ac.uk/mediaservices/pageflip/CWA_Evaluation_%20Report_2019/

Kendig, H., & Browning, C. (1997). Positive ageing: Facts and opportunities. *Medical Journal of Australia*, *167*(8), 409.

Kerschner, H., & Pegues, J. (1998). Productive ageing: A quality of life agenda. *Journal of the American Dietetic Association*, *98*(12), 1445–8.

Lak, A., Rashidghalam, P., Myint, P. K. et al. (2020). Comprehensive 5P framework for active aging using the ecological approach: an iterative systematic review. *BMC Public Health*, *20*, 33.

Malta, S., Williams, S. B., & Batchelor, F. A. (2018). An ant against an elephant: Retirement village residents' experiences of disputes and dispute resolution. *Australasian Journal Ageing*, *37*(3), 202–9.

McNiel, P., & Westphal, J. (2020). Cycling Without Age program: The impact for residents in Long-Term Care. *Western Journal of Nursing Research*, *42*(9), 728–35.

National Aboriginal Community Controlled Health Organisation (NACCHO). (2010). Constitution for the National Aboriginal Community Controlled Health Organisation. Retrieved https://www.naccho.org.au/governance

Oxford Advanced Learner's Dictionary (2015). Oxford University Press. Retrieved http://www.oxfordlearnersdictionaries.com/definition/english

Radford, K., & Garvey, G. (2021). Sovereignty at the heart of aging well for Australia's First Nations. *Nature Aging*, *1*(7), 569–70.

Rowe, J., & Kahn, R. (1997). Successful aging. *The Gerontologist*, *37*(4), 433–40.

Scharlach, A. E. (2017). Aging in context: Individual and environmental pathways to aging-friendly communities – The 2015 Matthew A. Pollack Award Lecture. *The Gerontologist*, *57*(4), 606–18.

United Nations (UN). (2002). Political declaration and Madrid international plan of action on ageing. Second World Assembly on Ageing, Madrid, Spain 8–12 April. UN.

——(2013). *World population ageing 2013*.

——(2019). *World population prospects 2019: Highlights* (ST/ESA/SER.A/423).

United Nations Population Fund & HelpAge International. (2011). *Overview of available policies and legislation, data and research, and institutional arrangements relating to older persons – Progress since Madrid.*

Wettasinghe, P., Allan, W., Garvey, G., Timbery, A., Hoskins, S., Veinovic, M., . . . Delbaere, K. (2020). Older Aboriginal Australians' health concerns and preferences for healthy ageing programs. *International Journal of Environmental Research and Public Health*, *17*(20), 7390.

World Health Organization (WHO). (2002). *Active ageing: A policy framework*. WHO.

——(2011). *WHO constitution*. Retrieved http://www.who.int/governance/eb/who_constitution_en.pdf

——(2015). *World report on ageing and health*. WHO. Retrieved http://www.who.int/ageing/events/world-report-2015-launch/en/

——(2017a). *Global strategy and action plan on ageing and health*. WHO. Retrieved http://www.who.int/ageing/WHO-GSAP-2017.pdf?ua=1

——(2017b). *Integrated care for older people: guidelines on community-level interventions to manage declines in intrinsic capacity*. WHO. Retrieved https://www.who.int/publications/i/item/9789241550109

——(2019a). *Integrated care for older people (ICOPE): Guidance for person-centred assessment and pathways in primary care*. WHO.

——(2019b). *Integrated care for older people (ICOPE) implementation framework: guidance for systems and services*. WHO.

——(2020a). *Decade of healthy ageing 2020–2030*. Retrieved https://www.who.int/initiatives/decade-of-healthy-ageing

——(2020b). *Decade of healthy ageing: Baseline report*. WHO. Retrieved https://www.who.int/publications/i/item/9789240017900

——(2021a). *Global report on ageism*. WHO.

——(2021b). *World health statistics 2021: monitoring health for the SDGs, sustainable development goals*. WHO.

The health inequities of people with intellectual and developmental disabilities: Strategies for change

18

Teresa Iacono and Christine Bigby

LEARNING OBJECTIVES

After studying this chapter, you should be able to:

1   describe the health inequities of people with intellectual and developmental disabilities
2   explain the effects of health inequities on people with intellectual and developmental disabilities
3   identify contributors to the health inequities for this group
4   identify strategies that can be adopted by health and human service professionals to reduce health inequities.

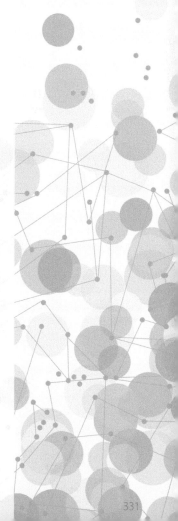

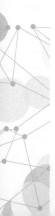

Intellectual and developmental disabilities (IDD) – lifelong disabilities that arise during the developmental period (up to 18 years) and result in problems in learning and/or daily functioning. They include intellectual disability, and other forms of developmental disability such as cerebral palsy and autism. Different terms have been used over time and in different countries to refer to intellectual disability, such as 'learning disabilities' in the United Kingdom.

Health inequity – the disparities in the health status of some individuals and groups. Inequality disproportionately affects the health of the most disadvantaged members of society, particularly in poorer nations.

Biological factor – a factor inherent to the person in terms of a genetic or other identifiable cause of their disability.

Social determinants of health – the social and economic conditions in which people are born, grow, live, work, play and age, and which influence their health, such as poverty, unemployment, social and civic participation and social relationships.

Introduction

People with **intellectual and developmental disabilities (IDD)** vary in terms of the nature and severity of their disabilities, but for all, their disability is lifelong. They also share the experience of **health inequities** in the form of higher rates of poor health, when compared with the general population. Together with **biological factors** relating to impairment or genetic factors, adverse **social determinants of health**, such as inadequate support for a healthy lifestyle, social exclusion, poverty, poor access to health services and unresponsive systems of care all contribute to their high rates of comorbid and secondary conditions that account for their poor health (Cooper et al., 2015; Hussain et al., 2020; Koritsas & Iacono, 2011; see also Chapter 7). Their needs are easily overlooked by health services due to the poorly understood and often invisible nature of their impairments. There is a human rights imperative to address their health inequities through broader social change to reduce their socio-economic disadvantages, and systemic changes to healthcare systems to ensure they are afforded the same access to quality care as others in the community (see also Chapter 11).

This chapter is focused on healthcare systems rather than broader social change. It explores the nature of the health inequities of people with IDD and identifies factors contributing to their poor health. The chapter ends with a review of strategies that show promise in addressing existing health problems, preventing the onset of poor health and improving healthcare systems.

The effects of health inequities

A large body of research has drawn attention to the health inequities of people with IDD, beginning with an early Australian study by Beange and colleagues (1995) . They documented a high rate of health problems among patients with IDD of a general practice clinic, who had health problems and risk factors that had been undiagnosed or misdiagnosed and/or were poorly managed. This study was a catalyst for numerous studies demonstrating that health inequities were endemic for people with IDD across high, middle and low-income countries, and shedding light on contributors and strategies to ameliorate the extent of health disparities (Robertson et al., 2015).

Mortality

Mortality, or rate of death, for people with IDD remains high, despite a dramatic overall increased life expectancy (Bourke et al., 2017; Florio & Trollor, 2015; Salomon & Trollor, 2019; Shooshtari et al., 2020). For example, Down syndrome – a common genetic cause of intellectual disability – life expectancy was 12 years in 1940, increasing to around 60 years by the early 21st century (Bittles et al., 2006); a recent Japanese study showed one in three persons with Down syndrome were living beyond 60 years (Motegi et al., 2021). Life expectancy for people with mild IDD is now similar to that of the general population, but remains much lower for people with more severe disability (Emerson et al., 2014).

> **Mortality** – the rate of death in a particular population.

High mortality rates have been found to arise from delays or problems with diagnosis or treatment, problems in identifying the person's needs and a failure to provide appropriate care as a person's needs change (Glover et al., 2017). People with IDD often die prematurely from causes that could be prevented by good-quality care (Glover et al., 2017; Trollor et al., 2017).

Comorbid conditions

People with IDD often have health conditions that are not related to their primary disability. In the United Kingdom, following a report documenting cases of the preventable deaths of people with intellectual disability in National Health Service hospitals (Mencap, 2007) and

> **Comorbid condition** – a disease process that co-occurs with, but is unrelated to, a disability, and has adverse effects on health.

a government-commissioned inquiry (Michael & Richardson, 2008), a health observatory was established to monitor health inequities, including rates of comorbid conditions. High rates were found by Emerson and colleagues (2011) for conditions that can be treated effectively through good-quality care (e.g. gastric ulcers and lymphoma caused by *Helicobacter pylori* bacteria, coronary heart disease and respiratory disease). These high rates of comorbid conditions contribute to health inequities and poor quality of life for people with IDD.

Secondary conditions

Secondary condition – a health condition occurring after a primary condition and that is preventable.

Unlike comorbid conditions, **secondary conditions** are associated with a person's primary disability (Koritsas & Iacono, 2011). They can also be prevented through appropriate and timely health care, and they can increase the severity of the primary disability, thereby tightly restricting participation in activities (Koritsas & Iacono, 2011). For example, a person with cerebral palsy is likely to develop severe contractures (a permanent shortening of a muscle or joint), resulting in deformity, if appropriate seating, positioning and exercise programs are not provided from an early age.

SPOTLIGHT 18.1

Death by indifference

People with IDD are at particular risk of poor outcomes when in hospital. The United Kingdom report *Death by Indifference* (Mencap, 2007) documented seven cases of people who died due to the failure of hospitals to address their needs. The following is an extract from one of these accounts:

> Martin had a stroke and was sent to hospital. While there, he also contracted pneumonia. Martin had trouble swallowing after his stroke and so was visited by a speech and language specialist. But Martin's swallow reflex did not return. He could not take food or water orally and so was put on a drip. Martin did not tolerate this well and sometimes pulled the drip out. In the second week at the hospital Martin was still unable to eat and the drip was not providing him with adequate nutrition. He was visited and tested by the speech and language team several times. They recorded in their notes that he should remain 'nil by mouth' and that 'alternative feeding methods should be considered'. However, no action was taken. This situation continued into a third week.
>
> By this time, his veins had collapsed, which meant that the doctors couldn't get the glucose liquid from his drip into his body. So they decided they needed to insert a feeding tube into his stomach. This would have required a surgical procedure. However, by the time they had made this decision, Martin had been without nutrition for 21 days and his condition had deteriorated so much that he was in no state to undergo an operation. Five days later, Martin died.
>
> The hospital admit that they did not act on the information that Martin was assessed as being at 'high risk' on the Malnutrition Universal Screening Test (MUST) scale, and that they did not follow their own enteral feeding policy. This policy states that alternative feeding methods should be considered after seven days.

QUESTION
What events contributed to Martin's death? Could they have been avoided and, if so, how?

Reasons for health inequities

Several factors contribute to the poorer health and experience of poor health care by people with IDD. These include biological factors relating to the underlying impairment and its cause, which are mostly not amenable to change but are amenable to management. Additionally, this group is exposed to many negative social determinants of health, which do offer the potential for change or at least amelioration of their effects.

Biological factors

A person's underlying impairment may be associated with particular health problems, or may put them at risk of comorbid or secondary conditions. These factors may be associated with chromosomal abnormalities. Down syndrome, for example, results from three copies of all or part of chromosome 21, rather than the usual two. This abnormality is responsible for intellectual disability, and may also result in congenital heart problems, respiratory problems, leukaemia, hearing impairment, dry skin conditions, instability in the cervical spine and early onset dementia (Vander Ploeg Booth, 2011).

Other, non-genetic causes of IDD, such as problems that occur before, during or soon after birth, can result in a primary disability as well as other health concerns. Deprivation of oxygen to the foetal brain prior to or during birth, for example, can result in cerebral palsy, as well as visual impairment and intellectual disability (Stanley et al., 2000). A person with cerebral palsy, which is a musculoskeletal disorder, will be at risk of severe difficulties with walking (and may rely on a wheelchair), communication impairment that may range in severity from being difficult to understand to being unable to use speech, and limb deformities through the development of contractures (Stanley et al., 2000).

The risk of comorbid and secondary health conditions can be reduced through appropriate health checks and screening, and early interventions and social supports. People with Down syndrome, for example, require blood tests to assess thyroid functioning, hearing and vision tests, and assessments of their respiratory, gastrointestinal and cardiovascular systems (Therapeutic Guidelines, 2012). As they approach their 50s, baseline assessments of their cognitive functioning and adaptive behaviour should be used to provide a means of determining decline, should dementia be suspected (Torr & Davis, 2007).

Negative social determinants

People with IDD are at high risk of many adverse social determinants of health that fall under the broad umbrella of social disadvantage, including poverty, unemployment and social isolation. People with disability and their carers have been described as being among the most economically and socially disadvantaged groups in the community (Emerson et al., 2011).

Poverty

Contributing to economic disadvantage of people with IDD is limited opportunity for employment. Internationally, very few people with IDD (around 26 per cent) are in paid employment (Butterworth et al., 2013), resulting in many relying on financial support from government. Even with such support, poverty may be the most pervasive social determinant of health for people with IDD, with Emerson and Hatton (2007) reviewing research to indicate 24–31 per cent of the increased risk for poor health among children and adolescents with intellectual disabilities may be attributable to their relative socio-economic disadvantage (p. 31). They reported that, of 1273 people with intellectual disabilities in the United Kingdom who had participated in a survey (*n*=2898), indicators of social disadvantage were significant predictors of variation in health status of people with mild to moderate intellectual disabilities, over and above variation attributable to person characteristics and living circumstances.

REFLECTION QUESTION

In what ways would poverty contribute to poor health of people with IDD, even in countries with universal health care, such as the United Kingdom and Australia?

Social inclusion

There has been much research demonstrating the association between better health and being socially included (see Chapter 11), whether by having extensive or personal social networks, availability of informal social support, feeling connected to the community through locality, participation in the groups that make up civic society, or more broadly as having social capital (Wiesel et al., 2019). On this dimension, too, people with IDD are at high risk, often lacking diverse social relationships and community links. Despite policies of de-institutionalisation and community living, many people with IDD remain socially isolated in communities, living in a distinct social space, made up of family, peers with IDD and paid staff (Bigby, 2008; Wiesel & Bigby, 2014), and are given few opportunities for the social contact that they desire (Gjermestad et al., 2017). The link between health inequities of people with IDD and their low level of social and civic participation was demonstrated in a large-scale United Kingdom study by Emerson and colleagues (2014).

Healthy lifestyles

People with IDD have been found to have unhealthy lifestyles and to have limited engagement with health promotion activities (Scott & Havercamp, 2016). Unhealthy lifestyles can be attributable to lack of opportunities for self-determination (engaging in decisions about day-to-day activities) and consequent reliance on others, as well as communication and learning difficulties. Health promotion programs often fail to engage people with IDD, and there is little guidance on adapting programs to this group because usually they have been omitted from studies (Naaldenberg et al., 2013). As a result, it seems that people with IDD, who can benefit in terms of improved health and fitness from exercise and diet regimens, engage in little regular exercise and have poor nutrition (see reviews by Bossink et al., 2017; Scott & Havercamp, 2016). There are many barriers to their engagement, including poor health, financial constraints, limited support from family or paid support staff (Bossink et al., 2017), and difficulties in accessing sports and other physical activities and discriminatory practices, which may be exacerbated for culturally and linguistically diverse communities (Kappelides et al., 2021).

Ineffective health care

Deinstitutionalisation of people with IDD since the 1970s followed major policy reform across developed countries that marked a shift from a medical model of care. Instead, a social model of disability provided a framework to redress systematic discrimination and negative attitudes often evident within mainstream healthcare services (MacArthur et al., 2015). Key to this process and central to these reforms was that, rather than relying on specialist services provided within institutions, people with IDD would access community-based services. Since deinstitutionalisation, people with IDD have been frequent users of healthcare services. In Australia, for example, people with IDD who live in supported accommodation attended their GPs much more often than others in the community (Iacono & Sutherland, 2006). There is also evidence that people with IDD have longer consultations with their GPs, yet common health problems remain unmanaged (Weise et al., 2017). Similarly, people with IDD are high-end users of hospitals, being more likely to be admitted and remain in intensive care for conditions that could be treated elsewhere, such as primary health clinics, and to experience one or more complications during their stays (Iacono et al., 2020).

Quality of care

Unfortunately, research has shown that the quality of care for people with an IDD is poor in both primary health services (Cooper et al., 2018; Weise et al., 2017) and hospitals (Iacono, Bigby et al., 2014b; Tuffrey-Wijne et al., 2014). In particular, people with IDD experience difficulties when trying to access services and, as noted, have health conditions that have gone undiagnosed or been misdiagnosed, often as a result of **diagnostic overshadowing**, or their conditions have been mismanaged or poorly managed (Beange et al., 1995; Cooper et al., 2018; Weise et al., 2017). Hospital systems have been particularly problematic. Studies in the United Kingdom have indicated failure to accommodate their needs, such as through provision of accessible information, liaison with carers and adequate discharge planning (Iacono, Bigby et al., 2014a; Tuffrey-Wijne et al., 2014). There is promising evidence, however, of improvements in hospital care. A recent Australian study in which 50 adults with IDD were prospectively followed from entry to hospitals to discharge demonstrated more positive than negative experiences (Bigby, Douglas & Iacono, 2018), with emergency department staff spending time to arrive at a diagnosis (Iacono et al., 2020).

Diagnostic overshadowing – the tendency to attribute symptoms of ill health to an underlying primary disability, resulting in a failure to conduct the required diagnostic assessments or to dismiss health complaints.

Medication management

An example of mismanagement is the overuse and often inappropriate prescription of medications, with little review over time. People with IDD have been described as the most medicated population (Trollor & Salomon, 2016), which is only partially attributable to high rates of comorbid conditions, in particular epilepsy (McMahon et al., 2020). Of most concern is the high usage of psychotropic medications, which are appropriately prescribed for psychiatric conditions (NDIS Quality and Safeguards Commission, 2021; Trollor & Salomon, 2016) . For people with IDD, they have been overused to control challenging behaviour in the absence of a psychiatric diagnosis (Trollor & Salomon, 2016). Attempts to reduce these medications appears to be hampered by lack of access by people with IDD to appropriate psychiatric services, lack of knowledge about the dangers of multiple medications for this group by GPs, and poor relationships with disability services, which need to be involved in any planned approach to reducing medications, in particular those used to control challenging behaviours (Torr, 2013).

Barriers to care

Health practitioner knowledge

GPs have reported barriers in delivering health care to people with IDD, including their own lack of knowledge about this group. They have reported needing education in human relations and sexual health, behavioural and psychiatric conditions, dealing with the complex medical issues people with IDD often present, and knowing how to engage them in preventive health care (Phillips et al., 2004; Smith & Laurence, 2021). These needs may help to explain the inappropriate use of psychotropic medications , as well as an under-utilisation of sexual health screenings, including Pap smears and breast examination for women, and prostate tests for men (Iacono & Sutherland, 2006; Weise et al., 2017). GPs have also raised concerns about the additional time required to assess and treat patients with IDD, without additional remuneration (Phillips et al., 2004; Smith & Laurence, 2021).

Communication difficulties

A further barrier is the communication difficulties experienced by many people with IDD in terms of comprehension and expression, which healthcare practitioners may fail to accommodate (Doherty et al., 2020). As a result, healthcare practitioners are highly reliant on carers – usually paid support workers or family members – to complete case histories, report symptoms and ensure compliance with management strategies (Doherty et al., 2020). Paid support workers, in particular, may not be able to identify or interpret indicators of underlying health problems, and certainly lack training in providing support to address existing health needs or prevent ill health (Webber et al., 2016).

Siloed systems

The siloed nature of service systems creates barriers to health care, such that practitioners in mainstream services may believe that all the needs of people with IDD should be catered for by disability service providers (Whittle et al., 2019). In Australia, this belief can be seen in the difficulties in accessing mental health services for people with IDD or lack of knowledge about services that are appropriate for them (Whittle et al., 2019). In other countries, such as the United Kingdom, IDD teams often work in community health services (Redley et al., 2012), and psychiatrists can access specific training in IDD (Torr, 2013). However, the existence of specialist professionals, as well as laws requiring equal access to services, do not seem to mitigate against inequities in access to quality and timely health care (Redley et al., 2012).

As people with IDD are living longer, they are more likely to need specialist geriatric health or dementia care services but, as with other mainstream services, they often experience difficulty in accessing them (Carling-Jenkins et al., 2012). Furthermore, the increasing incidence of age-related conditions can challenge disability services whose staff lack the skills required to support ageing service users (Araten-Bergman & Bigby, 2021; Iacono, Bigby,

Carling-Jenkins et al., 2014; Webber et al., 2016). Access to aged-care and dementia services also has been limited because of distrust by disability support workers (Iacono, Bigby, Carling-Jenkins et al., 2014; McCarron et al., 2010), and limited knowledge or willingness on the part of aged-care and dementia services to meet the needs of this group (McCarron et al., 2010).

Negative attitudes and stigma

People with IDD experience negative attitudes from health services providers and stigmatisation (Pelleboer-Gunnink et al., 2017). Some in the United Kingdom have argued that there is institutional discrimination in the national healthcare system (Cooper et al., 2011; Redley et al., 2012); widespread discrimination has also been seen in other countries (see Pelleboer-Gunnink et al., 2017). Negative attitudes of healthcare providers have put patients with IDD in hospitals at risk of poor outcomes, with the potential to contribute to premature deaths (Cooper et al., 2011; Mencap, 2007).

REFLECTION QUESTION

There is some controversy about the need for a specialist healthcare system for people with IDD versus provision of health care by mainstream providers. From a social inclusion perspective, what arguments can be made for mainstream health care for people with IDD?

SPOTLIGHT 18.2

Max

Max has Down syndrome and has lived in his group home for nine years, supported by disability support workers who know him well. Recently they have noticed that Max has lost interest in activities he usually enjoys and looks forward to, such as going ten-pin bowling on a Tuesday afternoon with others from his community day service, and shopping for the evening meal on a Friday, when it is his turn to choose the menu. Max has also become difficult to get out of bed in the morning, preferring to sleep late. The workers have also noticed that Max has become tentative in certain activities, requiring much coaxing and reassurance to do simple things like stepping into the shower. The house supervisor has made an appointment with Max's GP, who on hearing the concerns suggests that Max is showing signs of Alzheimer's disease. The GP has heard that people with Down syndrome more often than not develop this form of dementia early in life. However, the GP is not confident about making a firm diagnosis, and refers Max to a psychiatric clinic with expertise in IDD.

The psychiatrist who sees Max is sceptical that the changes are signs of dementia, given that he is only 35 years of age, around 15 years younger than when onset is usually seen in people with Down syndrome. She conducts a comprehensive medical examination, including a full blood test with a check of Max's thyroid function, and refers him to an ophthalmologist, as she notices that he is bumping into furniture in the clinic room and is very tentative when walking a long corridor. The psychiatrist's assessment also suggests possible mild to moderate depression, but she decides not to initiate any medications or other treatments until she has the results of the investigations.

The results of the various assessments indicate that Max's thyroid is underactive. In her letter to the GP, the psychiatrist recommends that Max be prescribed appropriate medication. Further, the ophthalmologist diagnoses cataracts in both eyes, and books surgery to have them removed. The psychiatrist sees Max for a review appointment six months after his surgery. By then, the signs of depression have disappeared, and the support workers report that Max is again interested in activities and is much more 'his old self'.

QUESTIONS
1 Why did the GP attribute Max's symptoms to early onset dementia?
2 What was the GP's diagnosis an example of?

Creating a responsive healthcare system

In the United Kingdom, Canada, the United States and Australia, legal and policy reform have provided the impetus for health care and support services to provide reasonable adjustments to ensure responsiveness to the needs of people with IDD; an effort to reduce their health inequities and thereby improve their quality of life. In Australia, there is a policy expectation that 'all health service providers have the capabilities to meet the needs of people with disability' (Commonwealth of Australia, 2011, p. 60). Reform of the disability service system through the National Disability Insurance Scheme (NDIS) and the National Disability Strategy is exerting additional pressure on mainstream services to make reasonable adjustments to ensure equality for people with IDD and to comply with international treaty obligations under the United Nations *Convention on the Rights of People with Disabilities* (United Nations, 2008).

Primary health care

Strategies to systematically improve responsiveness have been conceptualised in various ways. In respect of primary health care, Lennox and colleagues (2015) organised strategies under three broad groupings: regular health checks, support for primary healthcare professionals and system-level changes. Annual health checks, with prompts to guide practitioners to check for known risk factors and areas of health inequities (Lennox et al., 2015), have been policy in the United Kingdom since 2008 (Glover, 2015). Increased rates of health screening, health promotion and identification of conditions, including those considered life-threatening, which had previously been undetected, have been seen (Lennox et al., 2015). Support for primary healthcare professionals has been available in some Australian states through IDD academic and clinical centres that provide curriculum and training in undergraduate medical programs (Koritsas et al., 2012). System-level changes, such as addition of IDD specialists in secondary healthcare systems or extended consultation fees for patients with IDD, have also been implemented. However, this latter strategy was found to result in only limited uptake by GPs in Australia (Koritsas et al., 2012). Recently, the Australian government launched a 10-year plan of supports to GPs through primary care networks (Department of Health, 2019), but the success of this mainstream strategy will, as with past initiatives, rely on uptake by GPs.

Hospitals

In the context of hospital emergency departments, Lunsky and colleagues (2014) suggested three approaches to increasing responsiveness to people with IDD: improving recognition and identification of this group of patients; modifying the approach to care so it is more sensitive to their often-complex needs; and enhancing discharge processes and linkages to community care. Research in the United Kingdom into the use of Learning Disability Liaison Nurses (LDLNs) by MacArthur and colleagues (2015) demonstrated their value in supporting reasonable adjustments in positive outcomes for patients and their carers.

Other suggested reasonable adjustments include providing information tailored to the needs of people with IDD (MacArthur et al., 2015), such as through incorporating symbols and photos (Friese & Ailey, 2015); creating physical environments that are safe (e.g. free of noise, which can cause severe anxiety) and accessible (Friese & Ailey, 2015); and including carers and families in care processes and planning transitions across health services, such as through hospital discharge plans (Bigby et al., 2018).

A change in attitude

Promoting positive attitudes among service providers is key to ensuring a responsive health-care and support system. Despite widespread and systematic discrimination (Pelleboer-Gunnink et al., 2017), positive attitudes and willingness to support people with IDD have been found (Bigby et al., 2018; Smith & Laurence, 2021). In their recent Australian study of the hospital experiences of people with IDD, Bigby and colleagues (2018) found some hospital staff were skilled in accommodating the needs of this group, reflecting the application of general principles of good patient-centred care. Also evident were collaboration between hospital staff, disability support workers and family members. Problems found, however, were that such attempts at accommodation were inconsistent, and hospital staff often had little understanding of the role of families or disability support workers in the lives of people with IDD. These findings suggest a need for systemic attention to support and share good practice and reciprocal understanding between service systems, and between these systems and families. Inclusion of IDD in medical curriculum and providing opportunities for interacting with people with IDD during training can also engender more positive attitudes and greater understanding of the healthcare needs of people with IDD (Trollor et al., 2018).

SPOTLIGHT 18.3

Treating Annabel's foot wound

Annabel is aged 26 years and has a high tolerance for pain, which can result in delays by family and paid support workers in seeking medical care. Recently, she stepped on glass that was embedded in sand during an outing to the beach. The glass was stuck in her foot, but no bleeding was evident. Two days later, the support worker noticed redness and swelling under Annabel's foot and made an appointment with her GP. The practice had come to know Annabel and her needs that related to having intellectual disability and autism. She was given an appointment, but there was going to be a wait of 4 hours. In the meantime, a practice nurse rang the house and obtained details about the problem. The nurse realised that Annabel had a foreign object in her foot and should not walk, and was worried about possible infection. She organised for an ambulance to take Annabel to the local emergency department (ED). The nurse notified the ED of Annabel's needs, including to take her immediately to a quiet room as noisy and unfamiliar environments cause her severe anxiety and can make assessment and treatment difficult. The support worker accompanied Annabel, bringing along a soft cloth that Annabel liked to hold over her face when anxious. Upon arriving at the ED, Annabel was escorted directly into a small, quiet room. A nurse took her temperature and blood pressure. Annabel was soon seen by the registrar, who spoke gently, telling her that he was going to remove the glass. He sat for a few minutes chatting, and when he felt that she was calm asked her if it was okay for him to take the glass out of her foot, pointing to her foot as he spoke. The support worker sat with Annabel and talked gently to her during the procedure, and Annabel placed her cloth over her face. When the glass had been removed and the wound dressed, the support worker gently removed the cloth to show Annabel that the doctor had finished, and they could go home.

QUESTION

Can you list the reasonable adjustments made by the various service providers to support Annabel's care?

SUMMARY

This chapter has discussed the health of people with intellectual and developmental disabilities. By now, you would have learnt about the health issues that these individuals deal with in their everyday lives and within society. The salient issues are summarised here.

Learning objective 1: Describe the health inequities of people with intellectual and developmental disabilities.

People with IDD experience health inequities in terms of high rates of comorbid and secondary health conditions, poor access to quality and timely health care, and little participation in health promotion activities.

Learning objective 2: Explain the effects of health inequities on people with intellectual and developmental disabilities.

The effects of these health inequities include premature death, frequent hospitalisations and poor quality of life.

Learning objective 3: Identify contributors to the health inequities for this group.

Contributors to the health inequities experienced by people with IDD can include their underlying impairments, which may give rise to particular health risks or conditions. These problems can be managed or their effects reduced by addressing negative social determinants, including social and economic disadvantage; problematic attitudes of healthcare providers and society more broadly; and limited knowledge and negative attitudes by healthcare providers, which in turn are exacerbated by policy barriers that create service silos. In these ways, people with IDD can access and benefit from services available to other members of the community.

Learning objective 4: Identify strategies that can be adopted by health and human service professionals to reduce health inequities.

Several strategies can reduce health inequities experienced by people with IDD, largely through reasonable adjustments by service providers to meet their needs. To increase the potential for reasonable adjustments to be made, service providers need to be willing to develop an understanding of their needs and implement strategies.

TUTORIAL EXERCISES

1   Consider a situation in which you required the service of a healthcare provider. Were you satisfied with the service you received? If yes, what contributed to your satisfaction; if no, what contributed to your dissatisfaction?
2   Consider a person with IDD with limited communication skills attending the same healthcare provider, for the same reason. What reasonable adjustments do you think the person would require?
3   In light of your responses, how would you describe reasonable adjustments by healthcare providers?
4   How could addressing the health needs of people with IDD serve to improve health care for everyone?
5   How do the health inequities experienced by people with IDD compare with those experienced by other groups?

FURTHER READING

Bigby, C., Douglas, J., & Iacono, T. (2018). *Enabling mainstream systems to be more inclusive and responsive to people with disabilities: Hospital encounters of adults with cognitive disabilities report for the national disability research and development agenda*. Retrieved https://www.latrobe.edu.au/__data/assets/pdf_file/0004/1188760/Final-Report.pdf

Emerson, E., Baines, S., Allerton, L., & Welch, V. (2011). *Health inequalities & people with learning disabilities in the UK: 2011*. Improving Health and Lives: Learning Disabilities Observatory. Retrieved https://www.basw.co.uk/system/files/resources/basw_14846-4_0.pdf

NDIS Quality and Safeguards Commission (2021). Evidence summaries: Medications used for behaviours of concern in people with autism. Retrieved https://www.ndiscommission.gov.au/resources#evidence

Salomon, C., & Trollor, J. (2019). *A scoping review of causes and contributors to deaths of people with disability in Australia*. NDIS Quality and Safeguards Commission. Retrieved https://www.ndiscommission.gov.au/document/1881

REFERENCES

Araten-Bergman, T., & Bigby, C. (2021). Aging in place in group homes, an Australian context. In M. Putnam, & C. Bigby (Eds.), *Handbook of aging and disability* (pp. 334–46). Routledge.

Beange, H., McElduff, A., & Baker, W. (1995). Medical disorders of adults with mental retardation: A population study. *American Journal on Mental Retardation, 99*(6), 595–604.

Bigby, C. (2008). Known well by no-one: Trends in the informal social networks of middle-aged and older people with intellectual disability five years after moving to the community. *Journal of Intellectual & Developmental Disability, 33*(2), 148–57.

Bigby, C., Douglas, J., & Iacono, T. (2018). *Enabling mainstream systems to be more inclusive and responsive to people with disabilities: Hospital encounters of adults with cognitive disabilities report for the national disability research and development agenda*. Retrieved https://www.latrobe.edu.au/__data/assets/pdf_file/0004/1188760/Final-Report.pdf

Bittles, A. H., Bower, C., Hussain, R., & Glasson, E. J. (2006). The four ages of down syndrome. *European Journal of Public Health, 17*(2), 221–25.

Bossink, L. W. M., van der Putten, A. A. J., & Vlaskamp, C. (2017). Understanding low levels of physical activity in people with intellectual disabilities: A systematic review to identify barriers and facilitators. *Research in Developmental Disabilities, 68*, 95–110.

Bourke, J., Nembhard, W. N., Wong, K., & Leonard, H. (2017). Twenty-five year survival of children with intellectual disability in Western Australia. *Journal of Pediatrics, 188*, 232–39.

Butterworth, J., Smith, F., Hall, A., Migliore, A., Winsor, J., Domin, D., & Timmons, J. (2013). *Statedata: The national report on employment services and outcomes*. Institute for Community Inclusion, University of Massachusetts Boston. Retrieved https://book.statedata.info/12/

Carling-Jenkins, R., Torr, J., Iacono, T., & Bigby, C. (2012). People with down syndrome and alzheimer's disease in aged care and family environments. *Journal of Intellectual and Developmental Disability, 37* (1), 30–40.

Commonwealth of Australia. (2011). *National disability strategy 2010–2020*. Author.

Cooper, S.-A., Hughes-McCormack, L., Greenlaw, N., McConnachie, A., Allan, L., Baltzer, M., . . . Morrison, J. (2018). Management and prevalence of long-term conditions in primary health care for adults with intellectual disabilities compared with the general population: A population-based cohort study. *Journal of Applied Research in Intellectual Disabilities, 31*, 68–81.

Cooper, S. A., McConnachie, A., Allan, L., Melville, C., Smiley, E., & Morrison, J. (2011). Neighbourhood deprivation, health inequalities and service acces by adults with intellectual disabilities: A cross-sectional study. *Journal of Intellectual Disability Research*, *55*(3), 313–23.

Cooper, S. A., McLean, G., Guthrie, B., McConnachie, A., Mercer, S., Sullivan, F., & Morrison, J. (2015). Multiple physical and mental health comorbidity in adults with intellectual disabilities: Population-based cross-sectional analysis. *BMC Family Practice*, *16*, 110.

Department of Health. (2019). *National roadmap for improving the health of Australians with intellectual disability*. Australian Government.

Doherty, A. J., Atherton, H., Boland, P., Hastings, R., Hives, L., Hood, K., James-Jenkinson, L., Leavey, R., . . . Chauhan, U. (2020). Barriers and facilitators to primary health care for people with intellectual disabilities and/or autism: An integrative review. *BJGP Open*, *4*(3).

Emerson, E., Baines, S., Allerton, L., & Welch, V. (2011). *Health inequalities & people with learning disabilities in the UK: 2011*. Retrieved http://www.improvinghealthandlives.org.uk/

Emerson, E., & Hatton, C. (2007). Socioeconomic disadvantage, social participation and self-rated health of English men and women with mild and moderate intellectual disabilities: Cross sectional survey. *European Journal of Public Health*, *18*(1), 31–7.

Emerson, E., Hatton, C., Robertson, J., & Baines, S. (2014). Perceptions of neighbourhood quality, social and civic participation and the self rated health of British adults with intellectual disability: Cross sectional study. *BMC Public Health*, *14*(1), 1252.

Florio, T., & Trollor, J. (2015). Mortality among a cohort of persons with an intellectual disability in new south wales, Australia. *Journal of Applied Research in Intellectual Disabilities*, *28*(5), 383–93.

Friese, T., & Ailey, S. (2015). Specific standards of care for adults with intellectual disabilities. *Nursing Management*, *22*(1), 32–7.

Gjermestad, A., Luteberget, L., Midjo, T., & Witsø, A. E. (2017). Everyday life of persons with intellectual disability living in residential settings: A systematic review of qualitative studies. *Disability & Society*, *32*(2), 213–32.

Glover, G. (2015). Numbers and policy in care for people with intellectual disability in the United Kingdom [Review]. *Journal of Applied Research in Intellectual Disabilities*, *28*(1), 12–21.

Glover, G., Williams, R., Heslop, P., Oyinlola, J., & Grey, J. (2017). Mortality in people with intellectual disabilities in England. *Journal of Intellectual Disability Research*, *61*(1), 62–74.

Hussain, R., Wark, S., Janicki, M. P., Parmenter, T., & Knox, M. (2020). Multimorbidity in older people with intellectual disability. *Journal of Applied Research in Intellectual Disabilities*, *33*(6), 1234–44.

Iacono, T., Bigby, C., Carling-Jenkins, R., & Torr, J. (2014). 'Taking each day as it comes': Staff experiences of supporting people with down syndrome and alzheimer's disease in group homes *Journal of Intellectual Disability Research*, *58*(6), 521–33.

Iacono, T., Bigby, C., Douglas, J., & Spong, J. (2020). A prospective study of hospital episodes of adults with intellectual disability. *Journal of Intellectual Disability Research*, *64*(5), 357–67.

Iacono, T., Bigby, C., Unsworth, C., Douglas, J., & Fitzpatrick, P. (2014a). A systematic review of hospital experiences of people with intellectual disability. *BMC Health Services Research*, *14*(1), 505.

——(2014b). A systematic review of hospital experiences of people with intellectual disability. *BMC Health Services Research*, *14*(505).

Iacono, T., & Sutherland, G. (2006). Health screening and developmental disability. *Journal of Policy and Practice in Intellectual Disabilities*, *3*, 155–163.

Kappelides, P., Bould, E., & Bigby, C. (2021). Barriers to physical activity and sports participation for people with intellectual disabilities from culturally and linguistically diverse backgrounds [ePub]. *Research and Practice in Intellectual and Developmental Disabilities*, *8*(2), 157–69.

Koritsas, S., & Iacono, T. (2011). Secondary conditions in people with developmental disabilities. *American Journal on Intellectual and Developmental Disabilities*, *116*(1), 36–47.

Koritsas, S., Iacono, T., & Davis, R. (2012). Australian general practitioner uptake of a remunerated medicare health assessment for people with intellectual disability. *Journal of Intellectual & Developmental Disability, 37*(2), 151–4.

Lennox, N., Driel, M. v., & Dooren, K. v. (2015). Supporting primary healthcare professionals to care for people with intellectual disability: A research agenda. *Journal of Applied Research in Intellectual Disabilities, 28,* 33–42.

Lunsky, Y., Lake, J. K., Durbin, J., Perry, A., Bullock, H., Morris, S., & Lee, J. S. (2014). Understanding and improving care for individuals with intellectual and developmental disabilities in the emergency department. *International Review of Research in Developmental Disabilities, 47,* 1–37.

MacArthur, J., Brown, M., McKechanie, A., Mack, S., Hayes, M., & Fletcher, J. (2015). Making reasonable and achievable adjustments: The contributions of learning disability liaison nurses in 'getting it right' for people with learning disabilities receiving general hospitals care. *Journal of Advanced Nursing, 71*(7), 1552–63.

McCarron, M., McCallion, P., Fahey-McCarthy, E., Connaire, K., & Dunn-Lane, J. (2010). Supporting persons with down syndrome and advanced dementia: Challenges and care concerns. *Dementia, 9*(2), 285–98.

McMahon, M., Hatton, C., & Bowring, D. L. (2020). Polypharmacy and psychotropic polypharmacy in adults with intellectual disability: A cross-sectional total population study. *Journal of Intellectual Disability Research, 64*(11), 834–51.

Mencap. (2007). *Death by indifference: Following up the treat me right! Report.*

Michael, J., & Richardson, A. (2008). Healthcare for all: Report of the independent inquiry into access to healthcare for people with learning disabilities. *Tizard Learning Disability Review, 13*(4), 28–34.

Motegi, N., Morisaki, N., Suto, M., Tamai, H., Mori, R., & Nakayama, T. (2021). Secular trends in longevity among people with down syndrome in Japan, 1995-2016. *Pediatrics International, 63*(1), 94–101.

Naaldenberg, J., Kuijken, N., van Dooren, K., & H. (2013). Topics, methods and challenges in health promotion for people with intellectual disabilities: A structured review of literature. *Research in Developmental Disabilities, 34,* 4534–45.

NDIS Quality and Safeguards Commission. (2021). *Evidence review: Antipsychotics for behaviours of concern in children, adolescents and adults with autism.* Retrieved https://www.ndiscommission.gov.au/document/3136

Pelleboer-Gunnink, H. A., Van Oorsouw, W., Van Weeghel, J., & Embregts, P. (2017). Mainstream health professionals' stigmatising attitudes towards people with intellectual disabilities: A systematic review [Review]. *Journal of Intellectual Disability Research, 61*(5), 411–44.

Phillips, A., Morrison, J., & Davis, R. W. (2004). General practitioners' educational needs in intellectual disability health. *Journal of Intellectual Disability Research, 48*(2), 142–149.

Redley, M., Banks, C., Fopody, K., & Holland, A. (2012). Healthcare for men and women with learning disabilities: Understanding inequalities in access. *Disability & Society, 27*(6), 747–59.

Robertson, J., Hatton, C., Baines, S., & Emerson, E. (2015). Systematic reviews of the health or health care of people with intellectual disabilities: A systematic review to identify gaps in the evidence base. *Journal of Applied Research in Intellectual Disabilities, 28*(6), 455–523.

Salomon, C., & Trollor, J. (2019). *A scoping review of causes and contributors to deaths of people with disability in Australia.* NDIS Quality and Safeguards Commission. Retrieved https://www.ndiscommission.gov.au/document/1881

Scott, H. M., & Havercamp, S. M. (2016). Systematic review of health promotion programs focused on behavioral changes for people with intellectual disability [Review]. *Intellectual & Developmental Disabilities, 54*(1), 63–76.

Shooshtari, S., Ouellette-Kuntz, H., Balogh, R., McIsaac, M., Stankiewicz, E., Dik, N., & Burchill, C. (2020). Patterns of mortality among adults with intellectual and developmental disabilities in the Canadian province of Manitoba. *Journal of Policy and Practice in Intellectual Disabilities*, *17*(3), 270–8.

Smith, J. J., & Laurence, C. O. (2021). Attitudes and experiences of general practitioners who provided health care for people with intellectual disabilities: A South Australian perspective. *Research and Practice in Intellectual and Developmental Disabilities*, *8*(1), 25–36.

Stanley, F., Blair, E., & Alberman, E. (2000). *Cerebral palsies: Epidemiology and causal pathways* (Vol. 151). Cambridge University Press.

Therapeutic Guidelines. (2012). *Management guidelines: Developmental disability* (3rd ed.). Therapautic Guidelines Ltd.

Torr, J. (2013). Intellectual disability and mental ill health: A view of Australian research. *Journal of Mental Health Research in Intellectual Disabilities*, *62*(2), 159–78.

Torr, J., & Davis, R. (2007). Ageing and mental health problems in people with intellectual disabilities. *Current Opinion in Psychiatry*, *20*, 467–71.

Trollor, J., Eagleson, C., Turner, B., Tracy, J., Torr, J. J., Durvasula, S., . . . Lennox, N. (2018). Intellectual disability content within tertiary medical curriculum: How is it taught and by whom? *BMC Medical Education*, *18*(1), 182.

Trollor, J., & Salomon, C. (2016). Unnecessary psychotropic drug prescription in primary care for people with intellectual disability [Comment]. *Evidence-Based Mental Health*, *19*(2), 62.

Trollor, J., Srasuebkul, P., Xu, H., & Howlett, S. (2017). Cause of death and potentially avoidable deaths in australian adults with intellectual disability using retrospective linked data. *BMJ Open*, *7*(2), e013489.

Tuffrey-Wijne, I., Goulding, L., Giatras, N., Abraham, E., Gillard, S., White, S., Edwards, C., & Hollins, S. (2014). The barriers to and enablers of providing reasonably adusted health services to people with intellectual disabilities in acute hospitals: Evidence from a mixed methods study. *BMJ Open*, *4*, e004606.

United Nations. (2008). *Convention on the rights of persons with disabilities*. Retrieved http://www.Un.Org/disabilities/documents/convention/convoptprot-e.Pdf

Vander Ploeg Booth, K. (2011). Health disparities and intellectual disabilities: Lessons from individuals with down syndrome. *Developmental Disabilities Research Reviews*, *17*, 32–35.

Webber, R., Bowers, B., & Bigby, C. (2016). Confidence of group home staff in supporting the health needs of older residents with intellectual disability. *Journal of Intellectual & Developmental Disability*, *41*(2), 107–114.

Weise, J., Pollack, A., Britt, H., & Trollor, J. N. (2017). Primary health care for people with an intellectual disability: An exploration of consultations, problems identified, and their management in Australia. *Journal of Intellectual Disability Research*, *61*(5), 399–410.

Whittle, E. L., Fisher, K. R., Reppermund, S., & Trollor, J. (2019). Access to mental health services: The experiences of people with intellectual disabilities. *Journal of Applied Research in Intellectual Disabilities*, *32*(2), 368–79.

Wiesel, I., & Bigby, C. (2014). Being recognised and becoming known: Encounters between people with and without intellectual disability in the public realm. *Environment and Planning A: Economy and Space*, *46*(7), 1754–69.

Wiesel, I., Whitzman, C., Gleeson, B., & Bigby, C. (2019). The national disability insurance scheme in an urban context: Opportunities and challenges for Australian cities. *Urban Policy and Research*, *37*(1), 1–12.

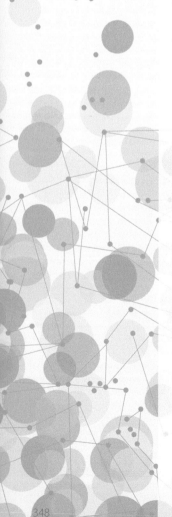

19

The health of indigenous peoples

Sharon Chirgwin and Diane Walker

Acknowledgements to Heather D'Antoine for contribution to the second edition.

LEARNING OBJECTIVES

After studying this chapter, you should be able to:

1 describe the factors that influence the health of indigenous peoples, using a public health framework
2 identify the factors that make indigenous peoples' health extremely complex in today's world
3 identify the characteristics of programs that have led to improvements in the health of indigenous peoples.

VIGNETTE

Voluntary isolation during COVID-19

When the COVID-19 pandemic swept through the world, isolation in the form of lockdown of whole communities was used by governments as a preventative measure in a range of ways. For example, all citizens of Wuhan and the Hubei province of China, where the virus was first identified, were subjected to 76 days of compulsory rigorous lockdown. Individual responses to the threat of the pandemic varied across the world according to worldview, education and sources of information.

On the advice of their leaders, selected indigenous peoples who had access to traditionally owned land chose to remove themselves and their families to more remote areas. This strategy was adopted, for example, by the Siekopai in Ecuador, the Navajo in the United States and the Rarotonga in the Cook Islands (Hausen, 2020).

Why did some indigenous groups seek this voluntary isolation? Even before the pandemic, indigenous peoples around the world were facing threats to their health, and many leaders of indigenous communities were aware that the pandemic could be one additional threat that some groups would not survive.

Introduction

Public health aims to limit avoidable disease, injury, disability and death in populations through preventative strategies (Public Health Association of Australia [PHAA], 2018). But the development of strategies cannot occur until the nature and extent of any issue is first identified and analysed, and research is carried out to identify causes. A public health framework involves an assessment of the roles of a range of non-health factors, known as social determinants, in the issue under consideration.

This chapter identifies the preventable health issues faced by indigenous people throughout the world before discussing some of the underlying determinants that make the causes of these issues extremely complex. While this may seem to be a 'deficits approach', and one frequently criticised by indigenous people, these initial steps are necessary because they provide a basis for a better understanding of what needs to be addressed, and the strategies that work, and why; these provide context for the success of programs identified in the final section. As we progress through the chapter, it should be apparent that indigenous people are best placed to find their own solutions and are beginning to do so, as the vignette at the start of this chapter illustrates.

Factors influencing the health of indigenous peoples of the world

Indigenous peoples – the descendants of the original inhabitants of a country or area who generally self-identify, are accepted by their community and have historical continuity with pre-colonial societies.

Before exploring indigenous health from a global perspective, it is first necessary to consider who the **indigenous peoples** of the world are. According to the United Nations (UN), there is no singular, authoritative definition for indigenous peoples (UN, 2013), but a range of characteristics distinguish indigenous peoples from other cultural groups where they live. A characteristic that is common to all is having a strong connection to their traditional lands, which in turn results in a strong sense of stewardship of its resources (Burgess et al., 2009; Lewis et al., 2020).

According to the United Nations Educational, Scientific and Cultural Organization (UNESCO, 2019) there are some 370 to 500 million indigenous peoples in the world, occupying 22 per cent of the global land mass. UNESCO also identifies that indigenous peoples represent the greater part of the world's cultural diversity and speak the major share of the world's 7000 languages. While it has taken a long time for recognition, indigenous peoples' traditional knowledge about the medicinal benefits of many plants, clays and other phenomena in the natural environment has resulted in a range of life-changing pharmaceuticals throughout the world. Their traditional approaches to environmental sustainability have been adopted globally in agriculture and land management (Lewis et al., 2020).

While indigenous peoples speak different languages, live on different continents and their traditional healers may have different approaches to healing, there is a commonality in their concept of wellbeing and health: that these are founded on a holistic approach (Commission on Social Determinants of Health [CSDH], 2008), which takes in the spectrum of spiritual, physical and cultural factors and in which all groups regard their maintenance of connection to land as essential to individual and community wellbeing.

Finally, a note on the use of the word 'indigenous'. The United Nations Permanent Forum on Indigenous Issues (n.d.) notes that for some, the term may have very negative connotations because of colonial-era policies and actions, and so many may not readily reveal or define their origin. Alternatively, some may prefer to be called by traditional names such as Adivasi, Janajati, Navajo or Māori. But preferences may also exist for broader groupings. For example, in Canada, indigenous peoples frequently prefer to be called 'First Nations people', while in Australia terms commonly used by individuals and organisations include 'Aboriginal and Torres Strait Islander' (Lowitja Institute, 2021), 'Aboriginal', 'Indigenous' and 'First Nations'. It is important to respect how individuals and communities choose to be identified.

A global snapshot of indigenous health

The fact that there is no singular, authoritative definition for indigenous peoples has been recognised as one of the challenges in collecting accurate and truly representative data about the state of indigenous health globally (Chino et al., 2019). The best data available comes from those countries with well-developed statistical systems, such as Australia, Canada, Aotearoa New Zealand and the United States (Chino et al., 2019). Health data collected in Canada, for example, identifies that when compared to the broader population, indigenous peoples (including those who identify as First Nations, Métis and Inuit) have elevated rates of:

- infant and child mortality
- infectious diseases
- malnutrition
- accidents
- suicide
- obesity
- cardiovascular disease

- diabetes
- diseases caused by environmental contamination (Lines & Jardine, 2019).

Despite the lack of reliable data from many of the countries where indigenous groups live, recent research reviewing the health and wellbeing of one million indigenous peoples in the Arctic regions (Young et al., 2020) and the summary of the health of indigenous peoples in Mexico (Pelcastre-Villafuerte et al., 2020) indicates that many indigenous groups throughout the world face similar health issues. Likewise, although there have been recent improvements in some areas in Australia (Lowitja Institute, 2021) and Aotearoa New Zealand (Ministry of Health, 2019; Nelson et al., 2021) similar gaps persist.

At first glance, the health issues listed above may seem to have quite different causes; some from specific organisms (pathogens), some from poor nutrition, others from environmental factors. However, the poor physical, mental and spiritual health of indigenous peoples throughout the world has its foundation in changes that occurred to their way of life when their countries were colonised. Present-day factors beyond their control also effects in addition to historical factors. These include the changing social, economic and political environments in which they live, and the lack of appreciation by policymakers of very different and sometimes diverse worldviews on what constitutes good health and what is required to sustain it.

SPOTLIGHT 19.1

Who are the Métis?

There are innumerable indigenous groups throughout the world whose names immediately associate them with the countries or areas of countries in which they live. For example, the Navajo with the United States, the Bantu with sub-Saharan Africa and the Māori with New Zealand. The Métis in Canada and the United States, however, have an indigenous status that is not as straightforward.

During colonisation of northern America in the 1700s, French and Scottish fur traders married indigenous women, which resulted in successive generations of people with both indigenous and European ancestry. These descendants have developed their own distinct cultures and collective nationhoods, although they inhabit three Prairie Provinces as well as parts of Ontario, British Columbia, the Northwest Territories and northern United States (Government of Canada, 2020). With such a differing range of connections to Country, there has been confusion with respect to who can claim to be Métis. In response, the Canadian government introduced the Powley test in 2003, to provide some clear criteria. This was a modification of an earlier test (the Van der Peet test) constructed to define the aboriginal rights of Indians (Métis Nation of Ontario, 2021).

QUESTIONS

The YouTube video: *Who are the Métis?* https://youtu.be/qUKcxc6-IDA introduces two Métis people who have quite different views about who can claim to be Métis. Watch it and consider the following:

1   How do the views of these two people differ?
2   How might the controversy affect the health of a person who cannot clearly prove their identity as Métis?

The effects of social determinants on indigenous health

Determinant of health – a factor within and external to the individual that determines their health; the specific social, economic and political circumstances into which individuals are born and live.

The social **determinants of health** are the structural factors or conditions that influence health and wellbeing (Lowitja Institute, 2021, p. 10). They include the conditions into which a person is born, lives and works (see Chapter 7).

Two important social determinants that lead to inequities in a population are the socio-economic and political contexts of the country in which those people live. These are two determinants that have had, and continue to have, an effect on the health of indigenous peoples globally (WHO, 2010). Since they highlight how many of the health issues indigenous people face today were, and continue to be, beyond their control, these determinants are the focus of this section of the chapter.

Social determinant 1 – traditional indigenous health beliefs (cultural and societal values)

Colonisation – the occupation of a country or area, whereby the occupiers take control of the land, resources and original inhabitants.

Prior to **colonisation**, the indigenous peoples of Africa, Australasia and the Americas had developed an understanding about their dependence on their environment for food, cures and shelter; knowledge of these was passed through generations (Montenegro & Stephens, 2006). Since many peoples moved according to seasonal supply, they avoided many of the infectious diseases, like cholera and typhus, that were common in the countries that colonised them (Healey, 2014; Hendry, 2014). Most had also developed a strong spiritual relationship with their surroundings and an understanding of cyclical events in living and non-living systems. Since they also expended energy to source and prepare natural food and water, they had few of the lifestyle diseases so common today (Rush et al., 2010). Infectious diseases and injuries were treated with plant and mineral remedies that had been developed over thousands of years; knowledge frequently held by select members of the group.

REFLECTION QUESTIONS

1 The nomadic lifestyle is generally seen as less 'civilised' than living in one place in an urban setting. However, what would be some of the healthier, preventative aspects of this lifestyle?
2 There are indigenous groups in the world that try to maintain their traditional nomadic lifestyles, such as the San of Africa, but this often meets with barriers because of the socio-economic and political context of the country. Consider some of the possible barriers.

Globally, some of the 370 million indigenous people continue to hold traditional beliefs about health and wellbeing, even though a proportion have adopted to varying extents some of the beliefs of the dominant culture. Some traditional health beliefs include that:

• Health is not merely the absence of illness.
• Health is holistic, incorporating family, the land or place where a person was born and the spiritual aspect.
• Good health requires all interrelated factors to be in balance (Nelson et al., 2021; Stoner et al., 2015).

In terms of the *causes* of ill health, it is again necessary to acknowledge considerable diversity according to the group, the knowledge they are permitted to hold and their degree of acceptance of the beliefs of the dominant culture. But unlike the biomedical view commonly held in developed countries, causes can include factors that are grouped as 'natural', from diet and emotions to 'not participating in important cultural ceremony' (Vukic et al. , 2011) and a range of spiritual or supernatural causes (Senior & Chenhall, 2013).

Some of these views are therefore markedly different from those of the cultures that colonised indigenous peoples, and because of the failure to recognise this difference and instead work with indigenous peoples to accommodate their views, cultural differences represent one of the structural determinants that has contributed to health inequities.

SPOTLIGHT 19.2

Connections and Puntu health

For most indigenous peoples, good health relies on maintaining connections. For example, good health (or *palya*) for the Puntu people who live in the remote desert of the Kimberley region in Western Australia depends on maintaining connections between physical, spiritual and social aspects that all contribute to the 'whole', with the social connectedness aspect being of particular significance for Puntu men. They believe that there are two aspects to the body – the 'outer' physical body and the 'inner' personal self – and they are connected. Many of the features of the inner self only become inscribed upon the body after a boy is initiated, and the strands of social life are bought together and the deeper meaning of the connections between individuals are disclosed, and new connections are established and reinforced. After initiation, involvement in rituals reinforces these social connections, in turn reinforcing spiritual wellbeing. The social aspect is also important for Puntu women because they provide healing as a group through 'women's business', frequently utilising bush medicines and traditional treatments. Even though the modern Puntu are pragmatic and do access mainstream health resources for the treatment of illness and injury, their beliefs about the importance of connections underlie their attitude to health (adapted from McCoy, 2008).

QUESTIONS

1   How could the beliefs of male Puntu about health assist in developing public health programs in mental health?
2   Can you identify any similarities in the Puntu connection approach to health and the way in which public health is viewed more generally?

Social determinant 2 – historical, global, social and political contexts

When colonial powers took over former indigenous lands, dispossession, disease and the introduction of harmful substances caused more premature deaths than any initial violent resistance (MacDonald & Steenbeek, 2015). Colonial powers regarded land as a valuable resource, as theirs by right of conquest or because they considered that indigenous peoples did not legally exist (Gilbert, 2016). They forced indigenous peoples from their lands, resulting in loss of traditional indigenous rights to food-gathering, farming practices, and hunting and fishing.

Such displacement caused dietary changes, in turn contributing to malnutrition in many populations, and ensuing higher maternal and infant mortality. Those children who did survive frequently experienced an extremely poor start in life. In Canada, it became policy to force indigenous children into church-run boarding schools (Gregg, 2018), while in other countries, such as the United States and Australia, whole populations were relocated into missions and reservations, where they were given rations of colonisers' food. As this was not as balanced as the diets they had enjoyed prior to colonisation, it led to specific nutritional deficiencies (Sebastian & Donelly, 2013).

Colonisers also brought with them a range of diseases such as measles, smallpox and tuberculosis, which had never been common in indigenous communities. Because indigenous people had never been exposed to these diseases, and therefore had no inherited resistance to them, they contributed to large-scale premature death in indigenous communities. For example, it is estimated that in South America, 100 years after first European contact and the introduction of smallpox and measles, the indigenous population had decreased from up to 150 million to 11 million (Montenegro & Stephens, 2006). In North America, an estimated 90–95 per cent of the population died between 1700 and the early 1800s (Wesley-Esquimaux & Smolewski, cited in Nutton & Fast, 2015).

The mental health of indigenous peoples also suffered when they were displaced from the lands to which they had strong ties. For their land was not only a source that met their physical needs, but also a conduit to their ancestors and spiritual wellbeing. This conduit gave them a sense of one-ness and belonging, and nurtured a powerful spiritual self-transcendence that offered a sense of purpose and meaning to their lives, essential to their overall health and wellbeing (Tse et al., 2005). Their beliefs and cultural practices were, however, seen as primitive by the colonisers. This frequently meant that they were forced to hide or neglect their beliefs, languages and customs, causing further emotional and psychological distress that added to, and exacerbated, physical health issues (Nutton & Fast, 2015).

Colonisation by Europeans also introduced alcohol, tobacco and, in some instances, opium (Brady, 2002), even though most indigenous peoples had their own psychoactive substances that they used for a range of healing and religious rituals (Steinberg, Hobbs & Mathewson, 2004). The new substances introduced by the colonisers caused physical, social and psychological damage to the users, adding another health burden, and also had wider effects on families and whole communities (Gracey & King, 2009).

Social determinant 3 – governance

Governance – 'the evolving processes, relationships, institutions and structures by which a group of people, community or society organise themselves collectively to achieve things that matter to them' (Smith & Hunt, 2008, p. 9).

Prior to colonisation, indigenous groups, irrespective of where they lived, had their own systems of **governance** (Ford et al., 2012; Nikolakis et al., 2019). However, displacement from traditional lands was accompanied by disruption to and displacement of many traditional structures in societies, including traditional governance. As Badger (2011) describes, the colonial governance and policies in place on many continents denied indigenous peoples their voice and control over their own lives, so poverty and reliance on government handouts became the norm.

This colonial disempowerment and dependence had physical effects as well as lasting psychological effects. From the early 2000s, many former colonies recognised this and adopted the policy of working toward indigenous self-determination (Nikolakis et al., 2019). However, the psychological traumas that previous generations suffered due to their treatment remains a factor in indigenous health today.

SPOTLIGHT 19.3

Communal governance of land in the South Pacific: Is it appropriate in today's world?

The mention of South Pacific life conjures images of happy people in grass skirts singing and dancing against a background of swaying palm trees and bright-blue skies. Prior to colonisation, those who lived on most islands of the South Pacific would have enjoyed a reasonable standard of living, due to the nature of the resources on land or sea, something economists have labelled as **subsistence affluence**. They would have shared resources in a communal or traditional family manner, with no single person or organisation being the rightful owner of land or fishing rights. Colonial governance complicated this traditional sharing of resources, by introducing the idea that if you cleared the land to grow crops, then it became yours.

> **Subsistence affluence –** having a good standard of living with little cash but self-reliance, based on what you can catch, collect, grow or barter.

In the past few decades, however, things have changed quite rapidly, due to high population growth, rapidly monetising economies, migration to urban areas and land degradation. These changes have placed considerable pressure on decisions and considerations about who owns the land in many South Pacific states. Economists believe that current levels of consumption are far above sustainable subsistence levels, and some propose that there must be a movement away from customary ownership, in the interests of certainty, economic prosperity and sustainability (Larmour, 2013).

QUESTIONS

1   List some effects the 'rapid changes' may have had on the diets and hence the health of those peoples used to 'subsistence affluence'.

2   Will there be any other possible health effects from the uncertainty these changes have caused?

The complexities of indigenous health in today's world

The global snapshot of data on indigenous health reveals that, even though it is over 200 years since the colonial powers first caused major disruption to the lives of indigenous peoples, there are still gaps remaining between the health of indigenous peoples and non-indigenous peoples (Lines & Jardine, 2019). While many countries, such as Australia, Canada and Aotearoa New Zealand, have tried to address the 'gaps' between indigenous and non-indigenous health in their respective countries, as noted by Gracey (2019) they have failed because of 'complex, interrelated factors', which include 'entrenched socioeconomic disadvantage, low educational standards, underemployment, high-risk health behaviours, and marginalisation from mainstream society' (p. 218). While these are but a proportion of the social determinants that are interacting, it is now recognised that the changes that have occurred to the genetic make-up of indigenous peoples due to past and continuing traumas, and that the double burden of infectious and lifestyle diseases have to be added to the mix.

The continuing effects of past historical trauma on the genes of indigenous peoples

Since the 1960s, evidence has been accumulating that the effects of genocides such as the holocaust, colonisation, war and slavery have affected the survivors as well as their offspring (Lehrner & Yehuda, 2018). This manifestation of intergenerational trauma is now thought to be due to two components: changes in genetic material prior to conception, including sperm and eggs, and the family environment and parental behaviours (Lehrner & Yehuda, 2018).

As described already, colonisation drove a large proportion of indigenous peoples from their traditional lands. Those that resisted were either killed or treated as criminals, and introduced diseases resulted in widespread deaths. While the loss of loved ones and imprisonment and institutionalisation were also traumatic, the dispersal and ensuing loss of spiritual connection to traditional land added to the distress. Added to the list of distressing factors was the forced adoption of the colonisers' food, dress, language, laws and governance (Reid et al., 2019). Even today, government policies and systemic racism in many countries continue cumulatively to compound intergenerational trauma (O'Neill et al., 2018).

The double burden of infectious and lifestyle diseases

The displacement of indigenous peoples from their traditional lands due to colonisation had adverse effects on their diet, frequently resulting in diseases of malnutrition. However, indigenous groups also encountered new infectious diseases, which as highlighted previously, killed more of them than any of the violent conflicts with the colonial invaders (Montenegro & Stephens, 2006). Over time, as biomedical knowledge has improved, infectious diseases such as smallpox, measles, tuberculosis and influenza are no longer the major causes of morbidity and mortality in the wealthier countries of the world. These disease have been overtaken by other diseases related to lifestyle (Gulis, 2017). However, many of these infectious diseases are still rife among those indigenous peoples who live in countries that have been colonised, due to poverty and poor living conditions. At the same time, like non-indigenous populations, they have also begun to suffer diseases related to diet, substance abuse and lack of exercise: the 'lifestyle diseases' that have overtaken infectious diseases as the cause of death in most developed nations. In today's world, indigenous peoples therefore frequently may experience a double burden of infectious and lifestyle diseases.

Can these complexities be addressed?

Even though many governments have made attempts to address the state of the health of indigenous peoples in their countries, this has frequently involved singling out specific issues for attention by non-indigenous strategists who have not completely understood the underlying complexities. Successes, however, have been noted when the approach has not been based on a biomedical and deficit approach that sees indigenous health as a problem to be solved, but instead has adopted a strengths-based, holistic approach (Nelson et al., 2021). Success has also been noted when indigenous peoples have taken charge and delivered services to their people by incorporating indigenous knowledges and protocols in the holistic indigenous manner.

While these programs are most usually delivered at the community level, Reid and colleagues (2019, p. 122) suggest that progress will be limited until some of the primary causes of the complexities are addressed at government policy levels, both internationally and nationally. While they have listed 12 projects that must be implemented before indigenous health will improve, some of the relevant projects include:

- the identification of racism as a global health determinant
- the immediate cessation of assimilationist state policies and practices that are forms of cultural oppression
- the right for indigenous voices to be heard in any decision-making process that affects indigenous lives
- the right to self-determination by indigenous peoples over their food sovereignty, health systems and models of care.

Spotlight 19.4 discusses in more detail the strengths-based approach, which is the basis for success at the community level.

SPOTLIGHT 19.4

Strengths-based approaches

The strength-based approach is increasingly being used in indigenous health research and, most importantly, in the delivery of programs at community level. If this approach is adopted more widely, it is proposed that progress toward closing gaps should be measured quite differently.

Strengths-based approaches have been utilised in many more disciplines than public health since the 1990s. But while there are some very positive results when used in specific public health programs in both urban and remote settings, there remain paternalistic attitudes and issues of power that must be overcome before strength-based practices can be more widely adopted (Askew et al., 2020).

To clarify: a strengths-based approach requires that, instead of coming from a perspective of what is wrong or what is not working, the reverse should be the starting point; that is, what is right and what is working. For example, instead of saying that 60 per cent of a community smokes tobacco, the positive is that 40 per cent do not smoke tobacco.

Askew and colleagues (2020) have identified clear guiding principles for a strengths-basedapproach in public health programs with indigenous groups. These include that:

- People and the relationships between people should always be the focus.
- The service provider needs to relinquish the idea that they are in charge and know best, to enable the participants to drive the program.
- Blame for underlying causes should not be the focus.
- Wherever possible, pride in being indigenous should be fostered.

Finally, it is suggested that, instead of performing 'statistical stock-takes of indigenous bodies and populations' what should be measured is 'the progress in the delivery of power and control ... into the hands of indigenous (people)' (Phioli, 2009, cited in Askew et al., 2020, p. 105).

Characteristics of successful programs and approaches

Three successful programs from Australia, Canada and Aotearoa New Zealand outlined in this section are examples of strength-based approaches that are multi-sectorial in their approach, use diversified activities and are indigenous-led.

Program 1: An indigenous approach to primary health in remote Australia

Schultz and colleagues (2018) found that where many other non-indigenous primary health care programs had limited success, a multi-sectorial approach of indigenous land management in Australia involving Indigenous people from select remote areas to care for and manage their traditional homelands had a range of benefits on the health and wellbeing of participants. These included:

- a strengthening of identity, empowerment and spiritual uplift (improved mental health)
- greater access to healthier traditional foods (improved physical health)
- the provision of enjoyable physical exercise (improved physical health)
- an escape from communities in which there were high levels of substance abuse (improved mental, physical and social health).

Program 2: A youth mentoring program in Canada

A multi-layered indigenous youth mentoring program developed in Winnipeg, Canada has been so successful that it has been extended to over 20 communities across the country. Young adult indigenous health leaders mentor high school students, and the high school students are then supported to mentor primary students. The mentoring consists of three components:

- physical activities
- cultural activities
- a healthy snack.

The program has become one of the most enjoyable parts of the week for many of the students, and it has also improved their emotional and mental wellbeing, built lasting relationships and leadership, improved nutritional knowledge and reduced the participants' waist circumference and body mass index (BMI), forming the basis for a healthier transition into adulthood (Ferguson et al., 2021).

Program 3: A whānau ora approach to health in Aotearoa New Zealand

Gifford and colleagues (2021) examined three successful programs in Māori communities that involved a program for young mothers, a community health well-being program and a service provider addressing chronic conditions. They found that the secret to the programs' success was a whānau ora, or a traditional Māori approach, which utilised the strengths in extended families. In all cases, priority was given to relationship-building before clinical intervention. After the relationships were established, the equal partners co-designed interventions that allowed for greater flexibility, and fewer time constraints. This resulted in greater commitment to, and uptake of, programs. This whānau ora approach has been adopted and become the driving force behind seven principles that identify the responsibilities of both the Māori people and the government when social and health services are delivered. According to Gifford and colleagues (2021), this approach 'has moved beyond being the ambulance at the bottom of the cliff to building a fence at the top' (p. 303).

Strengths-based approaches and the media

A final word about the presentation of strength-based solutions. Reporting successes receives less attention from the media than failures, so the deficit-based approach to reporting indigenous health 'problems' is still common (Hyett et al., 2019). Accordingly, while researchers have a role to play in improving indigenous health by investigating and highlighting what works, the media must report more positive outcomes. Promoting what can be achieved has the potential to engender optimism in indigenous people, encourage greater uptake of the approach and faster movement toward health parity.

SUMMARY

It is hoped that, as you have read this chapter, you have gained an understanding of the poor health that is a reality for so many indigenous peoples throughout the world and the complexity of the factors that underpin it, and that you have a more positive perspective on what can be done to improve indigenous health. Change will come with a strengths-based approach and will enable indigenous people steer us in the right directions.

Learning objective 1: Describe the factors that influence the health of indigenous peoples, using a public health framework.
While many determinants, such as socio-economic status, have their origins in historical and political events that occurred several generations ago, including displacement from traditional country and dispossession from resources, determinants such as governance and the nature of the health system can also be influential, as are racism, both institutionalised and personal. Key non-clinical factors therefore include poor physical conditions, such as where and how people live, and their nutrition, and also the emotional scars from a combination of injustices and lack of control over their lives that may lead to substance abuse.

Learning objective 2: Identify the factors that make indigenous peoples' health extremely complex in today's world.
Over the past two decades, post-colonial governments have allocated money and implemented programs to address many of the inequities in indigenous health, with limited improvements. This chapter has proposed that this is because in today's world indigenous health is complex, with several factors interacting. These factors include indigenous beliefs about health and illness, the continuing effects of trauma through generations, the living conditions that contribute to high rates of infectious diseases that are no longer a threat for the bulk of the population in affluent countries, and the changes to lifestyle and food that have led to additional burdens of chronic disease.

Learning objective 3: Identify the characteristics of programs that have led to improvements in the health of indigenous peoples.
While indigenous health may be complex, analysing the characteristics of programs that have been successful can provide some clues about how to tackle the complexities. In each of the three programs described in this chapter, the programs were delivered 'on the ground' in a local context, with appropriate local indigenous support, and have depended on the development of relationships. Thus, the characteristics of successful programs can be summarised by four words beginning with 'r': respect, reconciliation, relevance and relationships. In the first instance, there should be respect for indigenous knowledge and worldviews, and reconciliation of those views in an equal manner with non-indigenous. Similarly, they should also have local relevance by tailoring programs to the beliefs and needs of a specific indigenous group, and wherever possible they should utilise pre-existing relationships and have visible support from respected indigenous leaders.

TUTORIAL EXERCISES

1   Upon completion of this chapter, it is important that you reflect on what researchers call 'unconscious bias', with respect to people different from you . To first understand the basis for unconscious bias, go to the unconscious bias quiz (https://fsae.memberclicks.net/assets/DEI/Quiz-Unconcsious%20Bias.pdf) and complete the 10 short-answer questions (answers are provided).

2   If you were required to work with a specific group of indigenous people (even in an urban situation) on a health program, what should you find out even before any planning or interaction has occurred?

3   According to Reid and colleagues (2019), 'interventions for addressing health equity for indigenous peoples predominantly focus on purported risk factors at the person level and on changing indigenous behaviours rather than changing the unequal social and structural pre-conditions of those behaviours' (p. 123). What are the 'unequal social and structural preconditions'? What is necessary for major changes in these areas?

FURTHER READING

ANTaR. (2007). *Success stories in Indigenous health*. Retrieved https://antar.org.au/stories/success-stories-indigenous-health-a-showcase-successful-aboriginal-and-torres-strait

Godden, N. J. (2021). Community work, love and the indigenous worldview of buen vivir in Peru. *International Social Work, 64*(3), 354–70.

Hatala, A. R, Njeze, C., Morton, D., Pearl, T., & Bird-Naytowhow, K. (2020). Land and nature as sources of health and resilience among Indigenous youth in an urban Canadian context: a photovoice exploration. *BMC Public Health, 20*(1), 538.

Johnson, D., Parsons, M., & Fisher, K. (2021). Engaging Indigenous perspectives on health, wellbeing and climate change. A new research agenda for holistic climate action in Aotearoa and beyond. *Local Environment, 26*(4), 477–503.

REFERENCES

Askew, D. A., Brady, K., Mukandi, B., Singh, D., Sinha, T., Brough, M., & Bond, C. (2020). Closing the gap between rhetoric and practice in strengths-based approaches to Indigenous public health: a qualitative study. *Australian and New Zealand Journal of Public Health., 44*(2) 102–5.

Badger, A. (2011). Collective v. individual human rights in membership governance for indigenous peoples. *American University International Law Review, 26(2),* 485–514.

Brady, M. (2002). Health inequalities: Historical and cultural roots of tobacco use among Aboriginal and Torres Strait Islander people. *Australian and New Zealand Journal of Public Health, 26*(2), 120–4.

Burgess, C. P., Johnston, F. H., Berry, H. L., McDonnell, J., Yibarbuk, D., Gunabarra, C., Mileran, A., & Bailie, R. S. (2009). Healthy country, healthy people: The relationship between Indigenous health status and 'caring for country'. *Medical journal of Australia, 190*(10), 567–72.

Chino, M., Ring, I., Pulver, L. J., Waldon, J., & King, M. (2019). Improving health data for indigenous populations: The international group for indigenous health measurement. *Statistical Journal of the IAOS, 35*(1), 15–21.

Commission on Social Determinants of Health (CSDH). (2008). *Final report of the Commission on Social Determinants of Health*. World Health Organization.

Ferguson, L. J., Girolami, T., Thorstad, R., Rodgers, C. D., & Humbert, M. L. (2021). 'That's what the program is all about. . . building relationships": Exploring experiences in an urban offering of the indigenous youth mentorship program in Canada. *International Journal of Environmental Research and Public Health, 18*(2), 733.

Ford, L., Rowse, T., & Yeatman, A. (Eds.). (2012). *Between indigenous and settler governance*. ProQuest Ebook Central. Retrieved https://ebookcentral.proquest.com

Gifford, H., Cvitanovic, L., Boulton, A., & Batten, L. (2021). Chronic conditions in the community: Preventative principles and emerging practices among Māori health services providers. *Health*

Promotion Journal of Australia : Official Journal of Australian Association of Health Promotion Professionals., *32*(2).

Gilbert, J. (2016). *Indigenous peoples' land rights under international law: From victims to actors* (2nd rev. ed.). Brill, Brill Hes & De Graaf, Brill Nijhoff, Brill Rodopi and Hotei Publishing.

Government of Canada. (2020). *Métis Nation*. Library and Archives Canada. Retrieved https://www.bac-lac.gc.ca/eng/discover/aboriginalheritage/metis/Pages/introduction.aspx

Gracey, M. (2019). Closing the Aboriginal health gap. *The Lancet*, *394*(10194), 218.

Gracey, M., & King, M. (2009). Indigenous health part 1: Determinants and disease patterns. *The Lancet*, *374*(9683), 65–75.

Gregg, M. T. (2018). The long-term effects of American Indian boarding schools. *Journal of Development Economics*, *130*, 17–32.

Gulis, G. (2017). Changes in burden of disease and the epidemiological transition. *European Journal of Public Health*, *27*(Suppl 3), 31–2.

Hausen, T. (2020). *How COVID-19 could destroy indigenous communities*. BBC future. Retrieved https://www.bbc.com/future/article/20200727-how-covid-19-could-destroy-indigenous-communities

Healey, J. (2014). *Aboriginal and Torres Strait Islander health*. The Spinney Press. Retrieved http://ebookcentral.proquest.com/lib/cdu/detail.action?docID=1756105

Hendry, J. (2014). *Science and sustainability: Learning from Indigenous wisdom*. Palgrave Macmillan.

Hyett, S., Gabel, C., Marjerrison, S., & Schwartz, L. (2019). Deficit-based indigenous health research and the stereotyping of indigenous peoples. *Canadian Journal of Bioethics / Revue canadienne de bioéthique*, *2*(2), 102–9.

Larmour, P. (2013). *The governance of common property in the Pacific region*. ANU Press.

Lehrner, A., & Yehuda, R. (2018). Trauma across generations and paths to adaptation and resilience. *Psychological trauma: theory, research, practice, and policy*, *10*(1), 22.

Lewis, D., Williams, L., & Jones, R. (2020). A radical revision of the public health response to environmental crisis in a warming world: contributions of Indigenous knowledges and Indigenous feminist perspectives. *Canadian Journal of Public Health*, *111*, 897–900.

Lines, L-A., & Jardine, C. G. (2019). Connection to the land as a youth-identified social determinant of Indigenous Peoples' health. *BMC Public Health*, *19*(1), 176.

Lowitja Institute for the Close the Gap Campaign Steering Committee. (2021). *Close the Gap. Leadership and legacy through crises: keeping our mob safe*. Close the gap campaign report 2021. Close the Gap Campaign Steering Committee. Retrieved https://humanrights.gov.au/our-work/aboriginal-and-torres-strait-islander-social-justice/publications and https://antar.org.au/resources/issue/

MacDonald, C., & Steenbeek, A. (2015). The impact of colonization and western assimilation on health and wellbeing of Canadian Aboriginal People. *International Journal of Regional and Local History*, *10*(1), 32–46.

McCoy, B. F. (2008). *Holding men: Kanyirninpa and the health of Aboriginal men*. Aboriginal Studies Press.

Métis Nation of Ontario. (2021). *Establishing a Métis right*. Retrieved https://www.metisnation.org/registry/the-powley-case/establishing-a-metis-right-the-powley-test/

Ministry of Health. (2019). *Wai 2575 Māori Health Trends Report*. Ministry of Health, New Zealand.

Montenegro, R. A., & Stephens, C. (2006). Indigenous health in Latin America and the Caribbean. *The Lancet*, *367*(9525), 1859–69.

Nelson, V., Derrett, S., & Wyeth, E. (2021). Indigenous perspectives on concepts and determinants of flourishing in a health and well-being context: a scoping review protocol. *BMJ Open*, *11*(2), e045893.

Nikolakis, W., Cornell, S., Nelson, H. W., Pierre, S., & Phillips, G. (2019). *Reclaiming indigenous governance: Reflections and insights from Australia, Canada, New Zealand, and the United States*. University of Arizona Press.

Nutton, J., & Fast, E. (2015). Historical trauma, substance use, and indigenous peoples: seven generations of harm from a 'big event'. *Substance Mse & Misuse, 50*(7), 839–47.

O'Neill, L., Fraser, T., Kitchenham, A., & McDonald, V. (2018). Hidden burdens: A review of intergenerational, historical and complex trauma, implications for indigenous families. *Journal of Child & Adolescent Trauma, 11*(2), 173–86.

Pelcastre-Villafuerte, B. E., Meneses-Navarro, S., Reyes-Morales, H., & Rivera-Dommarco, J. Á. (2020). The health of indigenous peoples: challenges and perspectives. *Salud Publica de Mexico, 62*(3), 235–6.

Public Health Association of Australia (PHAA). (2018). What is public health? Retrieved https://www.phaa.net.au/documents/item/2757

Reid, P., Cormack, D., & Paine, S-J. (2019) . Colonial histories, racism and health – the experience of Maori and Indigenous peoples. *Public Health, 172*, 110–24.

Rush, E. C., Hsi, E., Ferguson, L. R., Williams, M. H., & Simmons, D. (2010). Traditional foods reported by a Māori community in 2004. *MAI Review, 2*, 1–10.

Schultz, R., Abbott, T., Yamaguchi, J., & Cairney, S. (2018). Indigenous land management as primary health care: Qualitative analysis from the Interplay research project in remote Australia. *BMC Health Services Research, 18*(1), 960.

Sebastian, T. ,& Donelly, M. (2013). Policy influences affecting the food practices of Indigenous Australians since colonisation. *Australian Aboriginal Studies, 2*, 59–72.

Senior, K. ,& Chenhall, R. (2013). Health beliefs and behaviour. *Medical Anthropology Quarterly, 27*(2), 155–74.

Smith, D., & Hunt, J. (2008). Understanding Indigenous Australian governance – research, theory and representations. In J. Hunt, D. Smith, S. Garling, & W. Sanders (Eds.), *Contested governance culture, power and institutions in Indigenous Australia*. (Research monograph 29). ANU Press.

Steinberg, M. K., Hobbs, J. J., & Mathewson, K. (2004). *Dangerous harvest: Drug plants and the transformation of Indigenous landscapes*. Oxford University Press.

Stoner, L., Page, R., Matheson, A., Tarrant, M., Stoner, K., Rubin, D., & Perry, L. (2015). The indigenous health gap: Raising awareness and changing attitudes. *Perspectives in public health, 135*(2), 68–70.

Tse, S., Lloyd, C., Petchkovsky, L. & Manaia, W. (2005). Exploration of Australian and New Zealand indigenous people's spirituality and mental health. *Australian Occupational Therapy Journal, 52*(3), 181–7.

United Nations (UN). (2013). Indigenous peoples and the United Nations Human Rights System. (Fact Sheet 9/Rev 2).

United Nations Educational, Scientific and Cultural Organization (UNESCO). (2019). *Indigenous peoples*. Retrieved https://en.unesco.org/indigenous-peoples

United Nations Permanent Forum on Indigenous Issues. (n.d.). Who are Indigenous Peoples? Indigenous peoples, Indigenous voices. Retrieved http://www.un.org/esa/socdev/unpfii/documents/5session_factsheet1.pdf

Vukic, A., Gregory, D., Martin-Misener, R., & Etowa, J. (2011). Aboriginal and western conceptions of mental health and illness. *Pimatisiwin: A Journal of Aboriginal and Indigenous Community Health, 9*(1), 65–86.

World Health Organization (WHO). (2010). *A conceptual framework for action on the social determinants of health*. Social Determinants of Health Discussion Paper 2. WHO. Retrieved https://www.who.int/sdhconference/resources/ConceptualframeworkforactiononSDH_eng.pdf

Young, T. K., Ragnhild Broderstad, A., Sumarokov, Y. A., & Bjerregaard, P. (2020). Disparities amidst plenty: A health portrait of Indigenous peoples in circumpolar regions. *International Journal of Circumpolar Health, 79*(1).

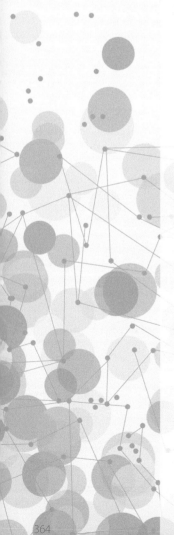

20

The health of migrants and refugees

Celia McMichael

LEARNING OBJECTIVES

After studying this chapter, you should be able to:

1   understand connections between migration and the social determinants of health
2   have knowledge of contemporary migration flows across the world
3   understand health issues across different stages of migration processes
4   understand developments in migrant health policy and practice.

Barthelemy: Refugee health

Barthelemy lives in Kakuma refugee camp in Kenya. In 2007, he and his family fled to Kakuma from conflict in the Democratic Republic of Congo (DRC). They left behind their home, livelihoods and family networks.

Kakuma refugee camp, established 1992, and the newly expanded Kalobeyei Settlement are home to 210 384 refugees from 22 different countries (UNHCR, 2021a). The largest populations are from Somalia, South Sudan and the DRC (UNHCR, 2019).

Refugee camps provide shelter from persecution that creates political refugees. They also present challenges, including threats to health. Conditions in Kakuma are grave, particularly as donor support has waned in recent years. The camp has limited resources, infrastructure and opportunities for employment and education. The threats to health include malnutrition and infectious diseases.

Barthelemy reports that he and his family of four experience water insecurity, food insecurity, poor housing, interpersonal violence and risk of infectious diseases such as cholera and COVID-19. Every few days, they line up early in the morning to obtain water from a tap or, when tap-water is unavailable, walk long distances to look for water in the bush. Every month, the UNHCR provides Barthelemy and his family with 8 kilograms of sorghum, 2 kilograms of yellow peas and a ration of oil. This food assistance is crucial yet inadequate; Barthelemy and his children are often hungry and have poor nutritional status. Their home offers limited protection from the wind and rain. They have experienced violent attacks and have moved within the camp in search of safer living conditions.

While responsibility for their care lies with the Kenyan government, the UNHCR and other organisations provide services including health care. There are two health facilities in Kakuma (UNHCR, 2019).

Since the beginning of 2019, 100 cases involving 423 individuals from Kakuma have been submitted for consideration for resettlement; 229 people departed for resettlement in 2019 (UNHCR, 2019). Barthelemy and his family have registered with the UNHCR and have applied for resettlement but they have not yet been successful.

Introduction

Migration is a defining issue of our times (Orcutt et al., 2020). An estimated 281 million migrants (3.6 per cent of the world's population) were living outside their countries of origin in 2020 (International Organization for Migration [IOM], 2021). In 2020, more than 55 million people were internally displaced within their countries of origin due to conflict and violence (48 million) or disaster (7 million) (Internal Displacement Monitoring Centre [IDMC], 2021). Population movement is shaped by globalisation, economic trade, shifting capital, socio-economic disparities, skill shortages, demographic change, transnational migrant networks, environmental and climatic change, political crises and conflicts, and opportunities in work and education (McMichael, 2015).

Migration – the movement of people across an international border or within a state.

Human migration has consequences for health, but migration is not intrinsically unhealthy. Migrants can experience health benefits through increased economic and educational opportunities, and better access to health services in destination sites. Yet, some migrants, such as those migrating between low-income countries, those displaced by conflict or natural disaster and irregular migrants, experience heightened threats to their health.

Irregular migrant – a person who, owing to unauthorised entry, breach of a condition of entry or the expiry of their visa, lacks legal status in a transit or host country. The term 'irregular' is preferable to 'illegal' because it does not carry the connotation of criminality (IOM, 2011).

Social determinants of migrant health

Social determinants of health refer to 'the full set of social conditions in which people live and work' (Commission on the Social Determinants of Health, 2007, p. 4). Socio-economic and political conditions determine the distribution of power, money and resources, and ultimately affect health (Marmot, 2005; see also Chapter 7). As with many populations, the health of migrants is determined largely by factors outside the health system.

Social determinants of migrant health – the conditions in which migrants are born, grow, migrate, live, work and age and which are influenced by socio-economic and political contexts and ultimately affect health (WHO, 2010).

Social determinants of migrant health emerge from the conditions in which migrants travel, live and work (see Figure 20.1). Some migrants, particularly irregular migrants, may experience discrimination, violence, exploitation, poverty, breakdown of family and social relationships, and poor living and working conditions, which can have adverse effects on their physical and mental health. Forcibly displaced populations, such as refugees and internally displaced persons (IDPs), comprise only a small percentage of migrants; they are frequently in vulnerable situations with associated challenges to health and wellbeing. In new sites of residence, migrants may be exposed to diseases to which they have limited immunity (Hugo, 2013). Importantly, migrants frequently face legal and socio-economic barriers that restrict access to health and social services, or health services may not be culturally and linguistically appropriate (IOM, 2013).

Refugee – an individual who, owing to a well-founded fear of being persecuted, is outside the country of their nationality, and is unable to or unwilling to seek the protection of that country or to return because of fear of persecution (IOM, 2011).

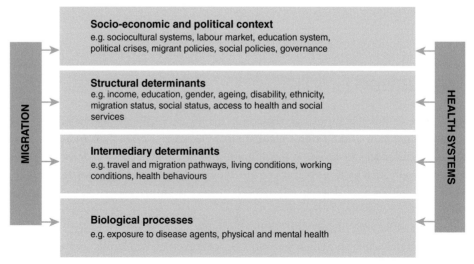

Figure 20.1   Framework for analysis of the social determinants of migrant health
Source: adapted from Commission on the Social Determinants of Health (2007).

SPOTLIGHT 20.1

The health of trafficked women in the United States

The United States is the second-largest destination for human trafficking globally (after Germany). Fifty thousand people are trafficked into the United States annually, many from Mexico and East Asia. Rosa, a 23-year-old woman from Oaxaca, Mexico, came to the United States as an unauthorised immigrant, with the assistance of a smuggler. She left her two young children with her mother, hoping they might eventually join her. The smuggler informed Rosa that she would find work in the United States and would be able to repay the $8000 she owed for passage across the border. Rosa speaks Mixteco and some Spanish, but no English. To cross the border, Rosa walked for days in the desert. She was taken to New Jersey to work as a nanny. Once there, she attended a private health clinic, reporting abdominal pain, painful intercourse and irregular menstrual bleeding. No one at the clinic spoke Mixteco. In the United States, non-citizen immigrants are more than three times more likely than citizens to be uninsured for health. Rosa does not have health insurance and has incurred out-of-pocket expenses for her health care (adapted from Dovydaitis, 2010).

QUESTION
With reference to Figure 20.1, identify some social determinants of Rosa's health.

Contemporary migration flows

Contemporary migration includes permanent, temporary, seasonal and circular movements, and ranges across a spectrum from forced to voluntary migration. While the percentage of international migrants relative to the global population has remained stable at around 2–3 per cent, in the past few decades their total number has increased in line with the growth in the world's population (IOM, 2017).

Migration estimates and types

Table 20.1 presents migrant types and recent global estimates. Some estimates are imprecise because of limited data collection and the challenges of counting irregular migrants (IOM, 2017).

Migrants often fit into multiple categories (such as 'irregular' and 'trafficked'), and their migration status can change over time (e.g. an 'asylum seeker' becomes a 'refugee'). From a population health perspective, the most important distinction is often whether a migrant is regular (documented) or irregular (undocumented). Migrants with irregular status comprise approximately 20 per cent of the global migrant population; these estimates are uncertain as few countries collect data on irregular migration flows (IOM, 2017). Irregular migrants are vulnerable to health risks – both physical and mental health – and have limited access to services when compared to those who travel through regular channels, such as skilled workers (Gushulak, 2000; Hugo, 2013; Steel et al., 2009).

For some migration pathways, women have higher rates of mobility than men, particularly for low-skilled labour opportunities, including domestic work, sex industry work or factory work (World Health Organization [WHO], 2010).

Table 20.1 Definitions and global estimates of migrant populations

Migrant category	Definition	Global estimates, year	Global estimate source
International migrants	Individuals who 'leave their country of origin, or the country of habitual residence, to establish themselves either permanently or temporarily in another country. An international frontier is therefore crossed' (IOM, 2011).	281 million (2020)	IOM, 2021
Internal migrants	'Individuals who move within the borders of a country – usually across regional, district or municipal boundaries – resulting in a change of usual place of residence' (UNDP, 2009).	740 million (2014)	IOM, 2017
International labour migrants	'Movement of persons from their home State to another State for the purpose of remunerated employment' (IOM, 2011).	164 million (2017), but likely to be underestimated	IOM, 2021
Irregular migrants	Individuals who 'owing to unauthorized entry, breach of a condition of entry, or the expiry of his or her visa, lacks legal status in a transit or host country' (IOM, 2011).	Reliable statistics on irregular migrants are not available	IOM, 2021
Trafficked people	'Persons recruited, transported, transferred, harboured or receipted, by means of threat or use of force or other forms of coercion, abduction, fraud, deception, abuse of power or of their position of vulnerability, or of the giving or receiving of payments or benefits to acquire their consent to be under the control of another person, for the purpose of exploitation' (IOM, 2011).	49 032 cases reported to UNODC by member states in 2018 (UNODC, 2020). Note, however, that data on trafficking beyond forms that come to the attention of authorities are limited.	UNODC, 2020
Internally displaced people	Individuals who have been forced to leave their usual place of residence, e.g. due to conflict, natural or human-made disaster, generalised violence, human rights violations – and who have not crossed an international border (IOM, 2011).	In 2020, 55 million people were internally displaced: 48 million by conflict and violence, and 7 million by disaster	IDMC, 2021
Refugee	An individual who 'owing to a well-founded fear of persecution for reasons of race, religion, nationality, membership of a particular social group or political opinions, is outside the country of his nationality and is unable or, owing to such fear, is unwilling to avail himself of the protection of that country' (IOM, 2011).	26 million (2019)	UNHCR, 2021b
Asylum seekers	'Persons seeking to be admitted into a country as refugees and awaiting decision on their application for refugee status under relevant international and national instruments' (IOM, 2011).	4.2 million (2019)	UNHCR, 2021b

Table 20.1 (*cont.*)

Migrant category	Definition	Global estimates, year	Global estimate source
Stateless people	'Individuals not considered as citizens of any state under national law. Stateless persons may or may not be migrants' (IOM, 2011).	4.2 million (2019)	UNHCR, 2021b
Development forced displacement and resettlement	Individuals who are compelled to move as a result of 'development' policies and projects: e.g. dams, roads, ports, urban clearance, mining, deforestation, agribusiness (Cernea, 2006).	15 million displaced per annum (2006 estimate)	Cernea, 2006
People displaced by environmental disasters	Displacement due to disasters associated with geophysical hazards such as earthquakes, volcanic eruptions, and weather-related hazards such as floods, storms, landslides and wildfires (IDMC, 2014)	30.7 million (2020), most in low and lower-middle income countries	IDMC, 2021

SPOTLIGHT 20.2

The health of migrant female domestic workers from Sri Lanka

There is extensive international labour migration from Sri Lanka; more than one million Sri Lankans work overseas. Women constitute approximately half of Sri Lanka's migrant worker population. Most are employed in domestic work in Middle Eastern countries. Sri Lankan 'housemaids' working overseas can experience exploitation, unpaid wages, breach of employment contracts, physical and sexual harassment, rape and torture, which in turn can lead to poor health, disability or even death (Human Rights Watch, 2017). Sri Lanka provides compulsory pre-departure orientation training for housemaids, with a focus on skills training, language and orientation. Internationally, a growing number of bilateral agreements and memoranda of understanding seek to protect the rights of migrant workers (Siriwardhana et al., 2015).

Kronfol and colleagues (2014) present the case of a 28-year-old woman from Sri Lanka working in Doha, Qatar. She arrived in Doha in summer and worked as a housemaid in conditions of extreme heat (over 45°C). The woman was brought to an emergency department after attempted suicide, having taken an overdose of paracetamol. The woman said she wanted to end her life because of the pressure of her job. Her sponsor agreed to end her contract but would not refund the money she had paid for her travel.

QUESTION

Consider the gender-related dimensions of health risks for some of the migrant categories listed in Table 20.1. Should women be understood as a 'vulnerable' category of migrant?

Health challenges and opportunities across stages of migration

This section examines migrant health according to stages of the migration process: pre-departure, transit, settlement in destination sites, interception and return (see Figure 20.2) (Gushulak & MacPherson, 2000; Zimmerman et al., 2011; IOM, 2013). Some of the distinct health risks and opportunities for different types of migrants, such as labour migrants and refugees, are highlighted.

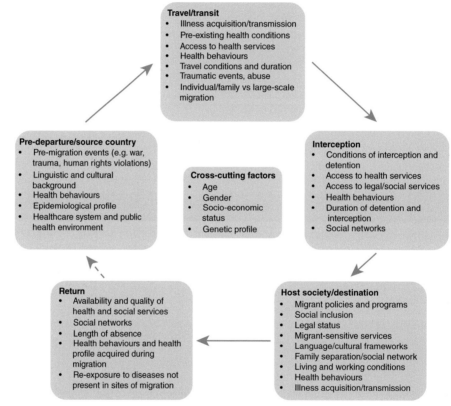

Figure 20.2   Stages of migration process and health determinants.
Source: adapted from IOM, 2013; Gushulak et al., (2010).

Pre-departure phase

Prior to migration, many factors affect health, including local disease risks, socio-economic contexts, environmental factors, health risk behaviours and access to health services. For example, Muslim Rohingya, a minority in Myanmar, have been seeking refuge for decades across the Thai and Bangladeshi borders. In Myanmar, they have no civil rights, are not allowed to travel without official permission, cannot own land and are often excluded from health care and education. Their health suffers; for example, acute malnutrition among Rohingya is 50 per cent higher than non-Rohingya in Rakhine State (Pocock et al., 2017). In 2012, communal violence erupted between Rohingya and Buddhist populations, and the

Myanmar government decreed that the Rohingya had no claim to citizenship. The UNHCR estimates that 140 000 people – mostly Rohingya – were displaced and over 800 000 people were without citizenship in 2014–15 (UNHCR, 2014). Over 600 000 Rohingya have fled to Bangladesh (Pocock et al., 2017). Both pre-migration experience and displacement have adverse effects on their psychological and physical health (see Figure 20.2).

For **regular migrants**, however, the pre-departure phase can offer an important opportunity to deliver health promotion (Zimmerman et al., 2011). Several countries with large numbers of labour migrants, such as the Philippines and Sri Lanka, have developed health education programs for outgoing migrants about health risks and health service entitlements. Most pre-departure health programs and policies focus on screening for transmissible infectious disease. For example, prior to arriving in Australia, humanitarian entrants undergo a 'visa medical', which may include a chest x-ray, HIV serology, syphilis serology and hepatitis B and C serology, as well as a medical examination. For successful humanitarian applicants, a pre-departure health check approximately three days prior to leaving includes treatment for parasites and infections, MMR (measles, mumps and rubella) vaccine and a malaria test (Victorian Foundation for Survivors of Torture, 2012).

Regular migrant – a person who migrates through recognised and authorised channels (IOM, 2011).

REFLECTION QUESTION

Mandatory HIV testing of refugees is controversial. UNHCR (2009) states that it contravenes human rights standards and can have significant effects on vulnerable refugees and their families. Can population health concerns for host communities justify mandatory HIV testing of asylum seekers and refugees? Why or why not?

Transit phase

Contemporary migration, particularly for irregular migrants, is rarely a linear process of movement from one country to another. Transit migration occurs as people move between places of origin and their planned destination, stopping for short or long periods (Zimmerman et al., 2011): for example, Mexicans who trek across the desert into the United States; Afghanis who flee by cross-border smugglers' routes through Thailand or India to Malaysia and Indonesia; people who enter North Africa or countries bordering the European Union (EU) and then attempt to cross to the EU by boat, foot or hidden in containers or trucks. There are multiple health risks during transit, particularly for irregular migrants (see Figure 20.2):

- Since 1996, the deaths of more than 75 000 people have been recorded on migration routes worldwide, over half while trying to reach Europe. This figure is a significant underestimate given the high numbers who go missing during transit, and because most of these migrant deaths are unrecorded (IOM, 2021; Singleton et al., 2017).
- Among refugees displaced to camp settings and peri-urban areas, there are health risks due to crowding, inadequate shelter, lack of food and water, inadequate public health services and disrupted social networks. In refugee camps, common infectious diseases include diarrhoea, measles, meningitis, acute respiratory infection, tuberculosis and malaria (Toole, 2006; McMichael, 2015). Population health strategies for COVID-19

prevention – for example, physical distancing and good hygiene – are difficult to follow in refugee camps. Importantly, in 2019 approximately 60 per cent of the world's refugees lived in urban environments in low-income and middle-income countries rather than camps: 'urban refugees' face challenges including lack of access to health services, poor living and working conditions, and xenophobic attitudes (UNHCR, 2020).

- Transit migration can expose migrants to infectious disease in new sites (McMichael, Barnett & McMichael, 2012). For example, people who migrate through or into malaria-endemic regions are at risk of infection (Rowland & Nosten, 2001). Migrants may also carry infections that spread to local populations. The resurgence of malaria in border regions of Asia, including drug-resistant falciparum malaria, has been attributed in part to population movement (Hugo, 2013). The Ebola crisis of 2016 was linked to poor disease surveillance and control measures along migration pathways across Guinea, Liberia and Sierra Leone (IOM, 2016).
- Human trafficking has adverse consequences for morbidity and mortality, including during the transit phase, which can entail high-risk transport, and physical, sexual and psychological violence (Gushulak & MacPherson, 2000).
- Health risks emerge due to the circumstances and duration of transit travel – including flight on foot or in boats or closed containers – which can lead to physical dangers, trauma, hunger and exposure to violence (IOM, 2013).

Border health

Border regions are often sites with substantial population mobility. Migration within and through border regions may include migrant workers (both regular and irregular), refugees and ethnic minority groups. Border health risks emerge from weak health systems, poor infrastructure, limited health referral and collaboration between neighbouring countries, limited access to treatment, use of substandard medicines and geographic isolation (Gushulak et al., 2010). Casual cross-border migration occurs in many countries in Asia, such as the movement of low-skilled workers to Thailand from Cambodia, Burma and Lao People's Democratic Republic. Communicable diseases such as malaria, tuberculosis (TB), and HIV/AIDS have been reported in border areas in the Greater Mekong Subregion (Ministry of Public Health Thailand, 2011). Incomplete and inconsistent treatment has increased drug-resistant strains of these diseases, particularly among mobile populations in border areas where counterfeit or substandard drugs are common (Ministry of Public Health Thailand, 2011).

Some health initiatives have been established for migrants and transit populations in border regions. For example, the 2nd Thai Border Health Development Master Plan 2012–16 aimed to improve the health of people in border areas (Thais, ethnic minorities, migrants, displaced people and asylum seekers) (Ministry of Public Health Thailand, 2011). The United States–Mexico Border Health Commission addresses public health concerns in the border region, including access to care and responsiveness to public health emergencies (Border Health Commission, 2020).

'Settlement' in destination sites

Settlement refers to temporary, long-term or permanent settlement in an intended location. The overwhelming majority of migration health research has focused on this phase, usually describing migrant health in high-income migrant-receiving countries (e.g., Australia, Canada, the United Kingdom and the United States) (Zimmerman et al., 2011).

A large body of research in high-income countries has identified the 'healthy migrant effect', which documents a migrant health advantage as compared to local-born citizens across multiple domains, including mortality, birthweight, self-rated health, non-communicable disease (e.g. obesity, hypertension, diabetes, cardiovascular diseases), teen pregnancy, suicide and tobacco and alcohol use (Kandula et al., 2004). The 'healthy migrant effect' is attributed to selective migration processes and pre-departure health testing. The migrant health advantage, however, dissipates over time due to adoption of unhealthy behaviours, inadequate living and working conditions, and low access to services (Delavari et al., 2013; Hugo, 2013).

The health concerns of migrants in low-income countries are less widely researched. Evidence suggests that many migrants in low-income countries experience poor health because they live and work in poor conditions, have limited access to health services, experience poverty, lack health education and information, and are often separated from family. For example, among migrant workers in low-income countries, TB transmission has been linked to poverty, poor housing, overcrowding, inadequate nutrition, exploitative working conditions, emerging multi-drug resistant TB, lack of access to health facilities and HIV–TB co-infection (Hugo, 2013; IOM, 2013). Some migrant workers in low-income settings – particularly female domestic and entertainment workers – are subject to violence and physical abuse, isolation and exploitative working conditions, and experience adverse health effects (Hugo, 2013). Many migrant workers are employed in dangerous sectors such as fisheries, mining and construction, with increased risk of occupational accidents and injury. Migrants to urban poor communities (e.g. Bangladeshis migrating from rural areas into the large slums of Dhaka) may be exposed to climate change-related effects that present threats to health, including water shortages, sea-level rise and flooding, and elevated rates of infectious diseases such as dengue (Banu et al., 2014). In summary, the characteristics of the migrant, pre-migration experiences and conditions of settlement in destination sites are all determinants of migrant health.

SPOTLIGHT 20.3

Declining migrant health in sites of settlement

Migrant women may experience elevated reproductive health risks and poor pregnancy outcomes (Bollini et al., 2009). Studies from Australia and Western Europe have documented higher rates of maternal mortality and morbidity, foetal and perinatal deaths, gestational diabetes mellitus and caesarean section among some immigrant women cohorts compared to women from the host country (see IOM, 2013; McMichael, Temple-Smith & Gifford, 2014). These disparities have been attributed to low awareness and underuse of health services such as prenatal and postnatal care. Migrants may also develop higher risk of non-communicable diseases compared to both local populations and those in places of origin. This risk is associated with dietary changes, acculturative stress, social isolation, increased health risk behaviours such as tobacco smoking and excessive alcohol consumption, and inadequate access to health services. A study of Somali women in

Australia found that, subsequent to their arrival, participants increased their consumption of pro-cessed foods (e.g. crisps, pizza and breakfast cereals), and substituted traditional bread for ready-baked bread and camel meat for lamb; 60 per cent of the sample was overweight or obese (BMI over 25) (Burns, 2004).

QUESTION

Given that migrants' health advantages can dissipate over time in sites of settlement, do migrants represent a burden on health services?

Interception and detention

Interception and detention occur for a small, highly vulnerable migrant population, including asylum seekers, undocumented workers and trafficked people (Zimmerman et al., 2011). They are linked to immigration and border control policies. For example, in the 1990s, the Australian government implemented a policy of mandatory detention for asylum seekers. Research globally has documented the adverse effects of immigration detention and inter-ception on asylum seekers' mental and physical health. Detained migrants may have inad-equate food and limited access to health care, lack social support, be exposed to violence and persecution, and may experience separation from family members (Rodriguez Pizarro, 2002; Sampson, Correa-Valez & Mitchell, 2007). Studies have found that detained asylum seekers have high rates of depression, anxiety and post-traumatic stress disorder (PTSD), and the extent of mental ill health is correlated with length of time in detention (Sampson et al., 2007). One study in the United States identified clinically significant symptoms of depression in 86 per cent of detainees, anxiety in 77 per cent and PTSD in 50 per cent, with one quarter reporting suicidal thoughts (Physicians for Human Rights, 2003). When detention is extended, the adverse health consequences become increasingly serious.

Return phase

Many migrants return to their place of origin, temporarily, indefinitely or permanently. People who return after exposure to serious human rights violations and exploitation, such as trafficked people, may experience persistent psychiatric morbidity. Return and repatriation of migrants with significant health conditions can increase the risk of long-term morbidity or mortality because services are not available or affordable (Zimmerman et al., 2011). Repatriated asylum seekers who are found not to be refugees may have limited access to health services in their countries of origin (Sampson et al., 2007). Many labour migrants, however, return with savings and remittances that enable them to afford a healthier lifestyle and improved access to health services for both themselves and their families (Zimmerman et al., 2011; IOM, 2013).

Policy and practice responses

It is important to support and ensure safe and healthy migration (Zimmerman et al., 2011). The health of migrants and mobile populations is significantly influenced by structural and political factors that determine the reason for mobility, conditions throughout migration processes, and living and working conditions in sites of destination. The right to health is enshrined in many human rights instruments. International agreements, such as the UN Global Compact for Migration and the UN Global Compact on Refugees, seek to ensure protection for the health of migrants and refugees (Abubakar et al., 2018).

There is growing global, regional and national commitment to developing **migrant-sensitive health systems** that are affordable, accessible and acceptable for migrants. Efforts to address the health needs of migrants will not only improve health outcomes; improved migrant health can also support settlement and integration, reduce health and social expenses, contribute to socio-economic development, and protect public health and human rights (IOM, 2013). Innovative migrant health policy and practice are increasingly focused on inclusion, social protection, rights-based approaches, universal health coverage and reduction of inequalities in health (WHO, 2010; McMichael & Healy, 2017). They move beyond protectionist approaches, such as infectious disease screening among migrants, and seek to recognise and respond to migrants' vulnerabilities and rights (see Betts, 2010).

> **Migrant-sensitive health system** – a health service that is culturally and linguistically appropriate, that has a workforce with the capacity to respond to migration-related health issues, and that delivers financially sustainable, comprehensive services (IOM, 2013).

The COVID-19 pandemic raises complex issues related to human mobility and infectious disease. COVID-19 has emerged in a world with local and international population mobility, including short-term mobility of tourists and workers as well as migration and displacement. With mobility along commercial and tourist routes, COVID-19 initially affected China's neighbouring countries, the United States and Europe. Efforts to prevent COVID-19 transmission have led to most countries tightening their borders and putting travel restrictions in place. These actions have affected refugees and migrants worldwide. For example, resettlement travel for refugees was suspended temporarily between March and June 2020 (Kluge et al., 2020). Some migrants and displaced populations may have heightened vulnerability to COVID-19 due to living and working conditions that increase exposure to the disease, difficulties implementing prevention strategies, barriers to health care access and challenges coping with the socio-economic effects of the pandemic. Research finds that migrants in some places are overrepresented among those who have been infected, hospitalised and died from COVID-19. Inclusive public health efforts that include migrants and displaced populations are important for effectively addressing the pandemic (Guadagno, 2020).

REFLECTION QUESTION

What are some of the links between human mobility and COVID-19? Consider aspects of disease diffusion, vulnerability and prevention.

The 2010 Global Consultation on Migrant Health proposed a framework of action on migrant health that built on the 2008 World Health Assembly's Resolution on the Health of Migrants. The framework called for:

1 improved monitoring and data on migrant health
2 adoption of national laws and practices that promote migrant right to health, equal access to health services and social protection for migrants

3 migrant-sensitive health systems that are culturally and linguistically appropriate, have enhanced workforce capacity to address migrant health issues, and deliver comprehensive and financially sustainable services

4 partnerships, networks and multi-country frameworks focused on migrant health (WHO, 2010).

In 2017, the Second Global Consultation on Migrant Health sought to further generate government support for action on migrant health, advance migrant health as a key global health agenda, develop monitoring frameworks, engage multi-sectoral partners and promote a research agenda to enhance migrant-inclusive policy (IOM, 2017).

While global frameworks for action, related international conventions, and multilateral agreements exist, responsibility for migrant-sensitive health policies and systems lies largely within nation states (Zimmerman et al., 2011). Governments are faced with the challenge of integrating the health needs of migrants into national plans, policies and strategies, and achieving universal health coverage, according to the 2030 Sustainable Development Goals. Many governments have acknowledged the need to address migrant health in their national plans, policies and strategies, and to remove access barriers to health services and resources (IOM, 2013). Several countries with high numbers of labour migrants have developed contributory social security schemes, tax-based schemes and employer-based health insurance, which aim to improve migrant access to health services and, accordingly, migrant health outcomes. Sri Lanka and the Philippines, for example, have developed insurance schemes for overseas migrant workers, and some migrants within the EU have access to portable healthcare benefits. Several migrant destination countries, such as Thailand, have compulsory migrant health schemes that ensure access to health service among registered migrants. Brazil, Spain and Portugal have developed policies that promote health coverage for migrants regardless of their legal status. Some countries provide targeted health services for migrant populations, such as the Refugee Health Nurse Program in Victoria, Australia, which was initiated in response to the poor and complex health problems of arriving refugees. Migrant-receiving countries, such as Australia, the United Kingdom and the United States, have developed migrant health-practice guidelines and resources that focus on health conditions of public health importance, migrant-specific health concerns, strategies to improve cultural competence and communication, and methods for comprehensive care delivery. These initiatives recognise the need to ensure the health of migrants as both good public health practice and as a human right (IOM, 2013).

SPOTLIGHT 20.4

Migrant health programs in Victoria, Australia

Studies in Australia and internationally have identified the potential for culturally competent healthcare systems to reduce health inequities and improve health outcomes among people from culturally and linguistically diverse (CALD) backgrounds, particularly migrant populations (Gill & Babacan, 2012). At the time of the 2016 Australian Census, 28 per cent of people living in the state of Victoria were born overseas (Department of Premier and Cabinet, 2017). The Cultural Responsiveness Framework: Guidelines for Victorian Health Services was launched in 2009 (Victorian Department of Health, 2009).

The framework aims to further improve the cultural responsiveness of health services in Victoria. It specifies six standards for culturally responsive health service practice: (1) a whole-of-organisation approach to cultural responsiveness; (2) leadership within health services around cultural responsiveness; (3) provision of accredited interpreters when required by patients; (4) inclusive healthcare planning such as responsiveness to dietary, spiritual, family and other cultural practices; (5) involvement of CALD consumers, carers and community members in planning and service review; and (6) staff professional development opportunities to enhance cultural responsiveness (Victorian Department of Health, 2009). Culturally responsive health systems aim to provide a political response to marginalisation of CALD communities and to address health inequalities (Johnstone & Kanitsaki, 2007).

QUESTION
Do cultural competence frameworks perpetuate cultural stereotypes?

SUMMARY

This chapter has discussed the health of migrants and refugees. Key points are summarised here.

Learning objective 1: Understand connections between migration and the social determinants of health.

Migration is not intrinsically 'unhealthy': migrants can experience benefits, including health benefits through, for example, increased economic and educational opportunities in destination countries. However, the conditions in which many migrants travel, live and work often present risks to health. Migrants, particularly irregular migrants, may experience discrimination, violence and exploitation, poor living and work conditions, and lack of access to services; these social determinants affect their physical and mental health and wellbeing.

Learning objective 2: Have knowledge of contemporary migration flows across the world.

Migration is a global phenomenon, with an estimated 281 million international migrants and 55 million internally displaced people. Contemporary migration flows are diverse and range across a spectrum from forced (e.g. refugees and victims of trafficking) to voluntary migration (e.g. documented labour migrants).

Learning objective 3: Understand health issues across different stages of migration processes.

Different migrant categories experience diverse health profiles, due in large part to the social determinants of migrant health. There are also different health risks and opportunities throughout the migration process. This chapter has examined health risks and benefits, and intervention opportunities, as they occur throughout different stages of migration, including pre-departure, transit, settlement in destination sites, interception and return.

Learning objective 4: Understand developments in migrant health policy and practice.

New approaches in migrant health policy and practice acknowledge the social determinants of migrant health and focus on inclusion, rights-based approaches, universal health coverage, and reduction of health inequalities. Universal health coverage, or 'leaving no one behind', is particularly high on the global health agenda and exists where there is access to affordable and effective health systems for all community members, including migrants. It is imperative to develop holistic and inclusive approaches to public health practice and policy that ensure that migration is safer and healthier for all.

TUTORIAL EXERCISES

1   What are 'social determinants of health' and how do they apply to migrants? Discuss, for example, irregular migrants in low-income settings and skilled migrants in high-income countries.
2   Historically, migrant health has been viewed through the lens of communicable disease control, with a focus on monitoring, screening and mobility control; more recently, rights-based approaches focus on migrant vulnerability and the right to health and health care. Apply these different lenses to the COVID-19 pandemic.
3   Do 'irregular migrants' have a right to health care in destination countries?
4   Can you identify 10 potential ways to ensure that health systems could be 'migrant-sensitive'? For example, consider laws or policies, location of health services, service delivery, financing and affordability, sociocultural acceptability and responsiveness.

FURTHER READING

Abubakar, I., Aldridge, R.W., Devakumar, D., Orcutt, M., Burns, R., Baretto, M.L. et al. (2018). The UCL–Lancet Commission on Migration and Health: The health of a world on the move. *The Lancet Commissions 392*(10164), P2606–54.

Castañeda, H., Holmes, S.M., Madrigal, D., DeTrinidad Young, M., Beyeler, N., & Quesada, J. (2015) Immigration as a social determinant of health. *Annual Review of Public Health*, *36*(1), 375–92.

Hossin, M.Z. (2020) International migration and health: It is time to go beyond conventional theoretical frameworks. *BMJ Global Health*, 5, e001938.

International Organization for Migration (IOM). (2017). *Health of migrants: Resetting the agenda*. Retrieved http://publications.iom.int/books/health-migrants-resetting-agenda

REFERENCES

Abubakar, I., Aldridge, R.W., Devakumar, D., Orcutt, M., Burns, R., Baretto, M.L. et al. (2018). The UCL–Lancet Commission on Migration and Health: The health of a world on the move. *The Lancet Commissions*, 392(10164), P2606–54.

Banu, S., Hu, W., Guo, Y., Hurst, C. & Tong, S. (2014). Projecting the impact of climate change on dengue transmission in Dhaka, Bangladesh. *Environment International*, *63*, 137–42.

Betts, A. (2010). *Migration governance: Alternative futures*. International Organization for Migration.

Bollini, P., Pampallona, S., Wanner, P., & Kupelnick, B. (2009). Pregnancy outcome of migrant women and integration policy: A systematic review of the international literature. *Social Science & Medicine*, *68*, 452–61.

Border Health Commission. (2020). *Healthy border 2020: A prevention and health promotion initiative*. United States–Mexico Border Health Commission. Retrieved https://aidsetc.org/sites/default/files/resources_files/res_2805.pdf

Burns, C. (2004). Effect of migration on food habits of Somali women living as refugees in Australia. *Ecology of Food and Nutrition*, *2*(3), 213–29.

Cernea, M. (2006). Development-induced and conflict-induced IDPs: Bridging the research divide. *Forced Migration Review*, Special Issue (December), 25–7.

Commission on the Social Determinants of Health. (2007). *A conceptual framework for action on the social determinants of health*. World Health Organization.

Delavari, M., Sønderlund, A., Swinburn, B., Mellor, D., & Renzaho, A. (2013). Acculturation and obesity among migrant populations in high income countries – a systematic review. *BMC Public Health*, *13*, 458.

Department of Premier and Cabinet. (2017). *Victoria's diverse population: 2016 census*. The State of Victoria. Retrieved https://www.vic.gov.au/discover-victorias-diverse-population

Dovydaitis, T. (2010). Human trafficking: The role of the health care provider. *Journal of Midwifery and Women's Health*, *55*(5), 462–7.

Gill, G. & Babacan, H. (2012). Developing a cultural responsiveness framework in healthcare systems: An Australian example. *Diversity and Equality in Health and Care*, *9*, 45–55.

Guadagno, L. (2020). *Migrants and the COVID-19 pandemic: An initial analysis*. Migration Research Series No. 60. International Organization for Migration.

Gushulak, B. (2000). Health determinants in migrants: The impact of population mobility on health. In P. J. van Krieken (Ed.), *Health, migration and return: A handbook for a multidisciplinary approach* (pp. 255–68). Asser Press.

Gushulak, B., & MacPherson, D. W. (2000). Health issues associated with the smuggling and trafficking of migrants. *Journal of Immigrant Health, 2*(2), 67–78.

Gushulak, B., Weekers, J., & MacPherson, D. W. (2010). Migrants in a globalized world – health threats, risks and challenges: An evidence-based framework. *Emerging Health Threats Journal, 2,* e10.

Hugo, G., (2013). Migration and health. In *Situation report on international migration in South and South-West Asia.* UNESCAP.

Human Rights Watch. (2017). *World Report 2017: Sri Lanka.* Human Rights Watch. Retrieved https://www.hrw.org/world-report/2017/country-chapters/sri-lanka#2d493c

Internal Displacement Monitor Centre (IDMC). (2014). *Global estimates 2014: People displaced by disasters.* IDMC. Retrieved http://www.internal-displacement.org/publications/global-estimates-2014-people-displaced-by-disasters

——(2021). *Global report on internal displacement 2021.* Retrieved https://www.internal-displacement.org/global-report/grid2021/

International Organization for Migration (IOM) (2011). *Glossary on migration.* IOM.

——(2013). *International migration, health and human rights.* IOM.

——(2016). *Health border and mobility management.* IOM.

——(2017). *Health of migrants: Resetting the agenda.* IOM.

——(2021). *Migration data portal.* IOM.

Johnstone, M., & Kanitsaki, O. (2007). An exploration of the notion and nature of the construct of cultural safety and its applicability to the Australian health care context. *Journal of Transcultural Nursing, 18,* 247–56.

Kandula, N. R., Kersey, M., & Lurie, N. (2004). Assuring the health of immigrants: What the leading health indicators tell us. *Annual Review of Public Health, 25,* 357–76.

Kluge, H.H., Jakab, Z., Bartovic, J., D'Anna, V., & Severoni, S. (2020). Refugee and migrant health in the COVID-19 response. *The Lancet, 395*(10232), P1237–9.

Kronfol, Z., Saleh, M., & Al-Ghafry, M. (2014). Mental health issues among migrant workers in Gulf Cooperation Council countries: Literature review and case illustrations. *Asian Journal of Psychiatry, 10,* 109–13.

Marmot, M. (2005). Social determinants of health inequalities. *Lancet, 365,* 1099–104.

McMichael, C. (2015). Climate change-related migration and infectious disease. *Virulence, 6*(6), 544–9.

McMichael, C., Barnett, J., & McMichael, A. J. (2012). An ill wind? Climate change, migration and health. *Environmental Health Perspectives, 120*(5), 646–54.

McMichael, C., & Healy, J. (2017). Health equity and migrants in the Greater Mekong Subregion. *Global Health Action, 10*(1), 1271594.

McMichael, C., Temple-Smith, M., & Gifford, S. (2014). The cultural and social shaping of sexual health in Australia. In M. Temple-Smith (Ed.), *Sexual health: A multidisciplinary perspective* (pp. 99–113). IP Communications.

Ministry of Public Health Thailand. (2011). *Border health development master plan 2012–16.* Bureau of Policy and Strategy, Ministry of Public Health. Retrieved http://searo.who.int/thailand/areas/borderandmigrant/en

Orcutt, M., Spiegel, P., Kumar, B., Abubakar, I., Clark, J., & Horton, R. (2020). Lancet Migration: global collaboration to advance migration health. *The Lancet, 395*(10221), 317–19.

Physicians for Human Rights (PHR). (2003). *From persecution to prison: The health consequences of detention for asylum seekers.* PHR and The Bellevue/NYU Program for Survivors of Torture.

Pocock, N. S., Mahmood, S. S., Zimmerman, C., & Orcutt, M. (2017). Imminent health crises among the Rohingya people of Myanmar. *British Medical Journal, 359,* j5210.

Rodriguez Pizarro, G. (2002). *Report of the UN Special Rapporteur on the human rights of migrants, Ms Gabriela Rodríguez Pizarro (para. 53).* UN Doc. E/CN.4/2003/85. United Nations.

Rowland, M., & Nosten, F. (2001). Malaria epidemiology and control in refugee camps and complex emergencies. *Annals of Tropical Medicine and Parasitolology, 95,* 741–54.

Sampson, R., Correa-Velez, I., & Mitchell, G. (2007). *Removing seriously ill asylum seekers from Australia*. Refugee Health Research Centre.

Singleton, A., Laczko, F., & Black, J. (2017). Measuring unsafe migration: The challenge of collecting accurate data on migrant fatalities. *Migration Policy Practice*, *7*(2), 4–9.

Siriwardhana, C., Wickramage, K., Siribaddana, S., Vidanapathirana, P., Jayasekara, B., Weerawarna, S., . . . Sumathipala, A. (2015). Common mental disorders among adult members of 'left-behind' international migrant worker families in Sri Lanka. *BMC Public Health*, *15*, 299.

Steel, Z., Chey, T., Silove, D., Marnane, C., Bryant, R. A., & van Ommeren, M. (2009). Association of torture and other potentially traumatic events with mental health outcomes among populations exposed to mass conflict and displacement: A systematic review and meta-analysis. *JAMA*, *302*, 537–49.

Toole, M. J. (2006). Forced migrants: Refugees and internally displaced persons. In B. Levy, & V. Sidel (Eds.), *Social injustice and public health* (pp. 190–204). Oxford University Press.

United Nations Development Programme (UNDP). (2009). *Human development report 2009: Overcoming barriers: Human mobility and development*. UNDP.

United Nations High Commissioner for Refugees (UNHCR). (2009). *Policy statement on HIV testing and counselling in health facilities for refugees, internally displaced persons and other persons of concern to UNHCR*. Retrieved https://www.unhcr.org/4b508b9c9.pdf

——(2014). *Myanmar: 2014-15 Global appeal*. Retrieved https://www.unhcr.org/publications/fundraising/528a0a32b/unhcr-global-appeal-2014-2015-myanmar.html

——(2019). Kakuma Camp and Kalobeyei Settlement Briefing Kit, May 2019. Retrieved https://www.unhcr.org/ke/wp-content/uploads/sites/2/2019/06/Briefing-Kit_May-2019-approved.pdf

——(2020). *UNHCR global trends: 2019*. United Nations High Commissioner for Refugees (UNHCR). Retrieved https://www.unhcr.org/5ee200e37/

——(2021a). *Total refugees and asylum-seekers in Turkana*. Retrieved https://data2.unhcr.org/en/country/ken/796

——(2021b). *Figures at a glance*. Retrieved https://www.unhcr.org/en-au/figures-at-a-glance.html

United Nations Office on Drugs and Crime (UNODC). (2020). *Global report on trafficking in persons 2020*. Retrieved https://www.unodc.org/documents/data-and-analysis/tip/2021/GLOTiP_2020_15jan_web.pdf

Victorian Department of Health. (2009). *Cultural responsiveness framework: Guidelines for Victorian health services*. Author. Retrieved http://www.health.vic.gov.au/__data/assets/pdf_file/0008/381068/cultural_responsiveness.pdf

Victorian Foundation for Survivors of Torture. (2012). *Caring for refugee patients in general practice: A desktop guide* (4th ed.). Author. Retrieved http://refugeehealthnetwork.org.au/wp-content/uploads/CRPGP_DTG_4thEdn_Vic_Online.pdf

World Health Organization (WHO). (2010). *Health of migrants – the way forward: Report of global consultation*. WHO.

Zimmerman, C., Kiss, L., & Hossain, M. (2011). Migration and health: A framework for 21st century policy-making. *PLoS Med*, *8*(5), e1001034.

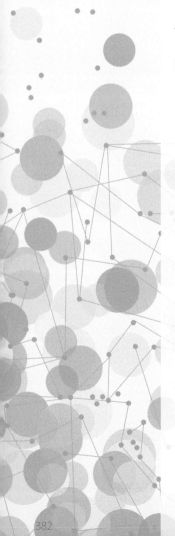

21

Understanding health in rural settings

Alan Crouch, Lisa Bourke and David Pierce

LEARNING OBJECTIVES

After studying this chapter, you should be able to:

1 understand the diversity of rural health
2 discuss the broader determinants of health with respect to their effects in rural settings
3 adapt the principles of health promotion and public health planning and practice to rural settings
4 understand the complexity of health systems in delivering accessible public health services to rural residents, especially with regard to consumer issues and health
5 demonstrate an appreciation of the role of power relations in influencing health outcomes in rural settings

VIGNETTE

The rural township of Riverdene

Riverdene is a (fictional) rural river town located on a regional border, with a population of 6000 people. An additional 1500 residents live in Bankstown, on the northern bank of the river. This jurisdictional river border separates communities in terms of their differing health system experiences. Bankstown residents have access to goods and services in Riverdene, which is located approximately 300 kilometres from the regional capital (population 2.9 million), the centre of government administration and specialised health services. The Riverdene township is the largest centre in the Riverlands local government area (LGA), covering 4000 square kilometres of mainly agricultural land and adjoining large tracts of agricultural land in the neighbouring region. Many people in Riverdene and Bankstown are employed in agriculture. Recently, differing restrictions and lockdown measures to contain the COVID-19 pandemic have had a significant effect on these cross-border communities. Farming communities and orchardists in the rural areas, which have been especially affected, now fear losses to their harvesting due to travel restrictions on the seasonal workforce. This is in addition to existing medical (farm accident, chemical exposure and chronic conditions), social and emotional health challenges. Residents are also subjected to significant disruption from time to time, as a consequence of differing regulations by the respective regional authorities. While confusion and resentment have been expressed through social media, firm evidence of residents' not complying with the respective health-focused restrictions has not been identified.

Approximately 2 per cent of the population of Riverdene is of First Nations heritage, 17 per cent speak a language other than English at home and 22 per cent was born overseas. The median age is 43 years, and 23 per cent of residents are aged 65 or older. In 2007, 90 refugees from countries in the Mekong River region were resettled in Riverdene and have since become active citizens in workplaces and community life. In terms of health and social indicators, and compared to the national population, Riverdene residents have:

- lower levels of participation in cancer-screening programs
- higher prevalence of tobacco and risky alcohol consumption, including among younger people
- lower levels of substance use (other than alcohol)
- higher mortality rates for diabetes, suicide and injury
- higher levels of unplanned teenage pregnancy/parenting
- lower immunisation coverage rates
- lower ratios of health professionals to population size
- higher levels of transgenerational welfare dependency
- higher levels of unemployment
- higher participation rates in sporting and recreational organisations and activities
- higher per-capita volunteering rates and service club membership.

Introduction

The health needs and experiences of rural residents are diverse. While some common themes, such as limitation of access to health services, are easily identified, also relevant is the diversity related to the geographic, social, economic and environmental factors that shape the character of a community.

There are diverse writings on rural health that inform public health practice. At the population level, evidence from epidemiological studies indicates variable mortality and morbidity from preventable acute and chronic conditions, both between rural and urban people and across the diversity of rural populations (Australian Institute of Health and Welfare [AIHW], 2020; Zahnd, Fogelman & Jenkins, 2018; Chandak, Nayer & Lin, 2018; Scheil-Adlung, 2015).

A preliminary analysis (AIHW, 2020) of national burden of disease data suggests that all-cause mortality, measured as fatal burden of disease (age-standardised rates of years-of-life-lost, or YLL), increases with increasing remoteness from major cities (Figure 21.1). Similar inequalities in morbidity, measured as non-fatal burden of disease (disability adjusted life years, or DALYs), have also been reported across remote areas, socio-economic groups and between Aboriginal and Torres Strait Islander peoples and non-Indigenous Australians (AIHW, 2021). Evidence from social epidemiological studies further suggests variation in the effects of social and structural determinants of health, based on geographic area (Penman-Aguilar et al., 2016; O'Campo & Dunn, 2012). In short, rural people have poorer health outcomes, poorer health behaviours, including drinking alcohol, smoking, levels of obesity (AIHW, 2017, 2018), and are more likely to experience disadvantage related to the social determinants of health, in particular lower incomes and education and being Indigenous (AIHW, 2019; Wakerman et al., 2017).

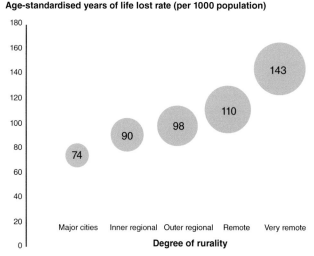

Figure 21.1   Influence of rurality on fatal burden of disease: Australia 2015
Source: adapted from AIHW (2015).

From the perspective of clinical practice and service provision, the availability and accessibility of services across the life cycle are key to understanding health in rural settings. Simple comparisons of the prevalence of a condition between urban and rural populations may not adequately characterise disease burden in rural communities. The limited health workforce, as well as the distance of services, appropriateness of models of service delivery, socio-economic disadvantage and overlapping relationships with health service staff all predispose rural residents to presentation for treatment at a later stage of disease (Murage et al., 2017).

Internationally, health outcomes associated with life in rural settings are not universally consistent, with differences identified between urban and rural settings, and between different rural settings within the same country. In Australia and Canada, for example, 'remote' is distinguished from 'rural' with each characterised as having different population demography, health needs and modes of service delivery (Wakerman, 2004).

A simple, dichotomous comparison of urban–rural may not reflect the respective populations' health experiences, with data from the United States suggesting that inner-urban and rural residents may experience higher levels of ill health than those in suburban areas and metropolitan centres (Eberhardt & Pamuk, 2004). The Canadian experience suggests there is an increasing health risk, if measured by mortality, in moving from urban to rural to remote areas, with the exception of those living in some rural areas that are close to, or influenced by, a larger metropolitan region (Ostry, 2009). Therefore, rurality plays a role in health outcomes. However, its effects are different for 14, 45 and 85-year-olds, for those with low incomes and above-average incomes, and for those who are accustomed to travelling to urban areas. There is great diversity within rural health and remote health, making explanation of the poorer health outcomes, workforce shortages and reduced access to care a complex task.

To provide a comprehensive perspective of rural health, this chapter employs a conceptual framework to assist in describing the complexity of rural health outcomes (see Figure 21.2). This framework was developed to understand the variation in health outcomes as due to a combination of structural constraints, geographic realities and individual, community and political actions. The framework's creators have argued that previous understandings of rural and remote health 'have been largely reactive to specific problems rather than systematically and comprehensively considering rural and remote health and identifying points of connection and change' (Bourke et al., 2012a, p. 319). The framework suggests that change can result in positive and negative rural health outcomes, and that individual, community and local actions can change health in a particular place. It further suggests that a change in one area of the framework affects other aspects of rural health. The framework acknowledges the geographical issues and the importance of local actions by health providers, health services and health consumers, as well as the role of policy, funding and broader social issues, such as racism. Specifically, the framework posits that **power relations** between stakeholders at the local, regional and national levels produce and reproduce health outcomes in rural areas. The framework also suggests that both action and inaction can explain rural health, and that continuing the status quo or resisting change is as much a response or expression of power as are new initiatives (see Bourke et al., 2012a).

Power relations – the negotiation of power across and within communities.

The framework proposes that the interrelationships of six concepts can be used to interpret issues and scenarios in rural and remote health (Bourke et al., 2012a). These concepts are:

- **geographical isolation** – with reference to the vignette at the start of this chapter, where Riverdene is located, its distance from other or larger centres, the local economy, environment etc.
- **the rural locale and the social interactions of people in the local area** – interactions between the residents of Riverdene about the pandemic to share information about the virus and associated restrictions, shape social connections during lockdown and alter employment, community participation and feelings of safety in the town
- **local health responses**, including local health services, consumer groups and local actions involving health care – in Riverdene, this includes the role of local health services

in responding to the pandemic, how the community respond to changes such as regulations on the wearing of masks, and changes in the workforce (e.g. a locum nurse practitioner posted to Riverdene for three months stayed for two years due to the pandemic)

- **broader health systems** that provide funding, health protocols, professional bodies and advocates, and the systems shaping health from outside the locale – such as governments implementing virus-testing clinics and telehealth programs in rural regions, and widespread, consistent public health messages about hand hygiene, number of visitors to the home, mask-wearing and access to health services
- **broader social systems** that shape life in rural and remote settings from outside, including social media, other media, cultural factors and the social determinants of health – including border closures separating Riverdene and Bankstown, financial support for those without work, and emerging views across the nation that rural places offer more space and safety than city suburbs
- **power relations** that drive the interaction of the other five concepts to produce particular health outcomes and issues – who gets to make the decisions, which voices are heard, who is not included, how interaction occurs, and the ways in which information and public health messages about the virus and associated restrictions spread across Riverdene that results in who hears and/or adopts updated public health messages, who subscribes to messages of conspiracy (e.g. 'the virus is not real') and who is (or is not) compliant with restrictions (Bourke et al., 2012a).

Using the vignette at the start of the chapter and issues as described for Riverdene at the time of the pandemic, this chapter explores each of the six concepts in the framework to understand how public health measures at all levels can contribute to rural health outcomes (Bourke et al., 2012b).

A framework of rural health

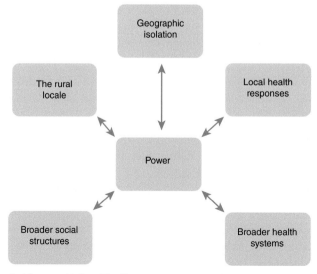

Figure 21.2   A conceptual framework of rural health

Geographical isolation

The local geography shapes the economy, population, use of natural resources and other social factors that influence health in a particular place (Bourke et al., 2012a). As an example, the distance from Riverdene to urban centres shapes the population's access to specialist care, which may differ according to life cycle, stage and needs. The National Rural Health Alliance (NRHA) has identified some specific effects of isolation that are related to high rates of injury in rural settings (NRHA, 2014). Other health issues relate to environmental contexts (e.g. snake bites), type of work (farm accidents) and travel (road accidents can be more severe as driving on highways is usually at high speeds). Geography also shapes the type of economy, which is often related to primary production (farming, fishing or mining) and, more recently tourism, which has implications for health.

Key to understanding rural health is the concept of **rurality**. Rurality varies between places like border-town Riverdene and surrounding smaller towns and hamlets. Some of the world's leading census and statistics agencies have used threshold-dependent characterisations of 'rural' (e.g. by defining 'rural' as a population of less than 500 people within an area of one square kilometre) for the purposes of their specific data analyses. However, given changes in technology and mobility, differences between rural and urban settings may have become less distinct. In this respect, recent developments in the definitions and measures of rurality have been premised on technological advancement in geographic information systems and machine learning, enabling wider application of fine-scale data collection and the definition of more complex indicators and measures of rurality (Doogan et al., 2018; Cohen et al., 2017).

Rurality – a condition characterising lived experience in places designated as 'rural'.

In Australia, there is a general trend that health, education and economic indicators for the population worsen according to rurality and remoteness (NRHA, 2017; Holden & Zhang, 2018; AIHW, 2019). Despite this general trend, a critical implication from categorisations of 'rurality' is the heterogeneous nature of the rural context. There is simply not one 'rural', but rather a multiplicity of locational, situational and social contexts that collectively comprise the lived experiences of the 'rural'. Considered in these terms, the geographic concept embodies distance from key services, travel time to access these services and the particular social, economic and terrain characteristics of the location.

SPOTLIGHT 21.1

How do jurisdictional differences influence isolation as experienced by the people of Riverdene and Bankstown?

The geography of Riverdene had a profound effect on both the town and the cross-border community of Bankstown during the first year of the COVID-19 pandemic. Lockdowns that confined all people to their places of residence had a greater effect on those living in town than those on farms with open spaces and where work continued. People who were not dependent on urban connection were affected to a lesser extent by the isolation mandates than those confined to their homes and separated from necessary services (e.g. specialist health care), family (e.g. not able to visit elderly parents) and employment-related needs (weekly trips to service small business needs). The effects of statewide policies varied for different rural places and different rural residents. Further, the isolation of these towns slowed the transmission of infection more effectively than in urban areas.

QUESTIONS

1 How did the geography of Riverdene affect the health, health needs and health services? What changes might have been seen during the pandemic, from the perspective of both the townships and local rural farming communities?

2 What approach would you take during a pandemic to develop a deep understanding of the geography of Riverdene (and in your own rural settings) as a key consideration in public health planning?

REFLECTION QUESTION

Reflect on recent global developments in geo-spatial and communications technologies, high-speed internet access in many countries, remote workforce practices, telemedicine and easy access to sources of global information. Thinking about Riverdene and your own country's rural locations, does geographical isolation have a critical influence on health outcomes?

The rural locale

The roles of local communities and the manner of their engagement in health have been characterised as a 'central tenet of public health policy and practice' (Preston et al., 2010; South & Smith, 2014; Wakerman et al., 2008). The rural locale concept includes embodiment of the social-in-place. It focuses on the actions and interactions of people in place that produce community norms, ways of doing things, access and inclusion (Bourke et al., 2012a).

In Riverdene, the interactions of people in formal groups, in sporting clubs and in conversations held on the main street influence what people know and do, and that in turn affects their health, fitness and wellbeing. Lockdowns during the pandemic altered these interactions and the social connections and flow of information within Riverdene.

The ability to influence the local community can be powerful (see Nolan et al., 2008). While this understanding applies universally, in small and isolated settings such as Riverdene and Bankstown, the effects of these attempts may be greater than in urban areas. For example, a proportion of Riverdene residents viewed the government-imposed restrictions during the pandemic as unnecessary and damaging to the local economy. As a result, these residents wore masks inappropriately (or not at all) and did little to restrict their social movements and interactions. This created tensions with other residents who were fearful of the virus, for reasons including that they worked in the healthcare sector, were older, or were carers of people at high risk of contracting the virus.

Such tension is consistent with Papa and colleagues' (2006) understanding of the dynamic processes and tensions in communities. These tensions provide opportunities for organising to achieve or resist change. Papa and colleagues (2006) have argued that, in their attempts to bring about change, individuals and communities experience 'contradictory tensions that both support and negate' change processes (p. 61). In Riverdene, the tension about restrictions affected community relationships and over time divided the community and created conflicting information.

SPOTLIGHT 21.2

Consumer activism affecting vaccine uptake

As vaccines were developed across the globe, there was discussion in Riverdene and Bankstown about their use, safety and whether they should be compulsory. A clustering of individuals with anti-vaccine beliefs organised to influence others to refuse immunisation when offered. This activism sparked community discussions in both Riverdene and Bankstown, between groups keen to have the vaccine (healthcare workers, older people, the local Aboriginal community and others in high-risk groups), others who opposed the vaccine, and many who were undecided. Letters to the editor in Riverdene's weekly newspaper were dominated by views on the vaccines for months before a vaccine was available.

As the anti-vaccine approach to exploiting vaccine hesitancy began to gain momentum in Riverdene, one woman approached the pharmacist to 'do something so that the town will consider vaccination'. With the support of the local business council, the woman and the pharmacist held a community meeting to present evidence on the safety of the vaccines in everyday language. This initiative allayed the fears of many present at the meeting who were hesitant about the vaccine, and a community action group was formed to disseminate the safety message through local businesses, clubs and community groups to the wider population. Consequently, a local norm evolved towards openness to a new vaccine in Riverdene. Power was effectively exercised among and between individuals within that community, thereby shaping conformity to the behavioural or social norm of vaccine acceptance.

However, across the river in Bankstown, residents were unable to attend this meeting or subsequent activities, and a strong anti-vaccine sentiment remained. As information crossed the border, this group was challenged but a strong norm of reluctance to be vaccinated ensued. This reinforces how networks and interactions in specific rural places can result in different responses.

QUESTIONS

Reflecting on your understanding of power relationships and **consumer activism** in the health disadvantage of rural people:

Consumer activism – action taken to assert consumer rights by users of health services.

1   How do you ensure effective distribution of public health messages in rural communities?

2   What other behaviours could community norms influence in relation to health in a rural community?

3   How does leadership influence public health in rural communities? Did the lack of public health leadership in Bankstown contribute to a different outcome? As a public health professional, how can you inspire local advocates to become leaders in rural towns?

Local health responses

Local health responses include the responses of health services, consumer groups, support groups, sporting clubs, schools and others who provide health information as well as other related actions that contribute to health, wellbeing and heath care in the rural locale (Bourke et al., 2012a). The model of health service is particularly important as models of care often differ between rural settings. Understanding the local model of care, including, for example, that many rural and remote hospitals are nurse-led, that specialist care can be accessed using telehealth technologies and that the local pharmacy is a key source of health information.

The reality of diminished consumer choice and control in rural settings critically underlies access issues. Specialist services are frequently provided intermittently, on a visiting basis, and although notionally 'accessible', are often not available in a responsive manner due to the high demand for appointments. In some Australian rural settings, health service planners have sought to respond creatively to medical workforce shortage-related elements of these access challenges by introducing nurse-led and pharmacy-led services into primary care systems, especially in screening and other prevention-oriented programs. In this context, these creative responses have acknowledged the essential inequality (compared with urban experience) in some elements of rural service provision, and have sought instead to achieve some degree of equivalence in the range, if not the depth, of accessible services. The use of this approach has aimed for greater **health equity**.

Health equity – a situation in which groups with different levels of underlying social advantage or disadvantage do not experience health inequalities associated solely with their social positioning.

In addition to these elements, and in the absence of private motor vehicle availability, distance to basic services and the lower levels of public infrastructure (compared to urban settings), including transport, present as perhaps the most frequently encountered dimension of the access barrier for low-income rural people in Australian settings. While many rural people are accustomed to travelling to services, the barrier occurs when cost, time and other priorities prevent travel.

In rural settings, the clients of health services may encounter more limited options in the choice of local care. This affects the health of farmers and agricultural workers who, while representing only a small proportion of the rural population, contribute disproportionately to the national economy. The access challenge for generalist rural health services is to better accommodate the needs of a diverse range of health service consumers (Terry et al., 2017).

Understandings of the complexities of access barriers should also be considered with respect to attitudinal and/or interpersonal factors (e.g. stoicism) that influence help-seeking behaviours and limit access for rural people (Pierce & Shann, 2012).

There is evidence for strengths in models of care, relationships and integration in the provision of health services in rural settings (Bourke et al., 2010; Malatzky & Bourke, 2016). Rural communities have, for example, initiated health responses to address local needs, such as consulting with the community, using community resources to address health issues and redesigning health services to meet the needs of the community and address their barriers to health care (Bourke et al., 2012b).

Wakerman and colleagues (2008) provide evidence that rural health services are more sustainable when they are primary health care-oriented, including health promotion, prevention and advocacy roles. These attributes contribute significantly to the lived experience of health in rural settings and are themselves determinants of health. The ways in which health systems operate influence how health services in the locale are funded, managed, monitored and held accountable. In turn, this shapes who is employed, what they do and which services remain unfunded. For example, while rural health services are funded to support travel by outreach services in small, outlying hamlets, they may not be funded to engage people with low health literacy or to promote health and wellbeing holistically.

SPOTLIGHT 21.3

Health service planning in Riverlands

Given Riverdene's role as a service centre for the local agricultural region, the health service was funded to provide a virus-testing centre during the COVID-19 pandemic. The testing centre was available to people from all towns and communities across the region. The new clinic was staffed by an immunisation-endorsed Nurse Practitioner and located in an unused small house at the edge of town, to ensure confidentiality and to distance the clinic from at-risk groups, including residents of the aged-care facility attached to the health centre. The private entrance to this property, along with a detailed and confidential process, encouraged local residents with symptoms to be present for testing.

A visitor to Riverdene was found to be positive to the virus, and contact-tracers identified locations within Riverdene and surrounding agricultural areas in which people may have been exposed to the virus. These included at a local café and supermarket in town and a caravan park used by seasonal fruit pickers servicing orchardists in the region. Residents and seasonal workers who had visited these places at similar times, together with their close contacts, were asked to be tested. The large number of residents, workers and contacts seeking testing exceeded the capacity of the small house at the edge of town, and consequently the local sporting club offered its premises for a short period to assist. Volunteers and community nurses undertook patient registration, and local businesses provided coffee, tea and water for those waiting to be tested. The community response enabled efficient testing in a short period of time. Fortunately, no local residents were found to be positive for the virus. Swift action, community cooperation and the sharing of resources enabled a large number of tests to rule out presence of the virus in Riverdene and enabled schools, businesses and others to re-open within days. In rural communities in other nations, such local response has not been supported with the necessary resources from broader health systems, forcing rural people to travel to urban areas for testing.

QUESTION

What are the advantages and disadvantages of a rural community developing local responses to health issues?

Broader health systems

In the framework, broader **health systems** refer to how health care is funded, monitored, lobbied for and organised (Bourke et al., 2012a). The World Health Organization (WHO) has described six key building blocks of the well-functioning health system. These include effective governance and leadership; sustainable financing; a health workforce fit for its tasks; appropriate and affordable health products; responsive service delivery; and health information and research capacity (WHO, 2015).

In the context of public health, review evidence (Kenny et al., 2013) suggests that key features of a well-functioning preventive and promotive health service include the legislative and regulatory mechanisms that enable decentralised, regional administrative and financial management structures, strategic planning functions and technical support services to bring executive control and decision-making closer to the points of service influence, thereby

Health system –
the organisation and coordination of human, institutional, material and financial resources for the delivery of health services.

enabling flexible regional responses to the influence of wider external factors. This requires the development of systems requiring:

- consumer participation in health service decision-making
- interdisciplinary and team-based modes of working (Rygh & Hjortdahl, 2007).

In addition, many countries have also developed a range of partnerships within their health systems, on the basis that these arrangements would strengthen service provision. Examples include partnerships with specialist research institutes and academic centres; partnerships with non-government agencies in the delivery of specialised services; and partnerships with Aboriginal Community Controlled Health Organisations (ACCHO). In Australia, the swift change in health funding for telehealth during the COVID-19 pandemic increased access to services for many rural residents and enabled people to access health care in their own homes. This provided support for older people, people living with chronic conditions and others who were restricted in their travel during the pandemic to have continued access to their healthcare providers. Thus, rural health needs broader health systems to be responsive to its needs and to enable local action as well as to require inclusion, health equity and innovation in addressing isolation. Sometimes these systems support local community action and sometimes they can challenge narrow social norms. Broader health systems that are not suited to rural health stifle models of rural health care and lead to inappropriate care that can reduce access for rural residents. For example, investment in or subsidy of private health services often disadvantages rural residents as there are fewer private health services in rural areas. On the other hand, rural workforce programs enable health services in rural settings. Broader health systems and government policies can limit services in rural areas or be proactive in supporting rural health care. Internationally, there is great variation in the support of rural health services, and in the rural workforce and funding for rural health, resulting in wide disparity among rural health across the globe.

Health promotion – initiatives that aim to enable healthy lifestyles and behaviours based on Ottawa Charter principles.

Other chapters in this book deal comprehensively with **health promotion**, its basis in the Ottawa Charter (WHO, 1986) and its focus on addressing the determinants of health (see chapters 3 and 7). Health literacy, the capacity to absorb and critically analyse health information from multiple sources, has been identified as a key determinant of health (Kickbusch, 2001) and there is strong evidence of health literacy disadvantage among rural Australians, especially men (AIHW, 2010). According to the WHO (2009), health literacy 'goes beyond a narrow concept of health education and individual behaviour-oriented communication, and addresses the environmental, political and social factors that determine health'.

Broader social systems

In many ways, rural Australians are not that different from urban Australians; they access the same (social) media and information, and are subject to the same laws, education systems, class structures and social systems (Bourke et al., 2012a). Throughout the COVID-19 pandemic, rural residents had access to global information and heard about the approaches taken in Aotearoa New Zealand with its strict lockdowns as well as those in the United States and Brazil, where government action was lacking. As such, broader social systems influence rural health. Residents of Riverdene access health information on the internet, are marginalised for undesirable behaviours, and are required to meet the same entry requirements for university study. These all affect their health or their socio-economic status, which is a key predictor of health. In rural communities, these markers can be more identifiable than in urban communities, so that local residents may shape what others know about them and how they portray themselves.

Other chapters in this book have comprehensively explored the wider social determinants of health (see chapters 5, 8 and 20). During the pandemic, these determinants altered for some residents of Riverdene. While many middle-class residents worked from home, maintained their incomes and often saved money due to reduced expenditure on leisure activities, many young, casual workers lost income while their living expenses remained fixed and their social connection was lower. The effects of the pandemic highlighted many inequalities, particularly for young people on low incomes.

There is debate about whether 'rurality' itself is a social determinant of health; some argue that rurality and remoteness are factors that negatively affect health, while others suggest that the higher prevalence of other social determinants in rural areas (such as socio-economic disadvantage) is the reason for poorer rural health outcomes (Beard et al., 2009). There is evidence that residents of rural and remote Australia generally have higher rates of smoking, alcohol use at risky levels and obesity than their urban counterparts (NRHA, 2013a, 2013b, 2014). Many of these risk factors are also correlated with lower-than-average annual household income and lower levels of education. So, while the question of rurality itself as a determinant remains unresolved, there is evidence that many individual and social factors contribute to poorer health in rural settings. There is also evidence that access factors, including the lack of services, lack of specialist services, costs of services, limited choice of services and the one-size-fits-all approach of some services, are important health determinants in rural areas (NRHA, 2011, 2016). Papa and colleagues (2006) have demonstrated the power and utility of dialectical approaches to precipitate transformative social change, which is of particular relevance in disadvantaged rural settings.

Addressing health inequity and the resulting **rural health differential** requires engagement with issues and systems outside of health. Acknowledging genetic, environmental and behavioural factors, the social determinants that are particularly relevant to rural and remote health include being Aboriginal and Torres Strait Islander (see Chapter 19), as well as income, education, housing, work status and type, social inclusion or exclusion, and access to social resources and health services (Marmot & Wilkinson, 2006).

Rural health differential – the difference in health outcomes attributable to rural living.

Power

Power can be both a constraining and/or an enabling factor in the health of rural residents (Bourke et al., 2012a). Power is key to the decisions that people make about health, including decisions at the local level about when to seek health care and how health professionals treat patients, through to political decisions about funding and depictions of rural health in media forums. These decisions shape information, knowledge, actions and interactions that improve, maintain or threaten rural health outcomes.

Through the actions and mobilising capacities of individuals and groups, the exercise of power can bring change to, for example, models of care and approaches to practice, mediated through innovation and entrepreneurship (Bourke et al., 2012a). The framework also notes that power explains the heterogeneity of the rural health experience, through its entrenchment in the actions of individuals and groups, and reflected through structural factors including funding and social determinants in specific places.

At broader systems levels, these authors note that power can be exercised by individuals through existing structures and channels, to advocate for greater political visibility of rural communities and for effective and equitable resourcing for health and social services in rural settings (Bourke et al., 2012a). As noted earlier, an understanding of tensions within the production of power at community levels can be used to organise change or to reinforce stasis, to produce new circumstances or to ensure the maintenance of the status quo. The example of Riverdene has highlighted how vaccination, testing and lockdown policies can be accepted, promoted, challenged, changed and/or maintained through the actions of individuals in rural places. Bourke and colleagues (2012a) note that power both permeates and intersects each of the other five framework concepts as it is embedded in all social relations and is continuously negotiated and re-negotiated. An important implication of this is that community based public health professionals and/or consumers can take actions to challenge existing power structures and relations that produce and reproduce rural health disadvantage. Examples of this in practice are explored by Papa and colleagues (2006) and other similar texts. Regardless, key to the framework is that all six of the concepts are at play in understanding rural health, both action and innovation as well as inaction and disadvantage.

REFLECTION QUESTIONS

The concept of power can used to understand the scenarios included in this chapter. Thinking about these situations is particularly interesting. Read through Spotlights 21.1, 21.2 and 21.3 and reflect on the following questions:

1 Who in Riverdene and Bankstown exercised power by seeking to shape social normative behaviour towards pandemic-control measures implemented by respective regional jurisdictions?
2 How could farmers and agricultural workers organise to expand the range of access options to essential services?
3 What strategies were used in these efforts and how was the development of these strategies influenced by the geography, locale, local health responses and by broader social and health systems?

SUMMARY

This chapter has sought to characterise the health of rural residents through a conceptual framework that encompasses the diversity of health actions and outcomes in rural areas. After studying this chapter, you will have gained insights into the theory and practice of public health in rural settings.

Learning objective 1: Understand the diversity of rural health.
This chapter explored the diversity of rural and remote health in Australia and the many factors that shape health outcomes in a particular place. The integration of geographical factors, along with the local social and health actions and the broader health systems and social structures – through the concept of power – lead to the ways in which health outcomes are produced and reproduced. Power relations identify which (and how many) of the other five concepts dominate to produce and reproduce a particular outcome.

Learning objective 2: Discuss the broader determinants of health with respect to their effects in rural settings.
The chapter examined the character of rurality, its conception as a determinant of health and the different attempts to establish its dimensions, the breadth of the concept, the significant lack of uniformity of its application in national and global contexts, and the critical need for good data and information at the local level to underpin effective public health planning and practice.

Learning objective 3: Adapt the principles of health promotion and public health planning and practice to rural settings.
The chapter reflected on the evidence that highlights the importance of health-seeking patterns of behaviour in understanding variable health outcomes in diverse rural settings. This provided a foundation from which to explore more deeply the insights from social theory on the dynamic tensions shaping the potential for change in communities; from sociology on power relationships and the social production and reproduction of rural disadvantage; and from understandings of the constructed nature of rurality and its meaning to different individuals and peoples. These underpin the planning and application to engage multiple voices, consider community norms and existing behaviours, and engage in community based health promotion initiatives in varying situations.

Learning objective 4: Understand the complexity of health systems in delivering accessible public health services to rural residents, especially with regard to consumer issues and health.
Considering the attributes of the well-functioning health system and the modes of its expression in addressing the needs to diverse populations of rural residents, the chapter provided insights into the critical importance of community and consumer participation and activism. It envisioned the complex interplay of all these factors and appreciated how these might be articulated within a framework for rural health that includes the internal and the external influences at the macro and micro levels, and the dynamic interactions between them that shape the lived experience of the health of rural residents.

Learning objective 5: Demonstrate an appreciation of the role of power relations in influencing health outcomes in rural settings.
Examining the determinants of health and their distribution highlighted the relationship between power, socio-economic factors, health-service access and poorer health outcomes. Census and other data from different countries, while pointing to a more variable relationship between rurality, socio-economic status and health outcomes, do not often account for the structures and influence of power in this context. The chapter provided some insights into the practical actions required to begin to shift the balance of power at the local level to promote beneficial change.

TUTORIAL EXERCISES

1   Based on the information provided in this chapter, develop a public health plan for Riverdene. What issues would you prioritise, how would you address public health needs and what attention would you give to the pandemic and to other health issues?

2   Based on the information provided in this chapter, develop a community health education and information program on pandemic control measures, targeting young people who believe that the COVID-19 pandemic affects only older people. In the rationale for your strategy, defend your choice of messages and media platforms, and the processes you will use to assess the effectiveness of your program.

3   Identify a rural community and consider all that you know about the community according to each concept in the framework. What is its geographic isolation? What do you know about the rural locale and its people? What do you know about local health services and all health responses in this locale? How is this locale influenced by broader health systems and social structures? How are power relations apparent or hidden in the health of this community? What else do you need to know about this place to understand its health and wellbeing?

4   Reflect on your answers to the Spotlight 21.1 questions. Several overseas governments paused the roll-out of a COVID-19 vaccine due to unexpected and potentially serious side-effects. This has caused growing resistance in Bankstown to receiving a vaccine shot. Brainstorm with a colleague on how you might address this situation from a public health planning and practice perspective. How might insights you gain in this exercise be useful in your own current or future professional situation?

5   Organise a debate that includes faculty members and students to explore the question: 'Is rurality a determinant of health and does geography matter?'

FURTHER READING

Daghagh Yazd S., Wheeler S.A., & Zuo A. (2019). Key risk factors affecting farmers' mental health: A systematic review. *International journal of environmental research and public health, 16*(23).

Liaw, S. T., & Kilpatrick, S. (2008). *A textbook of Australian rural health*. Australian Rural Health Education Network.

O'Campo, P., & Dunn, J. (Eds.). (2012). *Rethinking social epidemiology: Towards a science of change*. Springer.

Papa, J., Singhal, A., & Papa, W. (2006). *Organising for social change: A dialectic journey of theory and praxis*. Sage Publications.

Taylor, J., Wilkinson, D., & Cheers, B. (2008). *Working with communities in health and human services*. Oxford University Press.

REFERENCES

Australian Institute of Health and Welfare (AIHW). (2010). *A snapshot of men's health in regional and remote Australia*. Rural health series No. 11. (Cat. No. PHE 120). AIHW. Retrieved https://www.aihw.gov.au/getmedia/c6068d06-1f98-4a97-b7b6-c069cbfffe76/10742.pdf.aspx?inline=true

——(2015). *Australian burden of disease study 2015: Fatal burden preliminary estimates*. Retrieved https://www.aihw.gov.au/reports/burden-of-disease/fatal-burden-2015-preliminary-estimates/contents/remoteness-areas

——(2017). *Risk factors to health*. Retrieved https://www.aihw.gov.au/reports/australias-health/biomedical-risk-factors

——(2018). *Rural and remote Australians*. Retrieved https://www.aihw.gov.au/reports-statistics/population-groups/rural-remote-australians/overview

——(2019). *Rural and remote health*. Retrieved https://www.aihw.gov.au/reports/rural-remote-australians/rural-remote-health/contents/summary

——(2020). *Rural and remote health*. Retrieved https://www.aihw.gov.au/getmedia/838d92d0-6d34-4821-b5da-39e4a47a3d80/Rural-remote-health.pdf.aspx?inline=true

——(2021). *Australian burden of disease study: Impact and causes of illness and death in Australia 2018*. Retrieved https://www.aihw.gov.au/getmedia/5ef18dc9-414f-4899-bb35-08e239417694/aihw-bod-29.pdf.aspx?inline=true

Beard, J., Tomaska, N., Earnest, A., Summerhayes, R., & Morgan, G. (2009). Influence of socioeconomic and cultural factors on rural health. *Australian Journal of Rural Health*, *17*, 10–15.

Bourke, L., Humphreys, J.S., Wakerman, J., & Taylor, J. (2010). From 'problem-describing' to 'problem-solving': Challenging the 'deficit' view in remote and rural health. *Australian Journal of Rural Health*, *18*, 205–9.

——(2012a). Understanding rural and remote health: A framework for analysis in Australia. *Health & Place*, *18*(3), 496–503.

——(2012b). Understanding drivers of rural and remote health outcomes: A conceptual framework in action. *Australian Journal of Rural Health*, *20*(6), 318–23.

Chandak, A., Nayar, P., & Lin, G. (2019). Rural-urban disparities in access to breast cancer screening: A spatial clustering analysis. *The Journal of Rural Health*, *35*(2), 229–35.

Cohen, S. A., Cook, S. K., Kelley, L., Foutz, J. D., & Sando, T. A. (2017). A closer look at rural-urban health disparities: Associations between obesity and rurality vary by geospatial and sociodemographic factors. *Journal of Rural Health*, *2*, 167–79.

Doogan, N., Roberts, M., M., Tanenbaum, E., Mumford, E., & Stillman, F. (2018). Validation of a new continuous geographic isolation scale: A tool for rural health disparities research. *Social Science & Medicine*, 215, 123–32.

Eberhardt, M. S. &, Pamuk, E. R. (2004). The importance of place and residence: Examining health in rural and nonrural areas. *American Journal Public Health*, *94*(10), 1682–6.

Holden, R., & Zhang, J. (2018). *The economic impact of improving regional, rural & remote education in Australia*. The Gonski Institute for Education, UNSW.

Kenny, A., Hyett, N., Sawtell, J., Dickson-Swift, V., Farmer, J., & O'Meara, P. (2013). Community participation in rural health: A scoping review. *BMC Health Services Research*, *13*, 64.

Kickbusch, I. (2001). Health literacy: Addressing the health and education divide. *Health Promotion International*, *16*, 289–97.

Malatzky, C., & Bourke, L. (2016). Re-producing rural health: Challenging dominant discourses and the manifestation of power. *Journal of Rural Studies*, *45*, 157–164.

Marmot, M. & Wilkinson, R. (2006) *Social determinants of health* (2nd ed.). Oxford University Press.

Murage, P., Murchie, P., Bachmann, M., Crawford, M., & Jones, A. (2017). Impact of travel time and rurality on presentation and outcomes of symptomatic colorectal cancer: A cross-sectional cohort study in primary care. *British Journal of General Practice*, *660*, 302.

National Rural Health Alliance (NRHA). (2011). *An overview of the shortage of primary care services in rural and remote areas*. NRHA. Retrieved http://ruralhealth.org.au/sites/default/files/documents/nrha-policy-document/position/pos-summary-complementary-report-27-feb-11.pdf

——(2013a). *How many doctors are there in rural Australia?* NHRA. Retrieved http://ruralhealth.org.au/sites/default/files/media-files/mr19dechowmanydrsfinal.pdf

——(2013b). *Obesity in rural Australia*. NHRA. Retrieved http://ruralhealth.org.au/sites/default/files/publications//nrha-obesity-fact-sheet.pdf

——(2014). *Alcohol use in rural Australia*. NHRA. Retrieved http://ruralhealth.org.au/sites/default/files/publications/nrha-factsheet-alcohol.pdf

——(2016). *The health of people living in remote Australia*. Retrieved http://ruralhealth.org.au/sites/default/files/publications/nrha-remote-health-fs-election2016.pdf

——(2017). *Poverty in rural and remote Australia*. NHRA. Retrieved https://www.ruralhealth.org.au/sites/default/files/publications/nrha-factsheet-povertynov2017.pdf

Nolan, J., Schultz, P., Cialdini, R., Goldstein, N., & Griskevicius, V. (2008). Normative social influence is underdetected. *Personality and Social Psychology Bulletin*, *34*(7), 913–23.

O'Campo, P., & Dunn, J. (Eds.) (2012). *Rethinking social epidemiology: Towards a science of change*. Springer.

Ostry, A. S. (2009). The mortality gap between urban and rural Canadians: A gendered analysis. *Rural and Remote Health*, *9*, 1286–96.

Papa, J., Singhal, A., & Papa, W. (2006). *Organising for social change – A dialectic journey of theory and praxis* (pp. 29–62). Sage Publications.

Penman-Aguilar, A. Talih, M., Huang, D., Moonesinghe, R., Bouye, K., & Beckles, G. (2016). Measurement of health disparities, health inequities, and social determinants of health to support the advancement of health equity. *Journal of public health management and practice*, *22*(1), S33–42.

Pierce, D., & Shann, C. (2012). Rural Australians' mental health literacy: Identifying and addressing their knowledge and attitudes. *Journal of Community Medicine & Health Education*, *2*, 139.

Preston, R., Waugh, H., Larkins, S., & Taylor, J. (2010). Community participation in rural primary health care: Intervention or approach? *Australian Journal of Primary Health*, *16*, 4–16.

Rygh, G., & Hjortdahl, J. (2007). Continuous and integrated health care services in rural areas: A literature study. *Rural and Remote Health*, *7*, 766. Retrieved http://www.rrh.org.au/publishedarticles/article_print_766.pdf

Scheil-Adlung, X. (Ed). (2015). *Global evidence on inequities in rural health protection. New data on rural deficits in health coverage for 174 countries*. International Labour Organization.

South, J., & Smith, G. (2014). Evaluating community engagement as part of the public health system. *Journal of Epidemiology and Community Health*, *68*, 692–6.

Terry, D., Ervin, K., Crouch, A., Glenister, K., & Bourke, L. (2017). Heterogeneity of rural consumer perceptions of health service access across four regions of Victoria. *Journal of Rural Social Science*, *32*(2), 125–45.

Wakerman, J. (2004). Defining remote health. *The Australian Journal of Rural Health*, *12*, 210–14.

Wakerman, J., Bourke, L., Humphreys, J. S., & Taylor, J. (2017). Is remote health different to rural health? *Rural and Remote Health*, *17*(2), 3832.

Wakerman, J., Humphreys, J.S., Wells, R. et al. (2008). Primary health care delivery models in rural and remote Australia – a systematic review. *BMC Health Services Research*, 8, 276.

World Health Organization (WHO). (1986). *The Ottawa Charter for Health Promotion*. WHO.

——(2009). *7th global conference on health promotion. Track 2: Health literacy and health behaviour*. Retrieved http://www.who.int/healthpromotion/conferences/7gchp/track2/en/

——(2015). *The WHO health systems framework*. Retrieved https://www.who.int/healthsystems/strategy/everybodys_business.pdf

Zahnd, W. E., Fogleman, A. J., & Jenkins, W. D. (2018). Rural–urban disparities in stage of diagnosis among cancers with preventive opportunities. *American Journal of Preventive Medicine*, *5*, 688.

Drug use in Australia: A public health approach

22

Andrew Smirnov and Jake Najman

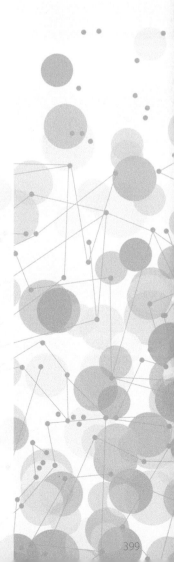

LEARNING OBJECTIVES

After studying this chapter, you should be able to:

1 distinguish between different drugs according to their effect types
2 describe four of the main factors that contribute to people's decisions to use drugs
3 describe the relative contribution of different substances to the burden of disease
4 explain ways in which social attitudes affect how we respond to drug use
5 identify possible changes to current policies that could reduce levels of drug-related harm.

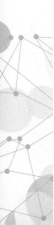

VIGNETTE

The marketing of drugs

A community's understanding of the use of legal and illegal (or 'illicit') drugs can be shaped by deliberate misinformation, sometimes false and misleading claims, and a wide range of prejudices. In the context of large corporations, there is a financial incentive to maximise sales of their products. The desire to maximise profits often leads companies to misrepresent the products they sell – in particular, to emphasise real (or non-existent) benefits (e.g. drinking **alcohol** or smoking cigarettes can make you a more attractive and better person, and you will have more fun with friends etc.). There is a related incentive to deny – or at least minimise – the harms attributed to a product.

The marketing of legal drugs contributes to their use. The alcohol industry has used marketing strategies that associate alcohol use with sport and sporting achievement, with improving friendship and popularity, and generally with having a 'good time'. When similar strategies were denied to the tobacco industry, the use of tobacco products declined. Understandably, the alcohol industry resists all efforts to limit the marketing and promotion of their products. To the extent that they find it possible, the alcohol industry engages in campaigns to mislead those who consume alcohol about the benefits and harms associated with its use. In some other countries (e.g. the United States), alcohol products carry warning labels; these varyingly acknowledge that alcohol causes cancer, heart disease and, when consumed by a pregnant woman, may lead to foetal alcohol syndrome in the child. Australian companies selling alcohol products in the United States carry these warning labels. These same Australian companies, selling the same product in Australia, often use no warning labels.

While in the past the most substantially misleading marketing and labelling practices have been in relation to tobacco and alcohol, there is concern about products that have recently been legalised, such as cannabis, will be subject to the same promotional pressures.

Alcohol – contains ethanol, which is carcinogenic. It comes in different forms, such as spirits, beer and wine, all of which are produced by fermentation of yeast and, for higher alcohol-content products, by subsequent distillation. Alcohol has a depressant effect on the central nervous system and impairs motor skills and cognitive functioning.

Introduction

In this chapter, we discuss drug use in Australia. We take a public health approach to the problems created in the use of drugs. Public health approaches focus on reducing the harmful consequences of substance use, irrespective of the type of substance being used (Csete et al., 2016). Reducing population-level harms related to substance use can be achieved by reducing the numbers of people who use drugs, and by reducing harmful patterns of use among those who choose to use them. These two goals can be compatible.

However, in some instances, policies aimed at achieving the first goal (reducing numbers) may work to the detriment of the second goal (reducing harm), if that policy is based on criminalising drug use (Csete et al., 2016). For example, laws criminalising heroin use may deter people from seeking help when an overdose occurs, for fear of being identified by police. The reverse might also be true for some policies that aim to reduce harm. For example, the legalisation of cannabis use could arguably increase rates of use, especially if the laws permitted the open marketing of cannabis products (Hall & Lynskey, 2016). Drug use can result in harm, but so can policies on drug use.

Public health responses to drug use acknowledge that some people will continue to use drugs regardless of legal or social sanctions. Consequently, policies aimed at reducing drug-related harm are central to a public health framework. Some public health policies (e.g. taxation) work by reducing both the numbers of users and the harmful patterns of use (Anderson et al., 2009).

Globally, policy approaches can be viewed along a spectrum. At one end, countries such as the Philippines have criminalised drug use to the extent that people who use drugs may be executed by the police if they do not surrender to authorities (Simangan, 2018). At the other end, many countries are shifting away from criminalisation. Portugal has decriminalised all drug use and has increased health services for people who use drugs (Goncalves, Lourenco & da Silva, 2015). In Australia, state and territorial government policies addressing substance use are heterogeneous and differ fundamentally according to the type of drug being targeted, even for legal drugs such as tobacco and alcohol (Hall & Weier, 2017). Despite the considerable variation in policy on illicit drug use among different countries, prohibition remains a cornerstone of policy internationally. A prohibitionist approach has been upheld through international treaties, including the 1961 *Single Convention on Narcotic Drugs* and the 1988 *Convention Against Illicit Drug Traffic in Narcotic Drugs and Psychoactive Substances* (United Nations Office on Drugs and Crime, 2013).

Types of drugs

Through recorded time people have used a variety of substances to enhance their mood or to treat perceived health problems. Drugs – including those now considered illicit drugs – represent one category of substance very commonly used in all societies over recorded time. Drugs are generally considered in terms of their primary effects, which vary according to dosage. While we adhere to this convention, there is a need to acknowledge that many people who use drugs use multiple drug types with sometimes differing, even conflicting effects (Zinberg, 1986). For example, people drinking alcohol may also use amphetamines. Alcohol may be used for its disinhibiting and sedating or relaxing effects, while amphetamines may be used as a stimulant. Mixing alcohol and amphetamines can increase the amount of time a person spends drinking, because the amphetamines override the sedative effects of alcohol (Leslie et al., 2016). Thus, discussing specific drugs as distinct substances may not do justice to actual behaviour. The three main categories of drugs are depressants, stimulants and hallucinogens. We consider each of these in turn.

REFLECTION QUESTION

In what ways are drugs that are illegal in Australia (e.g. heroin, methamphetamines) different from legal drugs (alcohol, tobacco) or drugs that are prescribed for medical use? Are there specific drugs whose classification as legal, illicit or medicinal may vary depending on the context and setting?

Depressants

Depressants are substances that depress the central nervous system and reduce the level of awareness and/or energy of the user (Julien, 2001). Depressants can reduce a person's physical coordination and awareness of their environment. Alcohol is the most frequently consumed depressant; others are heroin, morphine and benzodiazepines, other tranquillisers and petrol/ glue or paint (the latter usually sniffed).

Opioids – a class of drug that acts on the body's opioid receptors to produce powerful depressant effects on the central nervous system and euphoria. Opioids occur naturally as a product of the poppy plant (e.g. opium, morphine and heroin), in semi-synthetic forms (e.g. oxycodone, buprenorphine) and in synthetic forms (e.g. fentanyl, pethidine).

Heroin is an opioid, as are prescribed and other widely used **opioids** such as oxycodone and morphine. Opioids have pain-relieving and sedating effects. They suppress the rate of breathing, slowing the heart rate and increasing the risk that the heart stops functioning. One problem associated with opioid use is that the person using develops a tolerance over time and requires larger quantities to achieve the same benefit. Opioids are consumed orally, or they may be converted to a liquid and injected intravenously. While opioids are responsible for about 600 deaths in Australia each year, their harm to the vital organs of the body is generally low. Deaths that do occur are usually due to respiratory failure. While alcohol is a carcinogen and damages several bodily organs (e.g. liver, kidney, brain), the opioids are comparatively benign in their effects, with the important exception of respiratory failure (Julien, 2001).

Stimulants

Stimulants affect the central nervous system. Stimulants increase energy, alertness and activity. Commonly used stimulants are amphetamines, caffeine, nicotine and cocaine. Stimulants are widely used legally; for example, Ritalin, which is used to treat children with attention deficit hyperactivity disorder (ADHD), is an amphetamine. Members of the armed forces in World War II (and since) were supplied with amphetamines to enable them to stay awake at night or when long periods of continuous alertness were required (Julien, 2001). Stimulants increase central nervous system activity, they increase the heart rate and some-times create a feeling in the affected person that they can do more things than might otherwise be the case. Stimulants, particularly crystal methamphetamine ('ice') can be highly addictive. When taken by injection, amphetamines can cause users to feel a 'rush' of energy and euphoria. Similarly, the smoking of crystal methamphetamine can produce a rapid high. Amphetamines are also snorted (intranasal use) or swallowed, with more gradual onset of effects compared to injecting or smoking. There are some important harms associated with amphetamine use, including hallucinations, psychotic thoughts and violent behaviour. While most of the adverse symptoms associated with amphetamine use disappear once amphet-amine use has ceased, there may be more persistent harms depending upon the quantity and duration of amphetamine use. Most recent estimates of deaths attributable to amphetamine use are that between 100 and 200 Australians die each year (Australian Institute of Health and Welfare [AIHW], 2018).

Cocaine is a stimulant whose popularity in Australia has only recently begun to increase (AIHW, 2017). Drugs such as heroin and amphetamines have generally been sourced from Asia and South East Asia (Myanmar, China, Afghanistan). By contrast, cocaine is generally produced in South America (United Nations Office on Drugs and Crime, 2017), and conse-quently the importation of cocaine has involved a more difficult supply chain. Cocaine provides a rapid feeling of euphoria and, in some forms (e.g. 'crack' cocaine), is highly addictive. Cocaine is snorted through the nose, smoked, rubbed on gums or dissolved in fluid and injected. Cocaine use presents substantial public health concerns because of its immediate but short duration of effect (perhaps no longer than 30 minutes). Users may feel the need to continue using to maintain their feelings of euphoria. The health problems experienced by people who use cocaine may include hallucinations, paranoia and becoming malnourished, and include the normal risks of those who share injecting equipment or sexual partners. It is also possible to overdose on cocaine, with cardiovascular consequences that can be fatal (Julien, 2001).

Hallucinogens

Hallucinogens affect the nervous system by altering sensory perceptions and thought patterns. Visual hallucinations are a common effect (Julien, 2001). A wide variety of substances produce profound hallucinogenic effects, including naturally occurring substances such as psilocybin ('magic mushrooms'), ayahuasca and peyote, and synthesised drugs such as LSD (lysergic acid diethylamide) and PCP (phencyclidine). Sometimes, hallucinogens produce feelings of anxiety and paranoia (a 'bad trip'). The number of people using these drugs is relatively small, although the global popularity of traditional shamanistic drugs such as ayahuasca has recently increased. People who use hallucinogens tend to do so on an infrequent basis (Nichols, 2004).

Drugs with a mix of effects

Other drugs, including ecstasy (MDMA: 3,4-methylenedioxymethylamphetamine) and cannabis produce a variety of effects on the nervous system, and are more difficult to classify. Ecstasy produces a unique profile of stimulant and hallucinogenic effects, while cannabis can produce a mix of stimulant, depressant and hallucinogenic effects, which varies depending on the strain of cannabis being used (Green et al., 2003; Morgan et al., 2010).

Ecstasy is the most popular illicit stimulant in Australia (AIHW, 2017). Ecstasy is a 'ring-substituted' amphetamine derivative, which means that it differs in chemical structure from other amphetamines. Ring-substituted derivatives are like mescaline in their chemical structure, which contributes to their unique effects. Ecstasy is a powerful stimulant, and generally produces feelings of wellbeing, euphoria, empathy and social connectedness. The pharmacologist David Nichols (1986) introduced the label 'entactogens' (meaning 'to touch within') to describe the effects of ecstasy and similar amphetamine derivatives. In a cultural sense, there is a nexus between ecstasy use and electronic dance music; the use of this drug is common among people attending venues and events (such as raves) where electronic dance music is played (Reynolds, 2013; Smirnov et al., 2013). Due to the high demand for the drug and a fluctuating supply, a variety of synthetic stimulants and hallucinogens are sometimes sold as ecstasy. These drugs tend to be far more dangerous than ecstasy, and increase the risk of stimulant overdose (Rigg & Sharp, 2018).

Cannabis, the most widely used illicit drug in the world, may create feelings of being relaxed, a sense of increased appreciation of musical or artistic works, or of particular foods, and even feelings of being more creative. Cannabis users may experience these effects for hours after using. Notably, cannabis use, on its own, rarely leads to violent or aggressive behaviour (Wei et al., 2004).

Cannabis is usually smoked (frequently with tobacco), or it may be used to make food products (or as an oil) to be consumed orally. There are harms associated with the use of cannabis. Pregnant women who use cannabis have lower birthweight babies (Hayatbakhsh et al., 2012), and sustained use of cannabis over many years is associated with a range of more severe symptoms of mental illness (McGrath et al., 2010). Otherwise, short-term, occasional use of cannabis does not appear to be associated with adverse health outcomes.

The drug-related burden of disease

How big a problem is alcohol use in Australia?

Alcohol use in Australia is estimated to lead to 6000 deaths each year (AIHW, 2018). In addition to its effects on the foetus, such as foetal alcohol syndrome and less-severe foetal alcohol effects, alcohol consumption is a cause of bowel and breast cancer, mouth and pharyngeal cancer, oesophageal cancer, coronary heart disease, stroke, liver cancer, homicide and suicide (Boffetta & Hashibe, 2006; Wood et al., 2018).

Changes in disease burden over the period 2003 to 2011 have been attributed to alcohol. Overall, there was a slight decline in alcohol death rates in Australia between 2003 and 2011.

However, for the alcohol disease burden in Australia, more remote parts of Australia have a higher population adjusted burden compared to urban locations; for example, major cities had 9.0 per 1000 population deaths per year over that period, outer regional areas 11.9 per 1000 population deaths and very remote areas 21.5 deaths per 1000 population per year. Alcohol-related death rates in persons in very remote parts of Australia are 2.5 times those in persons living in major Australian cities. Also, persons living in the most economically disadvantaged parts of Australia have death rates about twice those experienced by people living in the most economically disadvantaged areas in Australia (Australian Bureau of Statistics, 2017).

Finally, it is worth noting that there are some deficiencies in the way alcohol consumption is reported in Australia. Self-reported alcohol consumed is an underestimate of the amount actually consumed. Looking at the total amount of alcohol sold and estimates of consumption from the National Drug Strategy Household Survey, only 80 per cent of the alcohol sold is reported in self-report surveys of alcohol consumption (AIHW, 2011). This has led researchers to recommend the use of an adjustment factor (of around 1.30) for these survey estimates of alcohol consumption (Livingston & Callinan, 2015; Stockwell et al., 2016).

SPOTLIGHT 22.1

Changes in alcohol consumption among Aboriginal and Torres Strait Islander peoples

Aboriginal and Torres Strait Islander peoples have historically had higher rates of abstinence from alcohol than non-Indigenous Australians, but have also been more likely to consume alcohol at levels that put them at risk of harm. However, the proportions of Aboriginal and Torres Strait Islander peoples drinking at harmful levels have significantly decreased over the past decade. The estimated proportion (aged 14 years or older) drinking at levels that increased their lifetime risk of harm from alcohol-related disease or injury decreased from 30 per cent in 2010 to 20 per cent in 2019. Similarly, the proportion engaging in risky single occasion drinking declined from 39 per cent in 2010 to 35 per cent in 2019. By comparison, in 2019 around 17 per cent of non-Indigenous Australians drank at levels that increased their lifetime risk and 26 per cent engaged in risky single-occasion drinking. Decreases in risky drinking have been driven by changing patterns among adolescents and young adults.

The historical differences in substance-use behaviour should not be considered in isolation, but as part of the broader problem of a gap in health status and life expectancy between Indigenous and non-Indigenous Australians. This gap is intergenerational, adversely affecting successive generations since British colonisation of Australia, and is linked with social and economic disadvantage (Zhao et al., 2013). Colonisation resulted in profound disruption of Aboriginal and Torres Strait Islander peoples' cultures. Family histories of traumatic events and the experience of racism have likely had a substantial effect on patterns of alcohol use (Ziersch et al., 2011).

Much of the public spotlight has been on alcohol misuse in remote communities, where problems of disadvantage, such as inadequate housing and employment, are especially evident. However, a majority of Aboriginal and Torres Strait Islander peoples live in major cities, where alcohol use and social stress are also major problems (Stevens & Paradies, 2014).

Reconnection with land (a person's Country), community and cultural traditions may be protective against harmful alcohol use; culture is integral to the programs run by Aboriginal Community Controlled Health Organisations (ACCHO), including health promotion programs such as Deadly Choices (Campbell et al., 2018; Canuto et al., 2021; see also Chapter 19).

In most cases, government policies responding to alcohol-related harms among Aboriginal and Torres Strait Islander peoples have not considered the specific needs of these populations, and have not been properly evaluated (d'Abbs, 2015). Similarly, there are few studies examining the effectiveness of alcohol treatment services (Brett et al., 2016; Leske et al., 2016). The available evidence suggests that the empowerment of Indigenous families and communities is a necessary element, for both population-level and treatment interventions. More research is required to understand what works in this area of public health policy.

QUESTION

Holistic approaches to health care involve caring for the person rather than simply treating an identified health problem. Describe some ways in which a culturally appropriate alcohol intervention for Aboriginal and Torres Strait Islander peoples might reflect a holistic approach.

How big a problem is substance use in Australia?

Figure 22.1 provides some details of the harms associated with the use of illicit drugs in Australia and how these have changed over the past 25 years. The histogram (bars) shows that the number of deaths in Australia, attributable to the use of drugs, was close to historic highs (in 2017 about 2000 deaths). Since Australia's population has increased over the 25-year period, the 'fairer' comparison is the age-standardised death rate. This death rate peaked in 1999, when the availability of heroin was high. Heroin availability declined in the years 2000–01; due to the war in Afghanistan, the production of heroin declined substantially and so did supplies in Australia. Since 2007–08, the drug-induced death rate has again increased and is now close to historic highs. This is despite periodic and repeated government campaigns to reduce the use of illicit drugs. In 2019, it was estimated that 9 million Australians (14 years and over) had ever used an illicit drug and 3.4 million Australians had used an illicit drug in the previous 12 months (AIHW, 2020). As Figure 22.1 indicates, the use of illicit drugs continues to be a major health problem in Australia.

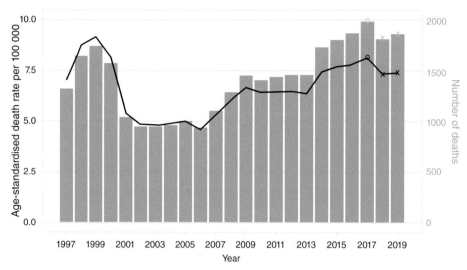

Figure 22.1   Number and age-standardised rate (per 100 000) of drug-induced deaths in Australia, 1997–2019.
Source: Chrzanowska et al., (2021).

Table 22.1 provides further details of the drugs used in Australia. Cannabis, ecstasy and meth/amphetamines have, over recent years, been the most commonly used drugs but cocaine use (and supplies) have now greatly increased (AIHW, 2020). The increasing use (and availability) of cocaine is of particular concern considering what is known about the harmful consequences of cocaine use in countries such as the United States. There is a possibility that the recent decline in rates of meth/amphetamine use may reflect its replacement with cocaine as a drug of choice.

Table 22.1   Use of illicit drugs in Australia, 2019

	Cannabis	Cocaine	Ecstasy	Meth/ Amphetamine
Lifetime ever use	36%	11%	12.5%	5.8%
Use in previous 12 months	12%	4%	3%	1.3%
Offered/opportunity to use past 12 months	23%	8.5%	7%	4.4%
Average (mean) age of first use	18.9 yrs	24.0 yrs	22.0 yrs	22.0 yrs
Of those using in 12 months, percentage who use frequently[*]	37%	17%	17%	16.9%

* Frequently for cannabis and meth/amphetamines is defined as weekly or more often;
for cocaine and ecstasy frequently is defined as monthly or more often.
Source: Based on AIHW (2020).

Two factors seem particularly important in the decision to begin using an illicit drug. The first is that persons who have not previously used a drug are offered a drug, usually by someone they already know. The second is that curiosity motivates many to accept the offer. In Table 22.1, we note that almost one in four Australians had been offered cannabis in the previous year and one in 12 had been offered cocaine. When we look at frequency of drug use, 37 per cent of cannabis and 16.9 per cent of meth/amphetamine users report using every week, while about 17 per cent of cocaine and ecstasy users report using once a month or more often (but not weekly). It is important to distinguish patterns of drug use in community samples (e.g. obtained from national population surveys) from patterns of use characteristic of those seeking treatment for a mental illness or problem with drug use, or both. The latter represent a relatively small subgroup of all users and tend to have much higher levels of use.

Patterns of drug use in Australia have changed over time and there have been important changes in the characteristics of those who use drugs (Table 22.2). It is relevant to distinguish those who have ever (in their lifetime) used an illicit drug from those who have recently (previous 12 months) used an illicit drug. Comparing 2001 and 2019 data, we see that lifetime ever-use of an illicit drug peaked in the 20–29-year age group in 2001 and the 40–49-year age group in 2019. By 2019, the majority of those aged between 20 and 59 years of age reported that they had ever used an illicit drug. When we look at drug use in the previous year (recent use), we see that in 2001 use was at a peak in the 20–29-year age group. This remained the case in 2019, although recent drug use in 2019 substantially increased in all groups aged 40 years and over. The increased recent use of illicit drugs by those aged 50–59 and 60+ years of age is particularly substantial. Data on those who die because of illicit drug use confirms that most deaths are in the middle age group (40–59 years). Australia is witnessing an ageing among those experiencing problems associated with their use of illicit drugs.

Table 22.2 Lifetime ever-use of an illicit drug by age, 2001 and 2019

Age group	2001		2019	
	Ever used (%)	Recent use (%)	Ever used (%)	Recent use (%)
14–19	38	26.0	22	15.1
20–29	63	32.3	50	28.8
30–39	53	17.4	52	17.6
40–49	42	9.4	55	13.4
50–59	22	3.5	50	10.6
60+	8	0.9	29	3.7

Source: Adapted from AIHW (2020).

The reasons for these changing age-related patterns are complex. To some extent they reflect an 'age cohort' effect, whereby a proportion of people who used drugs such as cannabis or opioids in early adulthood are persisting with some level of use in middle and older age (Kaur et al., 2021; Peterson, 2017). However, these changes also appear to reflect 'period effects', in which societal changes (e.g. liberalisation of attitudes to cannabis use; changes in analgesic prescription use) influence age-related substance use patterns.

The use of drugs by older persons poses a new set of challenges. Older persons are not generally a group who use illicit drugs to 'party' in the company of others. While little is specifically known about how the motivations of older users differ from those of younger users, it appears that the two main drug types leading to death (opiates and benzodiazepines) are used for the relief of symptoms involving pain and depressed mood. It is the use of prescribed drugs that leads to a fatal outcome for many older users of drugs (ABS, 2019). It is now the case that more persons die because they have used a prescribed opiate than those who die because they have used an opiate that has been obtained illegally (e.g. heroin) (Vadivelu et al., 2018).

The evidence concerning the harms experienced by those who use illicit drugs should also be considered. First, most people who use illicit drugs do so, perhaps, once a week or once a month, or even less often. There is little evidence that this level of use leads to lasting harms. On the other hand, the persistent use of drugs over an extended period likely leads to a variety of harms. These harms may increase in those who engage in polydrug use; that is, who use different drugs over the same time period.

Harms associated with the use of illicit drugs can be considered in one of three categories. Death or serious injury comprises one category of harm. Opiates and benzodiazepines are the main drugs leading to death, while some stimulants (meth/amphetamines, cocaine) appear to lead to violent or aggressive behaviour. A second category of harm involves seeking medical or hospital care when affected by illicit drugs, or being arrested for a drug offence. The use of cannabis or amphetamines comprises most of these latter harms (AIHW, 2020). A third category of harm involves a wide range of activities undertaken while under the influence of various substances (Table 22.3). Thus, it is not uncommon that people driving a car, swimming or at work are affected either by alcohol or illicit drugs. Only a small proportion of those affected by alcohol or drugs report verbally abusing someone, creating a disturbance, driving a boat or using machinery.

Table 22.3   Activities undertaken in past 12 months while under the influence of alcohol or illicit drugs

Activity	Alcohol (%)	Illicit drugs (%)
Went to work	8.7	9.9
Went swimming	15.4	12.4
Operated a boat or hazardous machinery	3.4	3.5
Drove a vehicle	18.5	15.1
Created a disturbance, damaged or stole goods	4.4	3.1
Verbally abused someone	6.8	2.8
Physically abused someone	1.0	0.6

Source: Based on AIHW (2016).

Medicinal cannabis

In recent years, we have witnessed a dramatic increase in the use of cannabis for medicinal purposes. This increase has been exemplified by successive states of the United States legislating for the prescribing of cannabis products for an extraordinarily wide range of conditions. Indeed, in several states the use of medicinal cannabis is very simple and only involves a doctor issuing a script at the request of the patient. To cater for this increased demand for 'legal' cannabis, cannabis shops (dispensaries) have proliferated (e.g. in California). One such dispensary, Med Men, advertises that it draws its inspiration from Apple computer stores. These cannabis stores have many different forms of cannabis available (e.g. cannabis that is grown organically grown or with higher concentrations of active ingredients).

While the evidence supporting the beneficial effects of cannabis is generally lacking, some support for the benefits of cannabis for certain health problems does exist. Interpreting this evidence requires a focus on two of the best-known ingredients of cannabis (cannabinoids); namely, THC (delta-9-tetrahydrocannabinol) and CBD (cannabidiol). THC is likely the main component of cannabis responsible for its intoxicating effects (i.e. feeling high). THC may be effective in treating chronic pain and anorexia and minimising the side effects of cancer treatments. By contrast, CBD does not have intoxicating effects but may be helpful in the treatment of some mental illnesses and epilepsy (Arnold, Nation & McGregor, 2020). Partly because CBD has no intoxicating effects, it is available as an over-the-counter product in some countries (not Australia). It is also important to note that therapeutic doses of THC are much lower than doses considered therapeutic for CBD (Arnold et al., 2020). The WHO has recommended that CBD not be a controlled product as its use presents no risk of abuse or dependence (O'Brien, 2020).

Medicinal cannabis may now be prescribed in every Australian state and territory except Tasmania. Pharmacists in Australia may dispense prescribed cannabis products; however, no cannabis products are subsidised on the Pharmaceutical Benefits Scheme (PBS). The most common symptoms leading to the prescribing of cannabis products are for arthritic, back and neck pain. These are typically conditions that are chronic and involve persistent pain that does not often respond well to minor analgesics. There are now several companies on the Australian stock exchange whose business is the production of cannabis for medicinal purposes (e.g. Cann Group, Zelira Therapeutics).

Of the estimated 600 000 Australians who used cannabis medicinally in 2019, only a very small proportion obtained a prescription, with the vast majority sourcing their cannabis through illegal markets.

Recreational use of cannabis

Countries in which it is legal to use cannabis as a recreational drug include Canada, Uruguay, the Netherlands, Spain and Switzerland. Cannabis use is also legal in 18 states of the United States. China is the largest exporter of cannabis in the world, despite the fact that cannabis use is prohibited in that country (O'Brien, 2020).

Recreational use of cannabis is legal in the Australian Capital Territory (ACT) for those 18 years of age and over (O'Brien, 2020). In Australia, it is illegal to drive a vehicle with any level of THC, even if the cannabis has been medically prescribed (O'Brien, 2020). It is, however, not known what level of THC in the body leads to impaired driving.

A general issue of concern must be the ambiguous legal status of cannabis, with its legality in some jurisdictions contrasted to its illegality in others. Many Australians are charged each year with offences relating to the use of cannabis. Once a person is convicted of a criminal offence, their future may be greatly affected. For example, they may be disqualified from employment in the public service or from travelling to some countries. The concern is that severe consequences may flow from laws that are variable.

Alcohol and illicit drugs – pleasure and prejudice

Alcohol and other drugs are the subject of heavily contested beliefs about what should be done to reduce their harms in society. Beliefs about alcohol and most drugs are subject to a range of often inaccurate stereotypes. These stereotypes are applied to almost all phenomena encountered by humans. For example, they may be racially based, gender-based or age-related. Here, it is important to note that these stereotypes are often inaccurate. Many of the same concerns are evident about people who use substances, both licit and illicit.

Table 22.4 reflects one way of understanding the values and beliefs that underpin how societies respond to problems posed by the use of licit and illicit drugs. The two main legal (licit) drugs used in Australia are tobacco and alcohol. The physical harm that is a consequence of the use of legal drugs is massive.

Table 22.4   Estimating the harms associated with listed behaviours

	Licit drug use (tobacco, alcohol)	Illicit drug use – more common (cannabis, ecstasy)	Illicit drug use – less common (opioids, ice, cocaine)	Petty theft (e.g. shoplifting)
Physical health harm to individual	Very high	Low	Moderate/high	Low
Mental health harm to individual	Low	Low	Moderate/high	Low
Physical harm to others	Moderate	Low	Moderate	Low
Harm to the broader society (economic, social)	Moderate/high	Low	Low	Low/moderate
Sanctions/punishments	Nil/low	High	High	Low

Note: Table based on estimates of substance-related mortality from the Global Burden of Disease Study (see Peacock et al., 2018; Rehm et al., 2006).

By contrast, the physical harm associated with use of cannabis and ecstasy is trivial; almost no-one dies in Australia as a consequence of using cannabis, while perhaps 10 Australians die each year as a consequence of using ecstasy. We have noted that over 600 Australians die each year due to the use of opiates (heroin as well as prescribed opiates for pain relief), and 100–200 Australians die as a consequence of using crystal or other forms of methamphetamine (ice) each year (AIHW, 2018). While these latter numbers are too high, they are low compared to the burden of deaths associated with the use of legal drugs. It is worth considering one other form of illegal behaviour (petty theft) to provide a contrast. Punishments for petty theft are appropriately minor. The issue here is that the penalties applied to those using illicit drugs appear to be disproportionate to the harms that are observed. The illegality of drug use may also be counter-productive due to **stigma** and concealment of drug-using behaviour (Leslie et al., 2018). Even the threat of severe punishment does not appear to 'work'. Compulsory incarceration does not seem to make a difference (there is a major problem with illicit drug use in prisons). A majority of people who are incarcerated begin using again after leaving prison, and repeated imprisonment is

Stigma – disapproval of a person on the basis of a trait such as substance use. Stigmatising a person involves attributing a set of negative characteristics to them (stereotypes), and can result in discrimination in health services and other everyday interactions. People may develop a sense of shame and worthlessness as a consequence of social stigma.

associated with higher levels of drug use and dependence (Smirnov et al., 2016). If, as appears to be the case, these penalties are also ineffective, then it is relevant to ask why they exist.

With regard to mental health harms, tobacco and alcohol are associated with a range of mental health problems, though there is uncertainty about whether these mental health problems precede or follow the use of tobacco and/or alcohol (Fluharty et al., 2017). In general, people who occasionally use cannabis and ecstasy are not affected by mental health problems – with the caveat that high and persistent levels of cannabis use have been found to lead to a range of mental health problems (McGrath et al., 2010). Mental health consequences are more readily observed in those who use opioids, crystal methamphetamine and cocaine.

Taking note of the known harms associated with the use of licit and illicit drugs, the ones causing the greatest harm (tobacco, alcohol) are legally accepted. By contrast, the use of some illicit drugs that cause comparatively little harm are subject to much more severe punishment.

REFLECTION QUESTION

What is a single policy measure that could help to reduce drug-related harm among young adults? Why do you think it would be effective? Would it be feasible to introduce this policy? Why or why not?

Why do people use drugs? What types of drugs do they use?

There continues to be a good deal of debate about why people use drugs, and this debate involves the use of both legal and illicit drugs. At one level the answer to why people use drugs is obvious: there is pleasure and reward associated with using drugs (Adinoff, 2004). The pleasure or reward may come either from the substance itself (relaxing or stimulant effects, experiencing a change in mood), or from the pleasures associated with the context in which drugs are used (e.g. meeting and socialising with friends, being a member of a social network who all use similar substances). For many, these are powerful motives to use that override the threat of possible harm likely to be experienced some time in the future. We argue that it is important to think of the use of drugs as a rational activity. All users have some understanding of the risks involved when using drugs. A good example is that cigarette smokers know that smoking may lead to lung cancer, as well as heart disease and other conditions. Despite this, a significant proportion of the population continues to smoke cigarettes. In this context, it is naïve to expect that those who are using drugs with fewer harms than tobacco will be dissuaded from using by the risks involved, even if those risks include criminal sanctions.

Regardless of the reasons people have for first using drugs, the reasons they continue to use may be different (Anthony et al., 1994). Thus, some drugs may lead to dependency more than others (nicotine is highly addictive), while the social context in which other drugs are used may provide a strong motive to continue to use; alcohol is often consumed by young people in a peer setting in which there may be encouragement to drink very heavily.

There are many reasons that people choose to use both legal and illicit drugs. These include that people may want to feel the effects of a drug (e.g. to relax), as a form of self-medication if they are distressed, or they may want to show they reject some societal constraints, or may wish to visibly demonstrate a degree of individuality (Boys, Marsden & Strang, 2001). Substance use may reflect a response to family breakdown or a particular pattern of parenting (Kuntsche et al., 2006). It may also be that some people are simply exposed to an environment of high drug use – they come into more frequent contact with some drugs than others (Wagner & Anthony, 2002). By contrast to the positive reasons for using, the negative reasons (e.g. health may be affected at an unknown period in the future), the cost to using, as well as the risk of police contact (generally evaluated as a low risk), may not weigh heavily when a decision is made to use a drug.

Another factor affecting decisions to use drugs involves their availability. Research conducted in the United States, using data from the National Household Surveys of Drug Abuse, has indicated that the population prevalence of drug use is proportionate to the prevalence of opportunities to try a drug (Van Etten & Anthony, 1999; Van Etten et al., 1997). This body of research also indicates that the propensity to try different drugs (i.e. to accept opportunities) differs by drug type. For example, 66.8 per cent of males and 65.5 per cent of females who had the opportunity to use cannabis eventually used this drug, compared to 50.6 per cent and 46.3 per cent for cocaine and 17.7 per cent and 25.6 per cent for heroin. This pattern suggests a lower propensity to accept opportunities for drugs that are less socially acceptable or perceived to be more dangerous. This highlights the role of rationality in decisions about drug use.

SPOTLIGHT 22.2

Technological change and substance use

The rapid development of the internet and other technologies has raised major issues for the control of substance use. These issues span the use of all substances including tobacco, alcohol and illicit drugs.

TOBACCO

Electronic cigarettes have recently proliferated and are increasingly popular in a number of countries, including the United States and the United Kingdom, although a majority of e-cigarette users are current or former smokers (Dai & Leventhal, 2019; McNeill et al., 2020). Like tobacco smoking, the vaping of nicotine is addictive. Access to liquid nicotine for use in e-cigarettes is currently restricted in Australia, although some people attempt to purchase through the internet to circumvent these restrictions. Access is limited through general practitioners who are willing to prescribe an unapproved medicine. Some researchers raise concerns about increasing e-cigarette use, including uncertainty about long-term harms, and the possibility that nicotine vaping could lead to cigarette smoking among young people or disrupt smoking-cessation attempts by current smokers (Chapman et al., 2019). However, others argue that the availability of e-cigarettes could have positive consequences as the vapour does not have the carcinogenic constituents of cigarette smoke. e-Cigarettes may serve as an important form of nicotine replacement for people who are highly addicted to tobacco smoking, leading some experts to call for increased access in Australia through appropriate regulation (Morphett, Hall & Gartner, 2021).

ALCOHOL

Technological changes associated with the sale and distribution of many food products (e.g. Uber Eats) has enabled the sale of alcohol through home delivery. Alcohol may be paid for prior to delivery and left at the front door without any direct contact with the purchaser, raising concerns about underage drinking, a lack of responsible service to those already intoxicated and also possible associated effects on domestic violence. Deliveries of alcohol to private homes where there may already be domestic conflict should not be a facilitated but unintended consequence of technological change. To date, legislative changes have not kept up with the behavioural changes brought about by the emergence of new technologies and ways of doing business.

ILLICIT DRUGS

Technological changes affect various aspects of the production, sale, distribution and use of illicit drugs.

The dark web

Many illegal products are advertised on websites that may be difficult to access and where interactions are encrypted. An analogy to illustrate: these sites function as online stores for illicit drugs. A seller, for example, may advertise a quantity and purity of heroin. Purchasers place competing bids and the highest bidder wins the auction. The site manager acts as an intermediary. Of course, governments (and law enforcement personnel) aim to close these sites as quickly as possible. People selling drugs on the dark web become effective at opening under new names and on new sites. Most recently, law enforcement agencies have adopted strategies of setting up their own sites on the dark web to capture those involved in illegal transactions.

New psychoactive substances

Partly to circumvent laws prohibiting the sale of drugs, people skilled in the manufacture of chemicals are manufacturing 'new' drugs (sometimes known as synthetic drugs, party drugs, bath salts or emerging drugs) that are intended to mimic the effects of drugs such as cannabis, amphetamines and cocaine. A new chemical drug has advantages in not being identifiable when a user is apprehended and where laws prohibiting its use may not have been enacted. In early 2020, some 120 countries worldwide reported the availability of 950 new psychoactive products. Monitoring and limiting the production and sale of new psychoactive drugs presents as an almost impossible task.

Social networking and illicit drugs

Knowledge about and experiences of the use of a wide range of illicit drugs is now widely shared over the internet. Regardless of which social media platforms people use to develop their own networking groups (D'Agostino et al., 2017) discussion of illicit drugs and their use is widely prevalent (Tao et al., 2016). Personal drug knowledge or anecdote is widely shared, including the effects of particular drugs, preferences, and strategies for dealing with the consequences of various patterns of drug use. In an important sense, every person using or intending to use a drug may now gain access to an extensive database of personal experiences. The effects of this type of knowledge on patterns of use and efforts to mitigate harm has not been adequately researched and is poorly understood.

QUESTION

In what fundamental ways do opportunities to procure drugs and drug-related information through the internet differ from more conventional opportunities to obtain and learn about drugs? What are potential implications of these differences?

Drug policies: A way forward

In reflecting on what has been done to reduce the harms associated with substance use, we need first to distinguish policies that are related to the use of legal drugs (tobacco, alcohol) from those needed to address the use of illicit drugs. We also consider a guiding principle (**harm minimisation**). Finally, we discuss some remaining concerns about illicit drug policies in Australia and the ways in which these policies have been implemented.

Harm minimisation – a policy approach acknowledging that some people will use drugs regardless of criminal and social sanctions, and consequently which includes a range of measures to reduce the harms associated with drug use.

The most effective initiatives to reduce tobacco and alcohol use in Australia have been focused on addressing two factors that contribute to use: the cost and marketing of products (see Burton et al., 2017 for a more detailed discussion). The substantially increasing cost of tobacco products has contributed to a decline in their use. There is convincing evidence that increasing the cost of alcohol would greatly influence its level of use, particularly among those who are most economically disadvantaged (Vandenberg & Sharma, 2016). A difference here between tobacco and alcohol policy has emerged. Thus, Australian governments have been unwilling to increase taxes on alcohol, presumably because of the way the industry functions in Australia. The alcohol-production industry involves several small farmers, and the industry exports a substantial proportion of its products (primarily to China, the United States and the United Kingdom). In Australia, bottled water may cost more than 'low-end' alcohol. Governments have not been persuaded to price alcohol in a manner consistent with the harm its use produces. In 2018, the Northern Territory government introduced legislation involving the minimum pricing of a unit of alcohol. Such a policy increases the price of the cheapest forms of alcohol but leaves the price of most other forms unaffected. The outcome of that initiative may determine whether other Australian states (or the federal government) follow.

A third type of strategy that has been successfully used to reduce alcohol consumption has been to reduce its availability (Burton et al., 2017). This involves reducing the number of alcohol outlets and reducing the hours that such outlets may sell alcohol. The alcohol industry has resisted these changes, and indeed, advocates for more outlets and longer hours of opening. Governments here are confronted with a choice between public health advocates who are committed to reducing the level of disease and death associated with the use of alcohol and an industry arguing that the tourism and recreational industries depend upon alcohol sales for their viability, and that the public health lobby is impeding the ability of people to enjoy a drink. Of greater concern is the extent to which the alcohol industry funds efforts to 'muddy the water'; that is, to discredit the findings of public health and other alcohol researchers (Mathews, Thorn & Giorgi, 2013). These same tactics were used (and, in middle- to low-income countries, continue to be used) by the tobacco industry. It is problematic that industries profit from the sale of their health-damaging products but are not required to contribute to the cost of medical care for those affected. There are efforts among public health advocates and policymakers internationally to begin recovery of healthcare costs from these industries (MacKenzie et al., 2017; Healton, 2018).

The Australian National Drug Strategy (Department of Health, 2017) is based on a harm-minimisation approach, and incorporates the three pillars of demand reduction (reducing demand for drugs), supply reduction (reducing drug availability) and harm reduction (reducing the harmful effects of drug use). With regard to policies to reduce the use of illicit drugs, the issues are very different from the policies that have been used for legal drugs. A core principle underpinning all drug policy has been that of harm minimisation. In broad terms, this principle accepts that policies need to be chosen on the basis that they make the largest contributions to reducing the harm created by using drugs. Harm minimisation can involve a choice between policies that all involve the potential for harm. For example, how would you respond when confronted by children in early or mid-adolescence who are injecting drugs? Recommended harm-minimisation responses include ensuring access to sterile needles and syringes and providing advice on safer injection practices (Dolan et al., 2005). A common argument against this public health response is that it facilitates the children's drug use behaviour. However, the social context of risk behaviour should be considered, as well as the consequences of not providing sterile injection equipment. For example, for children living 'rough' on the streets there may be no realistic way of stopping them from injecting drugs. If we cannot stop these children from injecting, then there is a public health imperative to keep them as healthy as possible until they do decide to stop (Des Jarlais & Friedman, 1987).

These types of strategies abound in the area of illicit drugs (Logan & Marlatt, 2010), and similar approaches can also be found for legal drugs. Harm-minimisation policies include:

1 providing an injecting room with a medical practitioner in attendance to reduce the risk of an opiate overdose death
2 providing facilities for pill-testing analysis at venues that are likely to involve illicit drug use to confirm the contents of the drug being used
3 providing clean needles to those who are injecting drugs, so that they do not become infected with hepatitis C or HIV
4 reducing taxes on low-alcohol products to encourage preference for their use over high-alcohol products
5 encouraging the sale of low-aromatic petrol in some communities, to reduce the level of petrol sniffing by young children in those communities.

While governments tend generally to endorse harm minimisation as a broad policy approach, there remain many in the community who disagree or who are unconvinced. Part of this reluctance is based on the view that there is a need to discourage people from using drugs altogether, and that the risk of incarceration or death is a necessary disincentive to use (Csete et al., 2016). However, a majority of those who use illicit drugs stop using after a period of time (Sobell, Ellingstad & Sobell, 2000; Klingemann, Sobell & Sobell, 2010), and punitive drug policies have not been found to achieve the desired result (Csete et al., 2016). The policy question here is whether public health or criminal justice policies are more effective in reducing the level of harm associated with the use of illicit drugs. The former is supported by a body of research while the latter has been largely discredited.

SPOTLIGHT 22.3

Decriminalisation of all illicit drugs in Portugal

In view of the conspicuous failure to reduce levels of illicit drug use in all economically advanced (and other) countries, the development of an alternative policy in Portugal is of worldwide interest (Greenwald, 2009). Like many other economically advanced countries, Portugal experienced a substantial increase in the use of illicit drugs, beginning in the 1970s and continuing until the 1990s. In the late

1990s, the Portuguese government initiated an enquiry into drug policies. The country's policy response was the decision to decriminalise all illicit drug use (but not drug dealing), starting in July 2001.

Decriminalisation needs to be distinguished from legalisation. Responsibility for illicit drug use was removed from the Portuguese criminal justice system and given to the health system. Drug use remains illegal and continues to be discouraged through persuasion and non-criminal penalties. The funds saved by not incarcerating drug users are redirected to provide more extensive drug treatment services. In general terms, the Portuguese policy trades off the cost of imprisonment, which is very high, with the cost of providing treatment services (Goncalves, Lourenco & Silva, 2015).

A person who is apprehended by police because they are found to be using an illicit drug may receive a fine (about equivalent to a parking ticket in Australia) or they might be required to attend a treatment service. There is little enforcement of these penalties.

An important component of the legal changes has been to approach drug problems as a health issue requiring support and encouragement. There is reduced stigma associated with those who use drugs, in part because they are no longer 'criminalised'.

When the legislation was implemented, there were predictions that illicit drug use would increase and that Portugal would become a magnet for drug users all over Europe. These have not occurred. The available evidence points to a decline in the use of illicit drugs in Portugal, particularly when compared to other European countries, where illicit drug use has increased over the same period. Further, for nearly every category of illicit drug, rates of use in Portugal are substantially lower than in Australia (for a review of the issues, see Greenwald, 2009).

Since the legislation was implemented in 2001, rates of drug use have remained relatively stable, declining for some (younger) age groups and increasing for some other groups (Moreira et al., 2007). Importantly, drug-induced deaths have declined, as has drug-related criminal offending. The decline in drug use by younger persons is particularly important as young age of first use is a characteristic of those who use illicit drugs when they become older. There is no evidence that the negative consequences predicted by those who opposed the decriminalisation have occurred.

QUESTION

Do you think the types of measures introduced in Portugal would be effective in Australia for reducing rates of drug-related harm? Provide three reasons to support your answer.

Decriminalisation – the removal of criminal penalties for the possession of drugs for personal use. Typically, criminal penalties for the production and supply of drugs are maintained. This distinguishes decriminalisation from legalisation, in which production and supply are legalised and regulated.

General policy issues

Estimates of the numbers in the community currently affected by substance use remain imprecise but are massive, irrespective of the way the estimate is derived. Better policies are needed in at least four areas. First, alcohol use continues to destroy lives, wreck families and contribute to violence and injury. Alcohol is causally related to over 60 diseases, it is a carcinogen and most recently has been convincingly shown to cause dementia (Boffetta & Hashibe, 2006; Wood et al., 2018). Yet, its use continues to be encouraged by mass advertising and promotion. The community has a right to be informed that alcohol use, particularly in large quantities, leads to disease and death. The known carcinogenic effects of alcohol need to be understood so that consumers can make informed decisions about using alcohol. There is a need for legislative change to reduce alcohol advertising, increase taxes on alcohol and reduce the number of alcohol outlets and the hours of opening. There is evidence that all these initiatives can make a difference and the cost of implementing them is low to negligible (Burton et al., 2017).

Second, laws that criminalise the possession and personal use of illicit drugs are not only ineffective, they increase the harms that are a consequence of illicit drug use (Csete et al., 2016). Life-course studies have demonstrated that the vast majority of people using illicit drugs cease using them without criminal sanctions or treatment (Klingemann et al., 2010). These studies show that illicit drug use generally begins at around 18–21 years of age and ceases at around 25–30 years of age. For the vast majority of those who use drugs, including many who abuse or become dependent on drugs, drug use is a life-course stage that is replaced by other activities (e.g. employment, intimate relationships, purchase of a house).

To criminalise these largely self-remitting behaviours is to 'make criminals'. People who use illicit drugs are too frequently the victims of not only their drug use but also of the societal response to this use. There is now a broad consensus in the field that current laws are not only ineffective but also counterproductive (Hall, 2018; Rogeberg et al., 2018; Vicknasingam et al., 2018). In Australia, drug-diversion programs have partly replaced a regimen of criminal sanctions. Even a conservative assessment of policy priorities would involve an expansion of drug-diversion programs. Drug use needs to be accepted as a health system issue and removed from the criminal justice system.

Third, the call for more drug treatment is the common and societally acceptable suggestion from many. However, evidence that drug treatment is effective and an efficient use of resources is not available. It is simply not possible to find a single national (or international) study that meets the criteria for a well-conducted community trial of drug treatment. Such a trial needs to meet minimal research standards, including an experimental and comparison group randomly selected from those affected (not self-selected), at least a one-year follow-up and adequate measurement of use and related behaviours preceding and following the trial. This observation, if it is correct, leads to the conclusion that hundreds of millions of dollars are being spent on treatment programs, none of which are supported by an adequate evidence base. To the obvious suggestion that it is impossible to improve treatment without a baseline knowledge of its outcomes, there is silence. There is a need to know what works and to increase support for treatment programs that work.

Finally, it is appropriate to be concerned about the drug and alcohol workforce. Most drug and alcohol counsellors are poorly trained and poorly paid. The drug and alcohol workforce is characterised by high staff turnover and a lack of higher-level (university) qualifications (Pidd et al., 2012). Part of the reason for this is that many agencies providing treatment services are poorly funded, with short-term contracts to provide services over what are sometimes large geographic areas. It could be proposed that if governments were serious about reducing the drug-induced burden of disease in Australia, they would commit to understanding what is currently happening, and to policies that have the best prospect of reducing the drug-induced burden of disease.

SUMMARY

Learning objective 1: Distinguish between different drug types according to their effect types.
Drugs can be classified according to the types of effects they have. Some have stimulant effects and others have depressant effects on the central nervous system. Alcohol is the most popular depressant drug. The effects of any drug can vary according to contextual factors, including the social environment in which it is being used and other drugs that are being used at the same time.

Learning objective 2: Describe four of the main factors that contribute to people's decisions to use drugs.
Decisions to use drugs are essentially rational: known risks and benefits are considered. The available information about drugs, and the way we respond to it, varies from person to person. People learn from those close to them, and no-one starts using a drug without having an opportunity to use it. The rewarding effects of drugs and the social environment in which they are used each contribute to continuation of drug use.

Learning objective 3: Describe the relative contribution of different substances to the burden of disease.
Tobacco and alcohol make the greatest contribution to the mortality burden in Australia. They are carcinogens and contribute significantly to years of life lost. Alcohol also contributes substantially to rates of assault and injury. Among the illicit drugs, heroin and other opioids are the leading contributors to mortality, primarily to due to drug overdose. Health and law enforcement policies can affect the likelihood of many drug use consequences.

Learning objective 4: Explain ways in which social attitudes affect how we respond to drug use.
Alcohol use, sometimes even excessive use, has a high degree of social acceptability in Australia. As a result, some of the harmful consequences of alcohol use are discounted at the individual and societal levels. Prevailing social attitudes inform our assumptions and expectations about a range of drugs. In the absence of knowledge about different drugs or the people who use them, negative stereotypes have a profound effect on our assumptions about appropriate responses to drug use.

Learning objective 5: Identify possible changes to current policies that could reduce levels of drug-related harm.
In contrast to the regulation of tobacco, the supply, promotion and use of alcohol is poorly regulated. There is a robust evidence base concerning cost-effective regulatory measures to decrease alcohol-related harm. With regard to illicit drugs, the criminalisation of use substantially increases the harmful consequences of use. Attention should be paid to experiences with alternative policy models of decriminalisation and legalisation.

TUTORIAL EXERCISES

1   Write down what you believe to be the five most harmful drugs and then rank them in order, from most to least harmful. Share everyone's answers with the group. Identify any differences in the drugs or rankings provided and discuss the rationale for these rankings. As a group, develop an agreed set of five drugs and an order of ranking.

2   What are some of the factors that influence the development of substance use policies? (Refer, for example, to the opening vignette). From a public health perspective, what strategies can be used to

develop better substance use policies? In your discussion, reflect on specific drug types (e.g. tobacco, alcohol and cannabis) and settings in which new policies have been developed.

3   A large proportion of people imprisoned in Australia are serving sentences for drug-related offences. It could be questioned whether people are less likely to use drugs after they have been in prison. What are the most promising strategies for improving health and social outcomes for people who are currently exposed to the criminal justice system due to their substance use? As a group, agree on the three most promising strategies.

4   Debate the proposition: 'In Australia, the legalisation of recreational cannabis use would reduce the levels of harm associated with the use of this drug.' In preparing for the debate, identify the types of factors that may influence changes in levels of harm.

FURTHER READING

Callinan, S., Room, R., Livingston, M., & Jiang, H. (2015). Who purchases low-cost alcohol in Australia? *Alcohol and Alcoholism*, *50*(6), 647–53.

d'Abbs, P. (2015). Widening the gap: The gulf between policy rhetoric and implementation reality in addressing alcohol problems among Indigenous Australians. *Drug and Alcohol Review*, *34*(5), 461–6.

Gonvcalves, R., Lourence, A., & da Silva, S. N. (2015). A social cost perspective in the wake of the Portuguese strategy for the fight against drugs. *International Journal of Drug Policy*, *26*, 199–209.

Melchior, M., Nakamura, A., Bolze, C., Hausfater, F., El Khoury, F., Mary-Krause, M., & Da Silva, M. A. (2019). Does liberalisation of cannabis policy influence levels of use in adolescents and young adults? A systematic review and meta-analysis. *BMJ Open*, *9*(7), e025880.

Siegfried N., & Parry, C. (2019). Do alcohol control policies work? An umbrella review and quality assessment of systematic reviews of alcohol control interventions (2006 – 2017). *PLOS One*, *14*(4), e0214865.

REFERENCES

Adinoff, B. (2004). Neurobiologic processes in drug reward and addiction. *Harvard Review of Psychiatry*, *12*(6), 305–30.

Anderson, P., Chisholm, D., & Fuhr, D. C. (2009). Alcohol and global health effectiveness and cost-effectiveness of policies and programmes to reduce the harm caused by alcohol. *Lancet*, *373*(9682), 2234–46.

Anthony, J. C., Warner, L. A., & Kessler, R. C. (1994). Comparative epidemiology of dependence on tobacco, alcohol, controlled substances, and inhalants: Basic findings from the national comorbidity survey. *Experimental and Clinical Psychopharmacology*, *2*(3), 244–68.

Arnold, J. C., Nation, T., & McGregor, I. S. (2020). Prescribing medicinal cannabis. *Australian Prescriber*, *43*(5), 152–9.

Australian Bureau of Statistics (ABS). (2017). *Measures of Australia's progress, 2010*. (Cat No. 1370.0 (4.1)). ABS. Retrieved http://www.abs.gov.au/ausstats/abs@.nsf/Lookup/by%20Subject/1370.0~2010~Main%20Features~Home%20page%20(1)

——(2019). *Causes of Death, Australia, 2018. Statistics on the number of deaths, by sex, selected age groups, and cause of death classified to the International Classification of Diseases (ICD)*. Retrieved https://www.abs.gov.au/statistics/health/causes-death/causes-death-australia/2018

Australian Institute of Health and Welfare (AIHW). (2011). *Measuring alcohol risk in the 2010 National Drug Strategy Household Survey: Implementation of the 2009 alcohol guidelines*. (Cat. No. PHE 152. Drug Statistics Series No. 26.)

——(2016). *National Drug Strategy Household Survey 2016*.

——(2017). *National Drug Strategy Household Survey 2016: Detailed findings*.

——(2018). *Impact of alcohol and illicit drug use on the burden of disease and injury in Australia. Australia Burden of Disease Study 2011*.

——(2020). *National Drug Strategy Household Survey 2019*. (Drug Statistics Series No. 32. PHE 270). AIHW.

Boffetta, P., & Hashibe, M. (2006). Alcohol and cancer. *The Lancet Oncology*, *7*(2), 149–56.

Boys, A., Marsden, J., & Strang, J. (2001). Understanding reasons for drug use amongst young people: A functional perspective. *Health Education Research*, *16*(4), 457–69.

Brett, J., Lee, K. S. K., Gray, D., Wilson, S., Freeburn, B., Harrison, K., & Conigrave, K. (2016). Mind the gap: What is the difference between alcohol treatment need and access for Aboriginal and Torres Strait Islander Australians? *Drug and Alcohol Review*, *35*(4), 456–60.

Burton, R., Henn, C., Lavoie, D., O'Connor, R., Perkins, C., Sweeney, K. . . . Sheron, N. (2017). A rapid evidence review of the effectiveness and cost-effectiveness of alcohol control policies: an English perspective. *Lancet*, *389*(10078), 1558–80.

Campbell, M. A., Hunt, J., Scrimgeour, D. J., Davey, M., & Jones, V. (2018). Contribution of Aboriginal Community-Controlled Health Services to improving Aboriginal health: An evidence review. *Australian Health Review*, *42*(2), 218–26.

Canuto, K. J., Aromataris, E., Burgess, T., Davy, C., McKivett, A., Schwartzkopff, K., . . . Brown, A. (2021). A scoping review of Aboriginal and Torres Strait Islander health promotion programs focused on modifying chronic disease risk factors. *Health Promotion Journal of Australia*, *32*(1), 46–74.

Chapman, S., Bareham, D., & Maziak, W. (2019). The gateway effect of e-cigarettes: reflections on main criticisms. *Nicotine and Tobacco Research*, *21*(5), 695–8.

Chrzanowska, A., Man, N., Sutherland, R., Degenhardt, L., & Peacock, A. (2021). *Trends in drug-induced deaths in Australia, 1997-2019*. Drug Trends Bulletin Series. National Drug and Alcohol Research Centre, UNSW.

Csete, J., Kamarulzaman, A., Kazatchkine, M., Altice, F., Balicki, M., Buxton, J. . . . Beyrer, C. (2016). Public health and international drug policy. *Lancet*, *387*(10026), 1427–80.

d'Abbs, P. (2015). Widening the gap: The gulf between policy rhetoric and implementation reality in addressing alcohol problems among Indigenous Australians. *Drug and Alcohol Review*, *34*(5), 461–6.

D'Agostino, A.R., Optican, A. R., Sowles, S. J., Krauss, M. J., Escobar Lee, K., & Cavazos-Rehg, P. A. (2017). Social networking online to recover from opioid use disorder: A study of community interactions. *Drug and Alcohol Dependence*, *181*, 5–10. Retrieved https://doi.org/10.1016/j.drugalcdep.2017.09.010

Dai, H., & Leventhal, A. M. (2019). Prevalence of e-cigarette use among adults in the United States, 2014-2018. *JAMA*, *322*(18), 1824–7.

Department of Health. (2017). *National drug strategy 2017–2026*. Australian Government.

Des Jarlais, D. C., & Friedman, S. R. (1987). HIV infection among intravenous drug users: Epidemiology and risk reduction. *AIDS*, *1*(2), 67–76.

Dolan, K., Dillon, P., & Silins, E. (2005). *Needle and syringe programs: Your questions answered*. Australian Government Department of Health and Ageing.

Fluharty, M., Taylor, A. E., Grabski, M., & Munafò, M. R. (2017). The association of cigarette smoking with depression and anxiety: A systematic review. *Nicotine & Tobacco Research*, *19*(1), 3–13.

Goncalves, R., Lourenco, A., & Silva, S. N. (2015). A social cost perspective in the wake of the Portuguese strategy for the fight against drugs. *International Journal of Drug Policy*, *26*(2), 199–209.

Green, B., Kavanagh, D., & Young, R. (2003). Being stoned: A review of self-reported cannabis effects. *Drug and Alcohol Review*, *22*(4), 453–60. doi:10.1080/09595230310001613976

Greenwald, G. (2009). *Drug decriminalization in Portugal: Lessons for creating fair and successful drug policies*. Cato Institute.

Hall, W. (2018). The future of the international drug control system and national drug prohibitions. *Addiction*, *113*(7), 1210–23.

Hall, W., & Lynskey, M. (2016). Why it is probably too soon to assess the public health effects of legalisation of recreational cannabis use in the USA. *Lancet Psychiatry*, *3*(9), 900–6.

Hall, W. D., & Weier, M. (2017). Reducing alcohol-related violence and other harm in Australia. *Medical Journal of Australia*, *206*(3), 111–12.

Hayatbakhsh, M. R., Flenady, V. J., Gibbons, K. S., Kingsbury, A. M., Hurrion, E., Mamun, A. A., & Najman, J. M. (2012). Birth outcomes associated with cannabis use before and during pregnancy. *Pediatric Research*, *71*(2), 215–19.

Healton, C. (2018). The tobacco master settlement agreement – Strategic lessons for addressing public health problems. *New England Journal of Medicine*, *379*(11), 997–1000.

Julien, R. M. (2001). *A primer of drug action: A concise nontechnical guide to the actions, uses, and side effects of psychoactive drugs* (9th ed.). Worth Publishers.

Kaur, N., Keyes, K. M., Hamilton, A. D., Chapman, C., Livingston, M., Slade, T., & Swift, W. (2021). Trends in cannabis use and attitudes toward legalization and use among Australians from 2001–2016: an age-period-cohort analysis. *Addiction*, *116*(5), 1152–61.

Klingemann, H., Sobell, M. B., & Sobell, L. C. (2010). Continuities and changes in self-change research. *Addiction*, *105*(9), 1510–18.

Kuntsche, E., Knibbe, R., Gmel, G., & Engels, R. (2006). Who drinks and why? A review of socio-demographic, personality, and contextual issues behind the drinking motives in young people. *Addictive Behaviors*, *31*(10), 1844–57.

Leske, S., Harris, M. G., Charlson, F. J., Ferrari, A. J., Baxter, A. J., Logan, J. M., . . . Whiteford, H. (2016). Systematic review of interventions for Indigenous adults with mental and substance use disorders in Australia, Canada, New Zealand and the United States. *Australian and New Zealand Journal of Psychiatry*, *50*(11), 1040–54.

Leslie, E. M., Cherney, A., Smirnov, A., Kemp, R., & Najman, J. M. (2018). Experiences of police contact among young adult recreational drug users: A qualitative study. *International Journal of Drug Policy*, *56*, 64–72.

Leslie, E. M., Smirnov, A., Cherney, A., Wells, H., Kemp, R., Legosz, M., & Najman, J. M. (2016). Predictors of hazardous alcohol consumption among young adult amphetamine-type stimulant users: A population-based prospective study. *Sage Open*, *6*(1).

Livingston, M., & Callinan, S. (2015). Underreporting in alcohol surveys: whose drinking is underestimated? *Journal of Studies on Alcohol and Drugs*, *76*(1), 158–64.

Logan, D. E., & Marlatt, G. A. (2010). Harm reduction therapy: A practice-friendly review of research. *Journal of Clinical Psychology*, *66*(2), 201–14.

MacKenzie, R., LeGresley, E., & Daube, M. (2017). Legal does not mean unaccountable: Suing tobacco companies to recover health care costs. *The Medical Journal of Australia*, *207*(10), 419–21.

Mathews, R., Thorn, M., & Giorgi, C. (2013). Vested interests in addiction research and policy: Is the alcohol industry delaying government action on alcohol health warning labels in Australia? *Addiction*, *108*(11), 1889–96.

McGrath, J., Welham, J., Scott, J., Varghese, D., Degenhardt, L., Hayatbakhsh, M. R., . . . Najman, J. M. (2010). Association between cannabis use and psychosis-related outcomes using sibling pair analysis in a cohort of young adults. *Archives of General Psychiatry*, *67*(5), 440–7.

McNeill, A., Brose, L.S., Calder, R., Bauld, L., & Robson, D. (2020). *Vaping in England: An evidence update including mental health and pregnancy, March 2020: a report commissioned by Public Health England*. Public Health England.

Moreira, M., Trigueiros, F., & Antunes, C. (2007). The evaluation of the Portuguese drug policy 1999–2004: The process and the impact on the new policy. *Drugs and Alcohol Today*, *7*(2), 14–25.

Morgan, C. J., Freeman, T. P., Schafer, G. L., & Curran, H. V. (2010). Cannabidiol attenuates the appetitive effects of Δ 9-tetrahydrocannabinol in humans smoking their chosen cannabis. *Neuropsychopharmacology*, *35*(9), 1879.

Morphett, K., Hall, W., & Gartner, C. (2021). The misuse of the precautionary principle in justifying Australia's ban on the sale of nicotine vaping products. *Nicotine & Tobacco Research*, *23*(1), 14–20.

Nichols, D. (1986). Differences between the mechanism of action of MDMA, MBDB, and the classic hallucinogens. Identification of a new therapeutic class: Enctactogens. *Journal of Psychoactive Drugs*, *18*(4), 305–13.

Nichols, D. E. (2004). Hallucinogens. *Pharmacology & Therapeutics*, *101*(2), 131–81.

O'Brien, K. (2020). Medicinal cannabis and its regulation in Australia – an update. *The Journal of the Australasian College of Nutritional and Environmental Medicine*, *39*(2), 3–9.

Peacock, A., Leung, J., Larney, S., Colledge, S., Hickman, M., Rehm, J., . . . Griffiths, P. (2018). Global statistics on alcohol, tobacco and illicit drug use: 2017 status report. *Addiction*, *113*(10), 1905–26

Peterson, G. (2017). Aged care: Substance abuse in the elderly: Yes, it does occur. *Australian Pharmacist*, *36*(5), 26–7.

Pidd, K., Roche, A., Duraisingam, V., & Carne, A. (2012). Minimum qualifications in the alcohol and other drugs field: Employers' views. *Drug and Alcohol Review*, *31*(4), 514–22.

Rehm, J., Rehm, J., Taylor, B., Rehm, J., Taylor, B., Room, R., . . . Room, R. (2006). Global burden of disease from alcohol, illicit drugs and tobacco. *Drug and Alcohol Review*, *25*(6), 503–13.

Reynolds, S. (2013). *Generation ecstasy: Into the world of techno and rave culture*. Routledge.

Rigg, K. K. & Sharp, A. (2018). Deaths related to MDMA (ecstasy/molly): Prevalence, root causes, and harm reduction interventions. *Journal of Substance Use*, *23*(4), 345–32.

Rogeberg, O., Bergsvik, D., Phillips, L. D., van Amsterdam, J., Eastwood, N., Henderson, G., . . . Nutt, D. (2018). A new approach to formulating and appraising drug policy: A multi-criterion decision analysis applied to alcohol and cannabis regulation. *International Journal of Drug Policy*, *56*, 144–52.

Simangan, D. (2018). Is the Philippine 'war on drugs' an act of genocide? *Journal of Genocide Research*, *20*(1), 68–89.

Smirnov, A., Kemp, R., Ward, J., Henderson, S., Williams, S., Dev, A., & Najman, J. M. (2016). Patterns of drug dependence in a Queensland (Australia) sample of Indigenous and non-Indigenous people who inject drugs. *Drug Alcohol Rev*, *35*(5), 611–19.

Smirnov, A., Najman, J. M., Hayatbakhsh, R., Wells, H., Legosz, M., & Kemp, R. (2013). Young adults' recreational social environment as a predictor of ecstasy use initiation: findings of a population-based prospective study. *Addiction*, *108*(10), 1809–17.

Sobell, L. C., Ellingstad, T. P., & Sobell, M. B. (2000). Natural recovery from alcohol and drug problems: methodological review of the research with suggestions for future directions. *Addiction*, *95*(5), 749–64.

Stevens, M., & Paradies, Y. (2014). Changes in exposure to 'life stressors' in the Aboriginal and Torres Strait Islander population, 2002 to 2008. *BMC Public Health*, *14*.

Stockwell, T., Zhao, J., Greenfield, T., Li, J., Livingston, M., & Meng, Y. (2016). Estimating under- and over-reporting of drinking in national surveys of alcohol consumption: identification of consistent biases across four English-speaking countries. *Addiction*, *111*, 1203–13.

Tao D., Roy, A., Chen, Z., Zhu, Q., & Pan, S. (2016). Analyzing and retrieving illicit drug-related posts from social media. *2016 IEEE International Conference on Bioinformatics and Biomedicine*. pp. 1555–60.

United Nations. (2017). *World drug report 2017*.

United Nations Office on Drugs and Crime. (2013). *The international drug control conventions*. United Nations.

Vadivelu, Kai, A. M., Kodumudi, V., Sramcik, J., & Kaye, A. D. (2018). The opioid crisis: a Comprehensive overview. *Current Pain and Headache Reports*, *22*(3), 1–6.

Van Etten, M. L., & Anthony, J. C. (1999). Comparative epidemiology of initial drug opportunities and transitions to first use: marijuana, cocaine, hallucinogens and heroin. *Drug Alcohol Depend*, *54*(2), 117–25.

Van Etten, M. L., Neumark, Y. D., & Anthony, J. C. (1997). Initial opportunity to use marijuana and the transition to first use: United States, 1979–1994. *Drug Alcohol Depend*, *49*(1), 1–7.

Vandenberg, B., & Sharma, A. (2016). Are alcohol taxation and pricing policies regressive? Product-level effects of a specific tax and a minimum unit price for alcohol. *Alcohol and Alcoholism*, *51*(4), 493–502.

Vicknasingam, B., Narayanan, S., Singh, D., & Chawarski, M. (2018). Decriminalization of drug use. *Current Opinion in Psychiatry*, *31*(4), 300–305.

Wagner, F. A., & Anthony, J. C. (2002). Into the world of illegal drug use: Exposure opportunity and other mechanisms linking the use of alcohol, tobacco, marijuana, and cocaine. *American Journal of Epidemiology*, *155*(10), 918–925.

Wei, E. H., Loeber, R., & White, H. R. (2004). Teasing apart the developmental associations between alcohol and marijuana use and violence. *Journal of Contemporary Criminal Justice*, *20*(2), 166–83.

Wood, A. M., Kaptoge, S., Butterworth, A. S., Willeit, P., Warnakula, S., Bolton, T., ... Burgess, S. (2018). Risk thresholds for alcohol consumption: combined analysis of individual-participant data for 599 912 current drinkers in 83 prospective studies. *The Lancet*, *391*(10129), 1513–23.

Zhao, Y. J., Wright, J., Begg, S., & Guthridge, S. (2013). Decomposing Indigenous life expectancy gap by risk factors: a life table analysis. *Population Health Metrics*, *11* (1).

Ziersch, A. M., Gallaher, G., Baum, F. & Bentley, M. (2011). Responding to racism: Insights on how racism can damage health from an urban study of Australian Aboriginal people. *Social Science & Medicine*, *73*(7), 1045–53.

Zinberg, N. E. (1986). *Drug, set, and setting: The basis for controlled intoxicant use*. Yale University Press.

Index

Aboriginal and Torres Strait Islander health workers and practitioners, 111
Aboriginal and Torres Strait Islander peoples. *See* Indigenous Australians
Aboriginal Community Controlled Health Service (ACCHS), 66–7
absolute rights, 204
access
 to essential medicines, 210
 to health services, 157–8, 337, 390
Active Ageing framework, 317
activism, 119, 389
adolescents
 and bullying, 306–8
 described, 298
 externalising problems, 299–301
 homeless, 298, 302–4
 internalising problems, 299–301
 and risk factors, 300, 302–3
 and substance use, 304–6
 victimisation, 306–8
 See also youth
advertising, 118
advocacy
 capacity building, 115
 definition, 113
 described, 113–14, 185, 193
 environmental health justice, 119–20
 ethical, 193
 ethics-based, 194–5
 in action, 118–19
 need for, 113
 political, 194
 theories, 116–18
 types of, 114
Advocacy Coalition Framework (ACF), 117
African Charter on Human and Peoples' Rights, 204
African Commission on Human and Peoples' Rights, 210
age-specific mortality rates, 243
ageing
 barriers and enablers to healthy, 325–6
 Decade of Healthy Ageing, 319–20
 definition, 316
 and environmental factors, 318–20
 First Nations Peoples, 320–1
 healthy defined, 317–19
 healthy redefined, 317–19

models of successful, 316
policy frameworks, 317
See also older people
agism, 325
Agreement on Trade-Related Aspects of Intellectual Property Rights, 191
alcohol
 availability, 195, 414
 costs, 414
 definition, 400
 marketing, 400
 sales, 413
alcohol advertising, 118
Alcohol Advertising Review Board (AARB), 118
alcohol use
 activities undertaken while under influence, 408
 adolescents, 304–6
 and amphetamines, 401
 and behaviour, 408
 beliefs about, 410
 burden of disease, 404–5
 harms associated with, 410–11
 Indigenous Australians, 404–5
 policies, 416
 reasons for, 305
 Russian-speaking immigrants, 221
 and treatment, 417
 youth, 152–3, 226–7
algae, blue-green, 259
alternative nicotine-delivery systems (ANDS), 44
altruism, 191
amphetamines, 401–2, 408
analytic studies, 240, 247
ancient Greece, 27–8
ancient Rome, 28–9
association
 in analytic studies, 247
 measures of, 252–5
asylum seekers, 367, 374
 See also migrants
attack rate, 243
attitudes
 changes, 341
 negative, 339
Australasian Faculty of Public Health Medicine (AFPHM), 112
Australian Council of Academic Public Health Institutions Australasia (CAPHIA), 110
Australian Health Promotion Association (APHA), 188

Australian Human Rights Commission, 133, 212
Australian Marriage Equality, 118
Australian Medical Association, 67
Australian National Drug Strategy, 414
Australian National Preventive Health Agency (ANPHA), 183
Australians
 health of, 5
 See also Indigenous Australians
autism, 272
autonomy, 98

behaviour
 choice, 166, 172–3
 and drug use, 408
 influences on, 167–8
 theories of individual, 168
 unacceptable, 299–301
behavioural change
 and advocacy, 194
 described, 151–2, 166
 interventions, 52, 169
 lifestyles, 283
 move to healthy public policy, 13
 stages of, 170–1
behavioural determinants of health, 148–9, 151–3
behavioural sciences, 4
behaviourism, 168–9, 176
beliefs about health, 352–3
benzodiazepines, 408
bioethics, 88
biological factors, 332, 335
biostatistics, 4
birth weight, 249
Black Lives Matter movement, 136, 193
'Body and Soul' program, 220
Bolivia
 childhood malnutrition, 72
border health, 372
Brazil
 'María da Penha Law', 201
Break It Off (BIO) campaign, 54
breast cancer
 living with, 224
breastfeeding
 HIV transmission, 2
BUGA UP (Billboard Utilising Graffitists against Unhealthy Promotions), 51
bullying, 306–8

burden of disease
    alcohol use, 404–5
    disability, 324
    environmental factors, 155
    mental illness, 12
    obesity, 8
    rural health, 384–5

Campaign for Tobacco-Free Kids, 51
cannabis, 401, 403–4, 406–8
    harms associated with, 410–11
    medicinal, 408–9
    and mental health, 411
    recreational use, 409
capability approach, 96
capacity building, 106–8
case-control studies, 248–9, 253
case management, 72
case reports, 246
case series, 246
cashless cards, 96–7
Chadwick, Sir Edwin, 31–2
Change the Record, 118
*Charter of Fundamental Rights of the
    European Union*, 205
chief health officers, 7
child care, 289
children
    coping strategies, 280
    in detention, 137–8
    human rights, 205
    lifestyle changes, 283
    and malnutrition, 72
    and mental health, 288–90
    obesity prevalence, 282
    obesity prevention, 281–3
    oral health, 283–6
    rights of, 280
    in same-sex parent families, 286–8
    and stressful events, 280
    See also adolescents
choice architecture, 174
choices
    and youth, 175
cholera, 30
chronic diseases, 323–4
civil society, 118
classical conditioning, 168
Climate and Health Alliance (CAHA),
    118, 188
climate change, 157, 183, 186
clinical ethics, 89
cocaine, 402, 407
Cochrane Collection, 192
coercion, 174
cognitions, 167
cohort studies, 249–50, 253
collective action in health, 31
colonisation, 352–5
Commission on the Social
    Determinants of Health, 207
communicable diseases, 29
communication difficulties, 338
communities
    Cycling Without Age, 315

driving initiatives, 282
and drug use, 305
health inequities, 76
health needs of, 263–4
health of, 130
and power, 393–4
role of rural, 388–9
community action
    challenges in creating, 52
    in tobacco control, 51–2
    strengthening, 50–1
community activism, 114
community based cluster randomised
    trials, 251
community development, 51, 114
community health
    definition, 63, 65
    origins, 64–5
    services, 66
    stakeholders, 66
community health workers, 74
comorbid conditions, 332–3, 335
competencies, 109–10
conditioning, 168–9
confounding, 249, 251
consciousness, 171
consequences
    immediate versus delayed, 174–6
consequentialist approaches, 89–91
constructivism, 222–3
consumer activism, 389
control groups, 248, 251
*Convention for the Protection of
    Human Rights and
    Fundamental Freedoms*, 205
*Convention on the Elimination of All
    Forms of Discrimination
    against Women*, 205
*Convention on the Rights of People
    with Disabilities*, 340
Convention on the Rights of the Child,
    205, 212, 280
cost of public health interventions, 265
Council of Europe, 205
counterconditioning, 171
COVID-19
    cases over time, 243–5
    described, 11, 237
    and face masks, 166
    impact, 176
    individual behaviour during, 165
    inequities, 120
    and migrants, 375
    and older people, 326
    and primary health care, 70
    voluntary isolation, 349
COVID-19 vaccines, 139, 191
critical race theory, 136–7
Croakey, 118
cross-sectional studies, 247, 253
crystal methamphetamine, 402
Cultural Responsiveness Framework:
    Guidelines for Victorian
    Health Services, 376
cumulative incidence (CI), 241, 253

cyberbullying, 306–8
Cycling Without Age, 315

Dandenong and District Aborigines
    Co-operative, 55–6
dark web, 413
data collection
    and case-control studies, 248–9
    cohort studies, 249
    epidemiological studies, 247
    methods, 223
    use of, 30
Death by Indifference report, 334
deaths
    causes of, 247, 323–4
    drug related, 405
    migrants, 371
    See also mortality rates
Decade of Healthy Ageing, 319–20
Declaration of Alma-Ata, 64
Declaration of Astana, 65, 70, 77–8
decriminalisation of drugs, 401,
    415–16
deinstitutionalisation, 337
delay discounting, 174–6
deliberate self-harm (DSH), 299
dental service use, 284
depressants, 402
depressive disorders, 8
descriptive knowledge, 88
descriptive studies, 246–7
detention of migrants, 374
determinants of health
    definition, 2, 54, 317, 352
    types of, 148–50
    See also social determinants of
        health
development forced displacement and
    resettlement, 367
developmental outcomes, 300
diagnostic overshadowing, 337
diet
    in ancient Greece, 27
    Indigenous peoples, 354
dietary recommendations, 317–19
disability
    burden of disease, 324
    causes of, 324
    definition, 322–3
    rates, 323
    See also intellectual and
        developmental disabilities
        (IDD)
disability-adjusted life years (DALYs),
    324
disciplines, 108
discounting, 174–6
disease
    chronic, 323–4
    and colonisation, 352–4
    global changes, 74–5
    incidence, 241–2
    natural history, 239–40
    occurrence, 240–3
    prevalence, 240–1

Divisions of General Practice, 68
domestic violence, 201, 229–30
Down syndrome, 333, 335, 339–40
downstream interventions, 149
drug use
    activities undertaken while under
        influence, 408
    adolescents, 304–6
    age-related patterns, 407–8
    and behaviour, 408
    beliefs about, 410
    harm minimisation, 414–15
    harms associated with, 408,
        410–11
    and health, 305
    and mental health, 411
    mortality rates, 405, 410
    numbers, 405–8
    older people, 407
    public health approaches, 305–6
    and punishment, 411
    reasons for, 305, 406, 411–12
    and technology changes, 413
    and treatment, 417
drugs
    and criminalisation, 400, 417
    decriminalisation, 401, 415–16
    new psychoactive, 413
    policies, 416–18
    and social media, 413
    types of, 401–4
    See also alcohol
Dubrovnik, Croatia, 29
Duncan, William Henry, 30

early childhood caries (ECC), 283
Ebola epidemic, 10
Ebola outbreak, 237, 372
e-cigarette use, 44, 412
ecological fallacies, 247
economic inequalities, 14
ecosystems, 150
ecstasy, 403, 406
education
    human rights, 211–13
    public health professionals, 110,
        112
electronic health records, 78
emotional problems, 299–301
emotions, 167, 171
empowerment
    and human rights, 211–13
Engels, Fredrick, 31
environmental and occupational
    health sciences, 4
environmental appraisal, 171
environmental determinants of
    health, 155–8
environmental factors
    and ageing, 318–20
    disproportionate effects, 156
    and mental illness, 8
    new hazards, 156–7
Environmental Health Australia
    (EHA), 112

environmental health justice, 119–20
environmental health officers, 112
environments
    challenges in creating, 50
    creating supportive, 48
    settings approach, 50
epidemics, 237
    definition, 9
    future of, 11
    individual behaviour during, 165
    origins, 28
    viruses, 10–11
epidemiological studies
    designs, 246–52
    ethical issues, 251
    measures of association, 252–5
    use of surveillance data, 252
epidemiologists, 111, 238
epidemiology
    analytic studies, 240, 247
    definition, 4, 238
    described, 238
    descriptive, 240, 243–5
    frequency of disease occurrence,
        240–3
    social, 130
epistemology, 222–3
equality, 95
equity, 94, 207
    definition, 95
ethical advocacy, 193
ethical issues
    epidemiological studies, 251
ethical principles, 89
ethics
    definition, 88
    frameworks, 98–9
    and vaccination, 87
ethics-based advocacy, 194–5
ethnic disparities, 135
ethnic groups, 135
Europe
    health in 19th-century, 29–32
    health in ancient, 27–9
European Convention on Human
    Rights, 205, 209
European Court of Human Rights,
    205, 209
European Union (EU), 205
evaluation, 260
    described, 269–70
    methods, 270–2
    public health interventions, 264,
        266, 268
    purpose of, 269
evidence, 228
evidence-based policy, 191–2
evidence-based public health
    described, 227–8
    and qualitative research, 227–30
experimental studies, 246, 250–1, 253
exposure, 247
externalising problems
    adolescents, 299–301
eye injuries, 232

face masks, 166
families
    same-sex parent, 286–8
    and substance use, 305
family resources workshops, 301
federal government
    and healthcare system, 187
    role in public health, 6
fires, 184
First Nations Peoples
    use of term, 350
    See also Indigenous peoples
fluoridation of water, 284
food, 153
food environments, 153–4
food prices, 119
food security, 119, 154
Forgotten Children report, 137–8
formative evaluation, 270
Foucault, Michel, 26
freedom, 92
funding
    general practice, 77
    primary health care (PHC), 69–70,
        77
    public health, 107–8
    research, 183

Galen, 28
general practice, 66
    funding, 77
general practitioners (GPs)
    definition, 66
    knowledge, 338
    numbers, 76
    in primary healthcare
        organisations, 68
    rebates, 69, 72
    role in public health, 7
    support from, 63
geographical isolation, 385, 387
geographical issues, 244
germ theory, 28, 31
gingivitis, 284
Global Charter for the Public's
    Health, 105, 107
global concerns
    disease, 74–5
    public health, 7–12
    vaccine equity, 139
Global Consultation on Migrant
    Health, 375
'Go for 2&5' fruit and vegetable
    campaign, 339–40
goals
    alternative terms for, 264
    public health interventions, 98–9,
        264
governance, 354–5
governments
    food environments, 154
    funding primary health care
        (PHC), 69–70, 77
    funding public health, 107–8
    and health football, 183

and healthcare system, 187–8
and human rights, 208–11
and migrants, 375
and 'nanny state', 48
and policies, 185
policy environment, 189–91
role in health, 185–7
role in public health, 6, 185
GP co-payment, 183
Greece, ancient, 27–8
'Grim Reaper' campaign, 194
gun control, 263

H1N1 viruses, 10
hallucinogens, 403
Hamilton, Alice, 31
harm minimisation, 414–15
harm-minimisation policy
    frameworks, 192
harm principle, 92–3, 99–100
Hawai'i
    'Body and Soul' program, 220
health
    in 19th-century Europe, 29–32
    in ancient Greece, 27–8
    in ancient Rome, 28–9
    of Australians, 5
    and bullying, 307
    as chosen or determined, 176–7
    collective action, 31
    definition, 3
    and homelessness, 303
    Indigenous Australians
        conceptualisations, 33
    and internalising problems, 300
    Māori conceptualisations, 33
    medical advancements, 35
    natural history, 239–40
    of older people, 322–5
    as political football, 183
    prerequisites for, 190
    and religion, 27
    responsibility for, 26
    right to, 371–2
    socio-ecological view, 150
    and substance use, 305
    where created, 132
    See also social determinants of
        health
health-adjusted life expectancy
    (HALE), 322
health belief model, 172–4
health beliefs
    traditional, 352–3
health checks, 371
health economics, 189
health equity, 202, 390
health expenditure, 76, 107–8, 188
health inequalities
    definition, 13–14
    and social justice, 14–15
health inequities
    Aboriginal and Torres Strait
        Islander peoples, 66

among disadvantaged
    communities, 76
definition, 13, 134, 193, 332
effects of, 333–4
environmental factors, 119–20
examples, 134–5
reasons for, 335–8
and social justice, 137–8
health literacy, 392
health needs of communities,
    263–4
health outcomes, 94
health problems
    responses to, 151
health promotion
    definition, 45
    settings approach, 50
health promotion scholarships,
    110–11
health services
    access to, 157–8, 337, 390
    administration, 4
    local, 389–90
    re-orienting, 54–6
    support from, 63
health status, 243, 324
    See also determinants of health
healthcare costs, 189
healthcare system
    Australian, 187–8
    barriers to care, 338–40
    creating responsive, 354–5
    migrant-sensitive, 374–7
    political susceptibility, 188
    and primary health care, 67
    quality of care, 337
    siloed systems, 338–9
    well-functioning, 391–2
healthcare workers
    knowledge, 338
    multidisciplinary care, 73–4
    and people with intellectual and
        developmental disabilities
        (IDD), 341
    skills and availability, 76
    training, 417
HealthPathways program, 78
healthy ageing. See ageing
healthy public policy, 13, 46, 48
heroin, 402, 405
Hippocrates, 28
HIV/AIDS
    epidemic, 9, 165
    transmission through breast milk,
        2
    in Uganda, 208
homelessness
    and adolescents, 298, 302–4
    risk factors, 302–3
hormone replacement therapy (HRT),
    249, 251
hospital outcomes
    people with intellectual and
        developmental disabilities
        (IDD), 334

hospitals
    and people with intellectual and
        developmental disabilities
        (IDD), 341
housing, 30, 321–2
human resources, 265
human rights
    accountability, 209–10
    described, 202–4
    and empowerment, 211–13
    holding governments to account,
        208–11
    importance of, 206, 340
    and Indigenous Australians, 211
    and multinational corporations,
        210
    national institutions, 205
    regional systems, 204–5
    and social determinants of health,
        206
    systems for monitoring,
        209–10
    universality, 204
    women and children, 205
Human Rights Council, 211
human rights education, 211–13
hygiene, origin of term, 27

I'll Walk with You (video), 208
illicit drugs. See drug use
illness
    risk of, 130
immigrants
    Russian-speaking, 221
immunisation, 389
    and autism, 272
    See also vaccination
impact evaluation, 271
incidence
    definition, 240
    described, 241–2
incidence rate (IR), 242
Indigenous Australians
    access to healthcare services,
        157–8
    ageing, 320–1
    alcohol use, 404–5
    conceptualisations of health, 33
    food prices, 119
    health, 33
    health and wellbeing, 320
    health inequities, 66
    and human rights, 211
    'Kick the Butt' initiative, 55–6
    life expectancy, 94, 134
    mortality rates, 243
    primary health care (PHC), 358
    Puntu people, 353
    Uluru Statement from the Heart,
        131–2
Indigenous health
    complexities of, 356–7
    gaps, 355
    global, 350–1
    social determinants, 352–5

Indigenous health (cont.)
strengths-based approaches,
357–60
and trauma, 356
Indigenous people
and colonisation, 353–5
Indigenous peoples
described, 349–50
and diseases, 356
and governance, 354–5
health beliefs, 352–3
health issues, 350–1, 354
social determinants of health,
352–5
terminology, 350
and trauma, 356
and voluntary isolation, 349
See also Māori people
individual determinants of health,
166, 172–3
See also behaviour
Indonesia
tobacco control, 44
inequities, 206
See also health inequities
infectious diseases, 356, 371
institutions, 106–7
integrated care, 73
integrated care for older people
(ICOPE) guidelines, 324
intellectual and developmental
disabilities (IDD), 332
See also people with intellectual
and developmental disabilities
(IDD)
intentions, 172
Inter-American Commission on
Human Rights, 209
interception of migrants, 374
interest groups, 118
Intergovernmental Panel on Climate
Change (IPCC), 183
internal migrants, 367
internalising problems
adolescents, 299–301
bullying, 307
internally displaced persons, 366–7
International Covenant on Civil and
Political Rights (ICCPR), 203
International Covenant on Economic,
Social and Cultural Rights
(ICESCR), 203, 207
international labour migrants, 367
international migrants, 367
interprofessional care, 72
intervention ladder, 99
intervention plans, 266–8
intervention studies, 246, 250–1
interventions, 149
evidence-based, 228
specifying, 261
See also public health
interventions
intrinsic capacity, 318
irregular migrants, 366–7, 369, 371–2

job insecurity, 141
justice, 94–5
theories of, 96

KAB (Knowledge, Attitude,
Behaviour), 52
'Kick the Butt' initiative, 55–6
knowledge resources, 265

Learning Disability Liaison Nurses
(LDLNs), 341
legislation, 46–7, 183, 185, 190
libertarianism, 97
described, 91–2
and objections to public health,
92–3
liberty, 91
life course, 317
life expectancy, 5, 94, 134, 333
definition, 316
healthy, 322
older people, 322–3
life experiences
early, 130
lifestyle choice, 152
lifestyle diseases, 356
lifestyles
changes, 283
choices, 176
and people with intellectual and
developmental disabilities
(IDD), 336
linkage studies, 252
Liverpool Building Act 1842 (Engl.),
30
living conditions
working class, 31
local governments
role in public health, 6
locus of control, 170
low birth weight, 249

Madrid International Plan of Action
on Ageing (Madrid Plan), 317
malaria, 372
malnutrition
in children, 72
Māori people
conceptualisations of health, 33
whānau ora approach to health,
359
marketing
licit drugs, 400
See also social marketing
campaigns
Marmot, Michael, 37
Master of Public Health, 110, 112
maternal and child health centres
(MCH), 71
maternal mortality, 134
Somaliland, 71
McKeown, Thomas, 36
measles, 87, 354
media, 118
and strengths-based approaches, 359

media campaigns, 53, 55
medical ethics, 89
medical officers and police, 29
Medical Research Future Fund, 183
Medicare, 69, 187
Medicare Locals, 68, 183
medication reviews, 73
medications
access to essential, 210
management, 337
men
with HIV/AIDS, 15–16
mental health
and children, 288–90
and drug use, 411
Indigenous peoples, 354
internalising problems, 301
prevalence, 8
protective factors, 289–90
risk factors, 8, 12, 289
support strategies, 289
methamphetamine, 402, 406
Métis, 351
#metoo movement, 133
miasma theory, 28, 31
migrant-sensitive health systems,
374–7
migrant studies, 246
migrants
case studies, 367, 369
estimates, 367
health at borders, 372
health during transit, 371–2
health in settlement sites, 372–4
health of detained, 374
health of returned, 374
health pre-departure, 370–1
policies and practice responses,
374–7
social determinants of health,
366
types of, 366–7
migration
described, 365–6
flows, 367
and health, 8–9
stages of, 370–4
Mill, John Stuart, 92
mining operations, 120
mobile phone use
by pedestrians, 173
models of care
effective, 71
integrated care, 73
multidisciplinary care teams,
72–3, 77
nurse-led, 73–4
patient centred medical homes
(PCMH), 74
moral reasoning, 97
moral values, 137
morbidity, 323–4
morning-after pill, 194
mortality, 323
maternal, 71, 134

mortality rates, 76, 134, 138, 243, 245, 333
drug use, 405, 410
mosquitoes, 28
multidisciplinary care, 72–3, 77
multimorbidity, 76, 323
multinational corporations, 210
Multiple Streams Framework (MSF), 117

'nanny state', 48, 93
nation-building, 35
National Aboriginal Community Controlled Health Organisation (NACCHO), 66, 320
National Disability Insurance Scheme, 340
National Health Priority Areas (NHPA), 187
national human rights institutions (NHRIs), 205
National Oral Health Plan 2015–2024, 285
National Preventive Health Strategy 2021–2030 (NPHS), 188
National Rural Health Alliance (NRHA), 387
National Suicide Prevention Strategy, 301
nationalism, 191
natural resources, 156
needs of communities, 263–4
negative attitudes, 339
negative liberty, 91
negative reinforcement, 169
neo-liberalism, 27
new public health, 3, 12–13, 225
See also social model of health
New Zealand public health history, 34–7
non-communicable diseases, 148, 237
normative claims, 88
Northern Territory goverment, 195
NOURISHING framework, 153–4
nudge, 174
Nuffield Ladder of Intervention, 190, 194
nurses, 73–4, 341
nutritional determinants of health, 149, 153–5
nutritional priorities, 154

obesity
and lifestyles, 283
prevalence, 7–8
prevalence rates, 282
prevention programs, 281–3
public health interventions, 268
obesogenic environments, 282
observational learning, 170
observational studies, 247, 251
occupational health sciences, 4
odds ratio (OR), 253

Office of the United Nations High Commissioner for Human Rights (OHCHR), 203, 207
old age, 316
older people
and COVID-19, 326
Cycling Without Age, 315
demographics, 315–16
drug use, 407
health of, 322–5
and healthy ageing, 316–17
and housing, 321–2
integrated care for older people (ICOPE) guidelines, 324
online interventions, 152–3
operant conditioning, 168
opiates, 408, 410
opioids, 402
opportunities
and outcomes, 96
oral health, 283–6
Organisation for Economic Co-operation and Development (OECD), 105
Ottawa Charter for Health Promotion, 45, 52, 206, 285
outcome evaluation, 270
outcomes
defining, 261
focus on, 90
and opportunities, 96
public health interventions, 98–9
validating, 261
overweight
prevalence, 7–8
See also obesity

palliative care
Sri Lanka, 75
pandemics
definition, 7, 9, 237
future of, 11
individual behaviour during, 165
parents
lifestyle changes, 283
Paris Principles, 205
partnerships, 392
paternalism, 93
patient centred medical homes (PCMH), 74
pedestrians
mobile phone use by, 173
peer factors, 305
Penha, María da, 201
people displaced by environmental disasters, 367
people from culturally and linguistically diverse (CALD) backgrounds, 376
See also migrants
people in rural areas
food prices, 119
people living with disability, 12

people with intellectual and developmental disabilities (IDD)
access to health care, 337
barriers to care, 338–40
and biological factors, 335
case studies, 332, 339–41
communication difficulties, 338
comorbid conditions, 332–3, 335
definition, 332
and health inequities, 333–4
hospital outcomes, 334
and lifestyles, 336
medication management, 337
mortality, 333
and poverty, 335
quality of care, 337
reasons for health inequities, 335–8
secondary conditions, 334–5
and social determinants of health, 335
and social inclusion, 336
People's Health Movement, 118
perceptions, 167
period prevalence, 241
personal characteristics, 243
personal skills, 52–4
Pharmaceutical Benefits Scheme, 69, 409
pharmacists, 73
physical resources, 266
place characteristics, 244
plagues, 29
planning, 260
See also public health planning
plumbing, 32
point prevalence, 241
policies
alcohol use, 416
context, 190
drugs, 416–18
economics, 190
evidence-based, 191–2
frameworks on ageing, 317
and governments, 185, 189–91
harm minimisation, 415
healthy public, 13, 46, 48
and migrants, 374–7
and practice gap, 192
political advocacy, 194
political determinants of health, 184, 353–4
political susceptibility, 188
political will, 186
Pomare, Maui, 34
population unit multipliers, 241
populations
estimates, 243
health status, 238
See also epidemiology
Portugal
decriminalisation of drugs, 401, 415–16

positive liberty, 91
positive reinforcement, 168
poverty, 141, 335
power relations, 385–6, 393–4
pre-departure phase of migration,
    370–1
prerequisites for health, 190
prevalence
    definition, 240
    described, 241
    mental illness, 8
    obesity, 7–8
    tobacco use, 14, 44, 46
prevention
    levels of, 4, 239
Prevention First, 118
prevention programs
    tobacco, 14
prevention science, 301
primary care, 64–5
primary health care (PHC)
    in Australia, 65–6
    challenges, 76–7
    comprehensive, 66
    costs, 69
    and COVID-19, 70
    definition, 63, 65
    funding, 69–70, 77
    future of, 77–80
    global, 70
    and global changes, 74–5
    and healthcare system, 67
    Indigenous approach, 358
    origins, 64–5
    and people with intellectual and
        developmental disabilities
        (IDD), 340
    priority actions, 70
    reforms, 68, 77, 183
primary health care organisations, 68
Primary Health Care Performance
    Initiative framework, 70
Primary Health Networks (PHNs),
    68
primary prevention measures, 4
process evaluation, 270
professional identity, 108
professions, 108
project teams, 260–1
protective factors, 151, 289–90
psychoactive substances, 413
public health
    in 19th-century Europe, 29–32
    in ancient Greece, 27–8
    in ancient Rome, 28–9
    Antipodean history, 34–7
    in Australia, 5, 105
    consequentialist approaches, 89–91
    definition, 3–4, 88, 105
    domains for building, 106–8
    global concerns, 7–12
    history of, 26–7
    justifiable restrictions on rights,
        207–8
    key social determinants, 140–2

new, 3, 12–13
    political priority?, 112–13
    and qualitative research, 224–7
    scope of, 88
    stronger systems, 105
Public Health Advocacy Institute, 115
Public Health Association of Australia
    (PHAA), 188
public health campaigns, 193, 282
    See also social marketing
        campaigns
public health disciplines, 4–5
Public Health Education and
    Research Program (PHERP),
    112
public health ethics, 88–9, 97–100
public health interventions
    aims, 260
    behavioural methods, 169
    bullying, 307
    cost, 265
    definition, 259
    determining appropriate, 264–6
    development, 260–1
    drug use, 305–6
    effective, 149
    evaluation, 264, 266, 268–70
    evaluation methods, 270–2
    externalising problems, 301
    goals, 98–9, 264
    homelessness, 303
    implementation, 268
    internalising problems, 301
    needs of community, 263–4
    oral health, 285–6
    outcomes, 98–9
    personal skills, 52–4
    plan for, 266–8
    planning principles, 260–1
    resources, 265–6
    review of steps, 266
    time, 265
public health models, 12
public health organisations, 6–7,
    105–7
public health planning
    principles, 260–1
    six-stage model, 262–9
public health professionals
    and advocacy, 115
    competencies, 109–10
    education, 110, 112
    and human rights, 206
    key, 111
    regulation, 110
    skills, 106
public health programs. See public
    health interventions
public health workforce
    described, 106, 108
Punctuated Equilibrium Theory
    (PET), 117
punishment, 169
    and drug use, 411
Puntu people, 353

qualitative methods, 223
qualitative research
    described, 221
    and epistemology, 222–3
    and evidence-based public health,
        227–30
    methodological frameworks,
        223
    and public health, 224–7
quality of care, 337
quantitative research
    described, 225
quarantine, 29, 31
    and SARS, 10
Queensland government, 188

racism
    structural, 136–7
randomised control trials, 228, 251
Real Time Prescription Monitoring
    system, 78
recall bias, 249
refugee health, 365
refugees, 366–7
    See also migrants
regular migrants, 371
regulation
    public health professionals, 110
reinforcement, 169
relative risk (RR), 253
religion and health, 27
research
    funding, 183
    See also epidemiological studies;
        evaluation; qualitative
        research
research ethics, 89
resilience in same-sex parent families,
    287
representation, 114
retirement villages, 321–2
returned migrants, 374
rights
    and health, 371–2
    justifiable restrictions, 207–8
    of the child, 280
    universality, 204
    See also human rights
risk factors
    and adolescents, 300
    described, 151
    homelessness, 302–3
    mental health, 289
    mental illness, 8, 12
risks
    of illness, 130
    perceptions of, 172–3
Riverdene (fictional town), 383, 387,
    391
Rohingya, 370
role models, 170
Rome, ancient, 28–9
Rose, Geoffrey, 130
rural health
    burden of disease, 384–5

and communities, 388–9
frameworks, 385–6
geographical isolation, 385, 387
local responses, 389–90
Riverdene (fictional town), 383,
   387, 391
and social determinants of health,
   393
rural health differential, 393
rurality, 387, 393
Russian-speaking immigrants, 221

same-sex marriage, 183
same-sex parent families,
   286–8
Samoan community, 220
SARS-CoV (severe acute respiratory
   syndrome), 237
scapegoating, 34
scholarships, 110–11
schools
   and bullying, 308
   and substance use, 305
screening programs, 189
seasonal patterns, 243
secondary conditions, 332,
   334–5
secondary prevention measures, 4,
   239
selection bias, 250
self-efficacy, 170
self-evaluation, 171
self-harm
   deliberate, 299
self-liberation, 171
self-monitoring of health, 78
self-regulation, 110
settings approach to health
   promotion, 49–50
settlement, 372–4
Severe Acute Respiratory Syndrome
   (SARS), 10
Sex Discrimination Commissioner,
   133
sexually transmissible infections, 29
siloed systems, 338–9
Siracusa principles, 207
six-stage model of public health
   planning, 262–9
smallpox, 354
smartphone applications, 78
Snow, John, 29–31
social and behavioural sciences, 4
social and emotional wellbeing
   (SEWB), 320
social capital building, 193
social democracy, 27
social determinants of health
   definition, 131, 281, 332
   described, 95
   and human rights, 206
   Indigenous peoples, 352–5
   key determinants of public health,
      140–2
   migrants, 366

and people with intellectual and
   developmental disabilities
   (IDD), 335
and rural health, 393
Solid Facts report, 140
Struggle Street (documentary
   series), 130
tobacco use, 37
social exclusion, 130
social factors
   and health inequalities, 14–15
   tobacco use, 14
social gradient in health, 138–9
social inclusion, 336
social inquiry. See qualitative research
social justice, 14–15, 137–8, 184, 201
social learning theory, 169–70, 176
social liberation, 171
social marketing
   definition, 53
social marketing campaigns
   'Go for 2&5' fruit and vegetable
      campaign, 339–40
   tobacco control, 53–4
social media, 51, 118, 194
   and drugs, 413
social model of health, 12–13
social policy reform, 114
social systems, 392–3
socio-ecological framework, 281
socio-ecological view of health,
   150
socio-economic status, 138
soft drinks, 94
Solid Facts report, 140
Somaliland
   maternal mortality, 71
Soul Buddyz, 212
Soul Buddyz Clubs, 212
South Africa
   human rights education, 212
South Pacific, 355
sovereign, 131
sport, 27
Sri Lanka
   palliative care, 75
Sri Lankans, 369
state and territory governments
   and healthcare system, 187–8
   role in public health, 6
stateless people, 367
stereotypes, 410
stigma, 37, 410
   definition, 287
   people with intellectual and
      developmental disabilities
      (IDD), 339
   same-sex parent families, 287–8
stimulants, 402–3, 408
strengths-based approaches, 357–60
   and media, 359
stressful events, 141
   and children, 280
structural determinants of health, 133
structural racism, 136–7

Struggle Street (documentary series),
   130
subjective norms, 172
subsistence affluence, 355
substance use. See alcohol use; drug
   use
sugar intake, 94
suicide, 299, 301
summative evaluation, 270
support services, 63
supportive environments, 48
surveillance data, 252
surveys, 247
Sustainable Development Goals,
   (SDGs), 65, 107, 243
swine-flu pandemic, 10, 244
systematic reviews, 228
systems approaches, 282
Szreter, Simon, 36

tax incentives, 187
te whare tapa wha, 33
team leaders, 267
technology
   development, 156
   for public health planning, 267
   use, 77–8
teenagers. See adolescents
Teeth Tales study, 285–6
telehealth, 78, 392
tertiary prevention measures, 4, 239
Thai women
   living with breast cancer, 224
theories, 168
theory of planned behaviour, 171–2,
   176
THRIVE alcohol intervention, 153
time
   and descriptive epidemiology,
      243–5
   and public health interventions,
      265
time discounting, 175
tobacco control
   in Australia, 46–7
   and community action, 51–2
   increasing cost, 414
   'Kick the Butt' initiative, 55–6
   and marketing, 400
   plain packaging, 47
   prevention programs, 14
   and public health, 44–5
   public health interventions, 268
   smoke-free work environments,
      49–50
   social marketing campaigns, 53–4
   World Health Organization
      Framework Convention, 14, 44
tobacco industry, 44–5
tobacco use
   adolescents, 304–6
   costs, 47, 53
   e-cigarettes, 44, 412
   harms associated with, 410–11
   and health belief model, 173

tobacco use (cont.)
    prevalence, 14, 44, 46
    as social determinant of health, 37
    and social factors, 14
Tobacco-Free Kids Action Fund, 51
trafficked people, 367, 372
transit migration, 371–2
translational research, 185
transport issues, 390
transtheoretical model, 170–1
trauma, 356
Triggs, Gillian, 137–8
truth-telling, 131
twin cities, USA
    health inequities, 135
two-by-two tables, 253
typhus, 30

Uganda
    HIV/AIDS in, 208
Uluru Statement from the Heart,
    131–2
unemployment, 140–2
United Nations (UN)
    and human rights, 202–4, 207
    Sustainable Development Goals,
        65, 107, 243
United Nations High Commissioner
    for Refugees (UNHCR), 365
*Universal Declaration on Human
    Rights* (UDHR), 202–3, 207
Universal Health Coverage (UHC), 65
upstream interventions, 149
urban refugees, 372
urbanisation, 12
utilitarianism, 89–91, 97, 99

vaccination
    and autism, 272
    beliefs about, 389
    and ethics, 87
    and utilitarianism, 91
vaccine equity, 139
vaccines, 139, 191
vector-borne diseases, 28
Venice, Italy, 29
victim blaming, 37, 152
victimisation, 306–8
violence
    and homelessness, 303
Virchow, Rudolph, 29–30
viruses
    epidemics, 10–11
vitamin D status, 254
vulnerability, 156
vulnerable people, 5–6
vulnerable populations, 5

water
    algae in, 259
    fluoridation, 284
    stagnant, 28
    supply systems, 28, 30, 32
water-borne diseases, 30
wellbeing
    dimensions of, 96
whānau ora approach to health,
    359
Whole of Systems Trial of
    Prevention Strategies for
    Obesity, 282
women
    human rights, 205

injuring intimate partners,
    229–30
migrants, 9, 373
with HIV/AIDS, 2, 9, 15–16
Woolworths supermarket chain, 195
working class
    living conditions, 31
working conditions, 31, 49
World Federation of Public Health
    Associations, 105
World Health Organization
    Active Ageing framework, 317
    and ageing, 324
    Closing the Gap in a Generation
        report, 134
    Decade of Healthy Ageing,
        319–20
    dietary recommendations, 153
    environmental factors, 156
    Framework Convention on
        Tobacco Control, 14, 44
    Global Health Observatory
        website, 247
    health promotion definition, 45
    and human rights, 205, 207
    Integrated Care for Older
        People (ICOPE) guidelines,
        324

youth
    alcohol use, 152–3, 226–7
    and choices, 175
    homeless, 302
youth mentoring programs, 358

Zika virus epidemic, 10